Recipes for Thought

MATERIAL TEXTS

Series Editors

Roger Chartier Leah Price
Joseph Farrell Peter Stallybrass
Anthony Grafton Michael F. Suarez, S.J.

A complete list of books in the series
is available from the publisher.

Recipes for Thought

Knowledge and Taste in the Early Modern English Kitchen

Wendy Wall

PENN

UNIVERSITY OF PENNSYLVANIA PRESS

PHILADELPHIA

Copyright © 2016 University of Pennsylvania Press

All rights reserved. Except for brief quotations used for purposes of review or scholarly citation, none of this book may be reproduced in any form by any means without written permission from the publisher.

Published by
University of Pennsylvania Press
Philadelphia, Pennsylvania 19104–4112
www.upenn.edu/pennpress

Printed in the United States of America on acid-free paper

1 3 5 7 9 10 8 6 4 2

Library of Congress Cataloging-in-Publication Data
Wall, Wendy, author.
 Recipes for thought : knowledge and taste in the early modern English kitchen / Wendy Wall.
   pages cm. — (Material texts)
 Includes bibliographical references and index.
 ISBN 978-0-8122-4758-9 (alk. paper)
 1. Food writing—England—History—16th century. 2. Food writing—England—History—17th century. 3. Cooking, English—History—16th century. 4. Cooking, English—History—17th century. 5. Formulas, recipes, etc.—England—History—16th century. 6. Formulas, recipes, etc.—England—History—17th century. 7. Medicine—Formulae, receipts, prescriptions—History. 8. Knowledge, Sociology of—History. 9. Renaissance—England. I. Title. II. Series: Material texts.
 TX645.W35 2016
 641.509—dc23   2015024750

For Leah Wall
And though she be but little, she is fierce

CONTENTS

Menu

PREFACE The Appetizer

ix

INTRODUCTION The Order of Serving

1

CHAPTER 1 Taste Acts

20

CHAPTER 2 Pleasure: Kitchen Conceits in Print

65

CHAPTER 3 Literacies: Handwriting and Handiwork

112

CHAPTER 4 Temporalities: Preservation, Seasoning, and Memorialization

167

CHAPTER 5 Knowledge: Recipes and Experimental Cultures

209

Coda

251

NOTES

257

WORKS CITED

283

INDEX

303

ACKNOWLEDGMENTS

311

PREFACE

The Appetizer

The Italians call the preface *La salsa del libro*, the sauce of the book, and if well seasoned it creates an appetite in the reader to devour the book itself.

—Isaac Disraeli

At dinner parties over the past few years, when I have admitted to writing a book on early modern English recipes, people have been amused if not aghast. But English cooking, with its soggy puddings and dry roast beef, is so notoriously boring, they would exclaim. And given the sophistication of Renaissance writing, why would one choose to investigate inelegant technical writing? Why indeed would anyone on earth devote time to thinking about the mechanics of English culinary writing?

Then, I drop the bombshell. In Shakespeare's day, English food was not very different from French or Italian cuisine. In fact, all of it was robust and highly seasoned. I have to repeat this point for it to sink in fully. Even the most knowledgeable "foodie" seems to find this information startling, though it is well known to culinary historians. From roughly 1200 to 1650, all European food—including English fare—relied on exotic seasonings to transform the natural flavors and textures of ingredients into dazzling combinations.[1] Indeed, the ability to alter the fundamental character, flavor, and texture of a foodstuff was a marker of civilized society. The basic international (though regionally inflected) European elite cuisine depended on spices imported from southern China, the Moluccas, Malaya, and India (including cinnamon, ginger, cardamom, nutmeg, mace, cloves, and grains of paradise). Imported by

Roman invaders, solidified by early trade with Italy and Spain, and made increasingly desirable during the Crusades, spices were at the center of the world economy that spurred discovery of the "New World" and colonial ventures. Spices were not prized because they could disguise the taste of spoiled meat, as legend has it, but instead were valued for their color, scent, medicinal properties, taste, and exclusivity.

The seventeenth century was when it all changed. European cuisine underwent nothing short of a seismic shift; the publication of Pierre La Varenne's 1651 *Le Cuisiner* heralded a definitive break with the cuisine of the past and set the template for a modern understanding of flavors. Instead of privileging profusion, abundance, and hybridity, the new French cuisine sought to showcase the natural flavors of ingredients. The keyword for the new palate was *delicacy*, which could be manifested by generating subtle butter-based sauces, removing sweeteners from savory dishes, reducing the number of seasonings in a single dish, increasing the ratio of herbs to spices, and developing techniques for concentrating natural flavors.

French recipe writers touted the ethical, aesthetic, and moral superiority of a "purist" cuisine over the former "transmutationalist" style of food:[2] "let the cabbage soup taste entirely of cabbage, a leek soup of leeks, a turnip soup of turnips, and so on," Nicholas Bonnefons wrote in criticizing French chefs who failed to move with the times, "leaving elaborate mixtures of chopped meat, diced vegetables, breadcrumbs and other deceptions."[3] Cutting-edge food was to divide artifice from nature as it identified "deceptions." Some writers expressed revulsion with the barbarousness of past tastes: "Doesn't it already make you shudder to think of a teal soup a *l'hypocra*s, or larks in sweet sauce?" A writer identified only as L.S.R. exclaims:

> Nowadays it is not the prodigious overflowing of dishes, the abundance of ragouts and gallimaufries, the extraordinary piles of meat which constitute a good table; it is not the confused mixtures of spices, the mountains of roasts, the successive services of *assiettes volantes*, in which it seems that nature and artifice have been entirely exhausted in the satisfaction of the sense, which is the most palpable object of our delicacy of taste. It is rather the exquisite choice of meats, the finesse with which they are seasoned, the courtesy and neatness with which they are served, their proportionate relation to the number of people and finally the general order of things which essentially contribute to the goodness and elegance of a meal (1674).[4]

The new table was to promote neoclassical values, balance art and nature, omit hybridity, and curb excess. Because of the decreasing credibility of the psycho-physiological theory of humoralism as well as the increased availability of spices (which gave them less cachet for culinary trendsetters), cookery across Europe was freed from the dictates of dietetic theory or traditional canons of taste.[5]

English recipe writers responded to this culinary shot heard round the world by rejecting the new cuisine as horrifically and quintessentially French. Initially they stubbornly held on to dishes with piquant flavorings and increased their attachment to older Arab-influenced pastry pies and puddings. Rather than developing emulsions and complex sauces (the foundation of French cookery), they gradually began to relegate strongly spiced concoctions to condiments used to garnish unseasoned joints of meat. Food became blander and blander. Age-old dishes that had formerly been surrounded by piquant foods began to be segregated out to take precedence: boiled pigeons, rabbit pies, black puddings, and mutton. Through the eighteenth century, English cuisine gradually modulated into the form that people today might recognize as modern British food: proteins roasted or boiled with simple seasonings. Beef, always associated with the English, emerged as the classic national dish.

In the eighteenth century, the idea that the English enjoyed a national cuisine became such a naturalized concept many people could not imagine it had ever *not* been the case. They erased their historical recipe traditions and forgot how decidedly foreign their food had so proudly been. In *The Art of Cookery*, John Thacker complained that the natural English bodily constitution simply could no longer tolerate the foreign, complexly spiced dishes intruding onto the realm; Thacker did not recognize that the dishes he found objectionable were standard fare in the English medieval diet.[6] Similarly, Joseph Addison urged readers of the *Tattler* to "return to the food of their forefathers, and reconcile themselves to beef and mutton. This was that diet which bred that hardy race of mortals who won the fields of Cressy and Agincourt."[7] By the time that William Hogarth placed a huge side of beef in the hands of an Englishman in his painting *The Gates of Calais*, this mythology had been fully entrenched. England became identified as the land of puddings, boiled meats, pies, plain vegetables, and roast beef.

And yet, my subject is *not* the history of diet at all, though this remarkable evolution provides a crucial backdrop for the stories I tell. My subject is the recipe of the past, which is as unexpectedly rich and surprising as the cuisine it recommended. To my mind, we have not yet accounted for the fact that England took the stage as the most active site of cookery publication in Europe between 1575 and 1650. Unlike other European countries, England got in the game of recipe publication early and with great intensity. Why, I wondered, were recipes were so popular in early modern England? What roles did they play in the cultural imagination, and what type of intellectual worlds did they provide for users? While we might situate these forms at the intersection of different histories—of food, manners, literacy, gender roles, the growth of the middle class, nationalism—I address the question of their function and appeal by reading the recipes themselves to extract from them more than a history of food. Rather than being a dull form of technical writing, recipes, I argue, register the creative, intellectual, and social exchanges of those in the early modern household who were negotiating "life on the ground," those people trying to make sense of their worlds. Throughout locations in England—in pulpits, schools, shops, theaters, taverns, noble estates, inns of court, and anatomy theaters—people energetically tried to figure out what it meant to be a person, animal, woman, social creature, sinner, performer, mortal being, maker, and/or experimenter. They received and conceived knowledge in active, highly embodied ways. We've only just begun to appreciate the fact that these debates-in-action were also taking place amid the pots, pans, quills, and papers of the kitchen.

After careful deliberation and in the interests of accessibility and uniformity, I have silently modernized early modern instances of *i, u, v,* and *vv*.

Recipes for Thought

INTRODUCTION

The Order of Serving

> Our Stationers shops have lately swarm[e]d with bookes of Cookery, Some in our Late Queenes name, Some from the Countesse of Kent, as if Selden had imployd his Antiquityes in her Kitchen.
> —John Beale, letter to Samuel Hartlib, 1659

Ingredients, Seasoning, Menu

I began this project with a simple curiosity about what recipes from the past could tell us about early modern culture. From previous research, I knew that early English recipes were a nodal point for attracting consumers to join an increasingly complicated global commerce system, one that stretched from the Spice Islands to Caribbean sugar plantations. I knew as well that people then, as now, used recipes to define social standing, national identity, and racialized categories.[1] But what I had not yet understood, and what this book attempts to bring to light, were the *intellectual* components involved in the creation, exchange, and use of a type of writing that we now consider distinctly unlearned. As I discovered a vast and understudied archive of English manuscript and printed collections produced between 1570 and roughly 1750, I began to dream up new and more specific questions: How could a recipe function simultaneously as scientific experiment and poetic exercise of wit? How might a recipe's mode of commemoration intersect with its use as a writing exercise pad for learning skills that crossed paper and food? How did recipes open doors so that people could reflect on concepts such as "knowledge," "wit," "literacy," "taste," and "time" even as they went about their everyday labors? In what precise ways did housewives contemplate figuration, natural philosophy, memory, and matter itself, even as they seemingly conformed to traditional and presumptively passive norms of female behavior? What did recipes allow people to explore, think, do, consider, make, and *taste* (in its meaning of "sample") in the early modern period?

"The cook must be neither a madman nor a simpleton," wrote Maestro Martino in a fifteenth-century Italian cookery book, "but he must have a great brain."[2] In this book I argue that early English recipes constituted and now bear witness to a rich and previously unacknowledged literate and brainy domestic culture, one in which women were predominantly, though not exclusively, involved. In scribal and print communities, recipe users circulated forms of fantasy and processed modes of thought that now appear to us to rest at the intersection of physiology, gastronomy, decorum, knowledge production, and labor. As I researched this book, it seemed to me more than incidental that the crafting and use of manuscript recipes involved the very "mechanic" skills taught in the collections themselves—how to sharpen a quill, make ink, inscribe meanings into surfaces, "read" by putting a hand to material, and experimentally test abstract notions. As Sara Pennell and Michelle DiMeo observe, "studying recipes helps to reinvest those quotidian activities of making, maintaining and mending with the significance they carried for early modern householders."[3] To my mind, these materials make legible the striking fusion of mental and manual early modern activities that lay at the core of domestic work. The recipe archive thus points us toward a highly substantial and practical mode of thinking concocted out of embodied action and textual engagement.[4]

Previous investigations of recipes have tended to be studies of practice, of which the recipe acts as a transparent window onto the past with little regard for the recipe form, its manner of transmission, or its relationship to modes of intellection.[5] Yet the story of recipes expands well beyond the history of puddings and pies, as it opens our view onto a household culture more complex, expansive, and speculative than previous accounts have acknowledged. Recipes, that is, tell a story in which what counts as "food," "writing," "taste," "nature," "letters," "matter," and "knowledge" are all profoundly in question and, as I shall argue, in flux. It is a story that adds domestic experiences to scholarship that has defamiliarized and historicized the very practice of early modern "reading," in part by taking seriously the materiality of representation.

Even as they functioned as sites of theoretical exploration, recipes also crossed households and other social spaces in ways that show us that domesticity was not a "private" sphere opposed to some reified public domain. Recipes were transit points that actively created and defined knowledge communities and networks of association. Exchanged as displays of skill, recipes could behave as forms of currency for moving up in the world and as tools for conspicuous acts of social and personal definition. Handed down to future generations as bequests or presented as tokens of affection, they were paper registers of bonds between people remote in time or space. While a recipe could provide a simple personal memorandum for workers in a kitchen, it was also simultaneously an assertion of existence ("I am here") and a community "message board" (or, in today's terms, a wiki) that collated responses and opinions for others to view. In fact, the term used in the early modern period, the *receipt* as opposed to our modern word *recipe*, signified this mobility and communal function: from the Latin *recipere*, meaning "to take back or receive," the receipt recorded a transaction. It functioned as what Pennell and DiMeo describe as a "palimpsest: the self and communities in 'conversation.'"[6]

We might start with a signature feature of recipes: they are founded on the transformation of natural elements into "made" worlds—through labor, contrivance, artifice, *techne*. They exist at the cusp of the movement from nature to art, from shapeless *materia* to cultural product, from the raw to the cooked. In their content, manner of address, format, and mode of exchange, recipes raised pointed questions about the stakes and meaning of that transformation; that is, they probed what it meant to be a maker, knower, creator, artist, artificer, worker, and preserver in early modern terms and within spaces that included the *domus*. I see the recipe genre, itself a striking syntactical and formal structure, as thus providing a case study for mapping domestic engagements with the intellectual and philosophical conundrums that emerged at the center of humanist thought in the Renaissance, a time in which poetry (*poiesis*) was understood as the art of "making," and scientific experimentation was taking place in artisans' shops as well as academies. Recipes asked readers outside formal sites of education to reflect on how something called "nature" was to be positioned in relation to the artifactual; they demanded that practitioners think about how and when to put natural materials in and out of time and how to evidence "truth." Reading and writing recipes, that is, offered practitioners the occasion for undertaking and scrutinizing nothing less than world making.[7]

But I have gotten ahead of myself. We first have to unthink modern definitions of the recipe in order to grasp its range and scope in the early modern period. A "receipt" was, as it is now, a formula for preparing something or achieving some end. Receipts did conform to our understanding of the term in offering advice on making edibles such as lemon creams, roast lamb, spinach fritter, gingerbread, boiled carp, almond butter, syllabubs, fricassees, salads, and calves foot jelly. But *receipts*, unlike recipes, were not only or primarily associated with food in their sixteenth-century incarnation (indeed this gradual shift in emphasis occurs over the period I trace). Receipts circulated a range of technical information: how to make cosmetics, inks, dyes, cures, salves, deodorants, pain relievers, herbal cordial waters, wines, confectionaries, perfumes, cleansers, pesticides, toothpastes, air fresheners, and lotions. They offered instruction for how to undertake surgical procedures, decorate objects, write letters, cultivate herbs, distill waters, and perform party tricks. These miscellaneous texts—in their earliest incarnation called "books of secrets"—proliferated within this first era of "how-to" knowledge in print.[8] Individual chapters of this book place different emphasis on the two central subjects of recipes—Chapters 1 and 2 concern themselves more with the culinary, Chapter 5 more with the medical—but on the whole, I am concerned with the fact that early modern recipe practice straddles what will only later fragment into disparate knowledges. Recipes register a world that had yet to divide into the modern regimes that we call the arts and sciences. Their sheer heterogeneity informs their meaning, and, by extension, the nature of domestic practice during this period.

Scholars have tended to work selectively with particular subsets of recipes to establish distinct histories of medicine, food, or manners. Three important large-scale narratives have emerged in these bodies of scholarship: (1) the rise of the medical profession, in which female-amateurs were gradually excluded as practitioners in the move toward male-dominated professionalization; (2) the evolution of the domestic sphere from a site of economic production to one of consumption, a movement that curtailed women's economic power in an emergent modern public sphere; and (3) the unfolding of the "civilizing process," which produced self-regulating subjects fit for a developing modern nation-state. Separating medical, household, and culinary recipes has been strategically important in these accounts, each of which illuminates critical social and economic formations. In failing to consider the entire range of activities included in what I call "recipe culture," however, these accounts have underemphasized the scope of domestic making, the role of the textual forms through which knowledge was mobilized, and the intellectual questions emerging from the juxtaposition of what are now seen as disparate practices. One result is that these accounts overstate the codification of restrictive (gender and other) identities in and through domestic activities.[9] Because these well-established histories have so greatly impacted our understanding of the early modern period, I do not rehearse them extensively. In fact, I feel free to *emphasize* the creative potential of the recipe world precisely because I know that my account will be read in tandem with these other vital and qualifying histories.[10] I offer a picture of what existing stories, dependent as they are on their particular objects of study, obscure—the role of the recipe as a form of thought that placed the user in relation to interwoven natural, social, and representational systems.

It's important to understand what recipes are and are not. First, they are not snapshots of what people daily concocted in their homes in the past. They do not thus readily lend themselves to the project of historical recovery.[11] Most of what people cooked or made was so familiar that it could be produced without consulting a book. Rather, recipes often recorded extraordinary meals or rare treatments—things precisely outside a maker's everyday repertoire. Attempting to read recipes as documentary evidence of women's lives is an important undertaking (and something that I engage in at points in this project), but it is made tricky by the fact that recipes were inflected by fantasy, shot through with dreams testifying to what people would ideally like to be (witness a celebrity recipe, such as King Edward's favorite preserved quinces, to appreciate the challenge of using these forms uncritically as evidence of use). If I sought to offer a history of English diet or a study of female labor, this book would look quite different: I would spend less time contemplating signs of culinary wit and the analyzing family genealogies scrawled among rosewater recipes and instead patiently sift account books, importation patterns, court documents, and guild records. Recipes, in my view, do not merely record practices, but testify to ways of speaking, persuading, and thinking.

It would be a mistake, however, to move in the opposite direction and view recipes as flights of fancy completely disconnected from practice. Corrections, annotations, and greasy stains show us that these texts were actively used in kitchens (Figure 1). Other documents provide extrinsic evidence that the dishes recipes recommended were, in fact, served. Recipes were, as Frances Dolan has recently reminded us in her important study of early modern evidentiary standards, as "fictional" and as "documentary" as materials traditionally used to establish history.[12] Readers today simply find recipes to be more transparent about the evidentiary and methodological challenges they pose. Elizabeth Spiller and Sara Pennell, to whom my work is especially indebted, navigate this problem by positioning recipes as neither categorically documentary nor prescriptive but instead as modes of transmission and circulation,

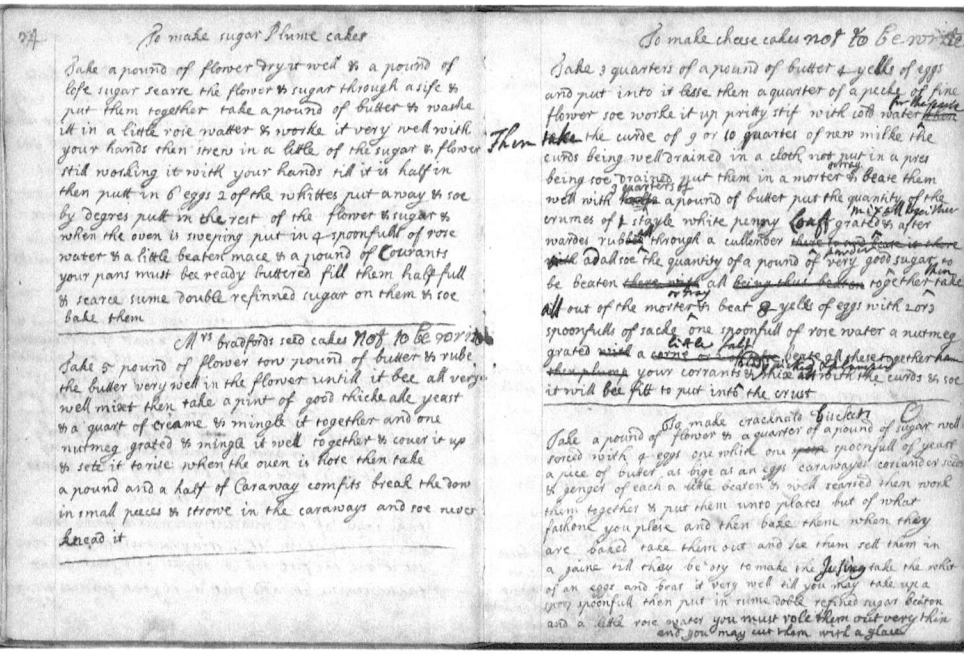

FIGURE 1. Signs of recipe use in Elizabeth Godfrey's *Collection of Medical and Cookery Receipts*, 1686, Wellcome Library, MS 2535, fol. 3.

important in generating networks of people, ideas, and acts.[13] In a given recipe book, compilers might intermix the familiar and the exceptional, the practical and the fanciful. Recipes might address readerships that did not exist, yet still bear practical information hungrily consumed by some readers. It is the fact that recipe books move so readily between the whimsical and the pragmatic that renders them so intriguing. They portray life, but not quite in the way that we might, at first glance, expect.

I frame my investigation of the intellectual stakes of recipe production and consumption within the broad story of their social use that I detail in my first chapter. This story begins in 1573, when popular author of science and history John Partridge introduced something that had not been seen in western Europe: a recipe book marketed to women and non-nobles. The only published English book devoted to culinary recipes, *A Proper New Booke of Cokery*, addressed servants in a noble household. While Italy had witnessed the 1475 publication of Bartolomeo Sacchi's regimen of health (*De Honesta Voluptate*), and France the 1560 *Grand Cuisiniere*, there was no efflorescence of the recipe genre in France, Spain, or Italy until much later. When continental recipe publications did eventually appear, they were not interested in cultivating a wide recipe readership, at least for two centuries. Only in England were women nominated in print to oversee a complex set of knowledges called "housewifery," which blended herbal cultivation, textile making, anatomy, water purification, chemistry, medical care, manners, butchery, the preservation of foodstuffs, and the manufacture of goods. England, for a brief time, became the most active site of cookery publication in Europe and the only country marketing recipe books for women; there would not be a comparable story to tell in other European countries for eighty years, and women would not be addressed as literate domestic worker-readers in other countries for another century.

The recipe books that flooded the book market in England in their first fifty years of popularity (1573–1630) identified expertise in cooking and medical care as an elite knowledge that print could disseminate to a wider population. These male-authored books sought to teach prosperous citizens, gentry and farmer's wives, to concoct medicines as well as modest versions of ostentatious foods displayed at noble feasts, including trompe l'oeil desserts called "conceits." Early titles advertised potential social prestige: *A Treasurie of Commodious Conceits, Delightes for Ladies, A Closet for Ladies and Gentlewomen, The Ladies Cabinet Opened*. Part of the pleasure that such texts afforded was the revelation of formerly exclusive puzzles that socially ambitious women could now master as they undertook manual work. In their domestic roles, women could script food-poems, surprise diners, and create things of beauty both fashionable and practical. They were tutored on how to shape sugar paste and extract natural dyes so as to produce culinary masquerades such as faux bacon and eggs.

Even as they emphasized the cultural capital to be gained by particular forms of labor, recipes insisted on the *practical* and fundamental work that the "lady of stature" undertook. Because food and drugs were not separated conceptually in these texts, even seemingly frivolous foods were connected to the utilitarian tasks of health care. Humoral physiology, as critics have explored, emphasized diet's importance in managing the instability of the four Galenic humors coursing through the body, each bearing different properties. In the last decades, scholars have thought extensively about how this theory shaped notions of subjectivity, interiority, and social relations. Because alteration of humors could occur through sleep, exercise, bloodletting, the outtake of substances, and—centrally—eating, humoral theory broadly underwrote recipe culture, with diet understood as the functional balancing of one ingredient (e.g., mutton) against another (e.g., ginger) as part of the overarching process of stabilizing the constitution of a particular diner. The reason to eat strawberry jam, recipe books assume, had less to do with the sheer deliciousness of the food and more with the fact that it could alleviate a temporary condition (such as an ague) or an ongoing predisposition (such as "a hot liver"). The work of culinary preparation—even the creation of foods that we see as luxurious—required that the household worker consider materials flowing in and out of bodies and environments. Individual recipes readily straddled multiple medicinal and culinary uses. In her collection, Susanna Packe recommended "preserved walnuts" "more for medisen then [a] banquit," with the word "more" interestingly signaling the dish's dual function as dessert and cough syrup.[14] In *The English Housewife*, Markham included his roasted leg of mutton within a cookery section, but he does not hesitate to declare that it was "both good in taste and excellent sovereign for . . . flux in the reins" (that is, it deliciously alleviated diarrhea).[15]

Sometimes transferring the properties of animals or plants into human bodies involved placing that body in relation to violent acts: larks and snails had to be killed in a precise manner, animals had to be split alive and butchered. In Markham's plague recipe, the reader was to transfer physical properties from bird to human by applying "a live Pidgeon cut in two parts or els a plaster made of the yolke of an egge, hony, herbe of grace chopt exceeding small, and wheat flower" to a wound (1615; 8). As I have discussed previously, household workers healed humans and nourished their humoral needs by managing flows within an economy of organicism in which living beings acted as *sites* of transactions. Culinary work was a subset of the "care of the body," the administration of a physical entity whose frailty, vulnerability, and mortality were always starkly on view. Food work, that is, strikingly made people aware of the grinding jaws of death. While recent scholarship has probed ways that humoralism saturated early modern thought and culture, we have not yet truly appreciated its effect on the conception of the household maker and the literate culture in which she was enmeshed. The elite leisure skills on view in early recipes endowed the housewife-cum-lady with the power to orchestrate a world pulsing with life and threatened with death.

As the seventeenth century wore on, recipe users' traditional way of establishing the truth of the natural world by creating products—producing what Antonio Pérez-Ramos has termed a "maker's knowledge"—became more visible and culturally noteworthy, largely because it was adopted and celebrated by reformers of natural philosophy.[16] Not only were similar chemical, herbal, and physiological inquiries undertaken across domestic and scientific domains, but acts of household manufacture, as well as their translation into written forms, invited a gender-inclusive group of people across the social spectrum to grapple with epistemological questions. In the household, practitioners actively engaged issues debated at the Royal Society: the nature of experience; the production of natural "facts" through imitation, art, and manipulation; and the quandary of how information could be converted into something called knowledge through attribution, documentation, and rhetorical formatting. Exchanging tips about how to preserve apricots or create indelible dyes not only made the household worker a chemical experimenter: it also forced her to think about protocols for evidencing "truth" in writing, a crucial problem within emerging cultures of experimentation.

By 1750, published English cookbooks would look very different: a primarily medicinal notion of food had transformed into a concept of cuisine; female writers had taken over the food-writing industry and had vested cookbook expertise in hands-on empirical knowledge rather than textual citation; and, after the culinary revolution of the mid-seventeenth century, national cuisines with less appreciation for artfulness emerged. Instead of delights for ladies, recipe books advertised utilitarian and national goals: *English Housewifery*, *The Compleat Housewife*, *The British Housewife*. The call for housewives and ladies to fashion playful edible representational worlds faded from view in light of calls for attending to civic duty. The pleasures of proving gentility and manipulating the natural world were subordinated to the need to manage a narrower sphere of home economics. With the devaluation of humoralism, a clearer line demarcated cooking from medical care, conceptually and practically. Domestic work was less involved with a cosmically imagined struggle against decay and mortality. Recipe books, no longer interested in vesting status in prestigious modes of *work*, were increasingly addressed to servants and housekeepers; ladies of "good taste" were to take only a managerial role in overseeing the creation of a thrifty and virtuous household.

Determining the readership of recipe books between 1550 and 1750 is a tricky business. Given that many early recipes call for costly ingredients such as sugar, pepper, gum arabic, and gold leaf, it seems unlikely that any but the extremely affluent could have been their real targeted audience. Because few men—and even fewer women—could read, it also seems unlikely that recipe books would have reached "all estates" as they claimed. Yet Partridge's inaugural *Treasurie of Commodious Conceits* was part of a cheap print market; it sold for four pence, the price of a quart of good ale. Despite low literacy rates for women—estimated (using traditional means that I discuss below) at between 5 and 10 percent around 1600—early recipe books were stubbornly addressed to housewives and ladies. While anyone might have bought these books, extant copies boast women's and men's signatures, including women of no rank. We can guess that affluent gentry, yeomen's wives, and merchant's wives read the earliest printed recipes. Over the course of the seventeenth century as literacy spread, these books reached those further down the social scale, including servants and actor's wives, and, in the eighteenth century, the target audience shifted to housekeepers and mistresses of households who shared their books with entrepreneurial cooks and servants. While our ability to determine the readership for such books increases over the period that I study, many assertions about early readership remain speculative. Barbara Ketchum Wheaton, in fact, sees the very existence of early recipe books as a mystery: "Why, indeed should there have been any? Who would have written them, and for whom?"[17] This is a good question, because literate early modern women are not typically now imagined to be interested in manual labor and early modern workers are not typically imagined to have been able to read. Rather than trying to solve the puzzle of readership empirically (which I am convinced cannot be done persuasively based on the evidence), I make the question of "literacy" and "readership" part of my inquiry, something that recipe books address and theorize.

In the wake of social, intellectual, and economic changes occurring in the late seventeenth and early eighteenth centuries, the smart and fashionable lady no longer valued domestic labor as an engine of knowledge and taste. The terms of recipe book fantasy thus evolved. Instead of promising the thrills of orchestrating domestic spectacles, managing flesh in a perilous world, and emulating elite lifestyles, recipe books began to celebrate national distinction and a certainty verified by the trial and error of handiwork delegated to servants. Between the starkly defined endpoints of my study—the advent of published recipe books in the 1570s and the consolidation of housekeeper's cookery books in the late eighteenth century—recipe texts air debates over the ideological meaning and stakes of household making.[18] Gathering recipes into collections, compilers and publishers cued readers to consider the boundaries of community, nation, and/or family. What did it mean when strangers began to share particular ways of skinning a rabbit, creating an edible coat of arms, or making a carrot pudding? Who controlled taste?

Setting the Table

I began this study with the desire to elaborate a more complex contextualization around those printed recipe books that I had analyzed in an earlier project, where I examined household-oriented texts including recipes, plays, and estate guides. Creating a wider contextual frame also required expanding the historical range of my reading so that it included recipes produced over the course of two hundred years. In order to get a sense of how readers responded to prescriptive advice, I pored through marginal annotations and signatures in printed collections. Then I discovered and began to read manuscripts. I was astounded to find a more extensive archive of manuscript materials than I had imagined: over 140 collections housed in the Wellcome Library for the History of Medicine, British Library, Folger Shakespeare Library, Szathmary Culinary Arts Collection at the University of Iowa, Whitney Cookery Collection at the New York Public Library, and Esther Aresty Collection at the University of Pennsylvania; and newly digitalized collections available on the database Perdita.[19] I discovered that manuscript recipe collections existed in a wide variety of physical forms: at one end of the spectrum were large folio texts bound in leather with gold-embossed family crests and initials (Figure 2). At the other were fragments of ragged working notebooks, some of which resembled hastily assembled scrapbooks. Almost all collections register signs of use, and almost all were collaboratively conceived and produced both materially and conceptually; that is, they were written in different hands over time and they cited numerous recipe donors and sources. Interspersed among recipes were other forms of writing: poems, accounting sums, Bible verses, French lessons, sermons, IOUs, practice artwork, family records.

Manuscript sources transformed the story that I had begun to tell. Most crucially, their indeterminate provenance made it impossible to generalize about their historical and material location. Even when signed with what appears to be a clear ownership mark, they often remain fully or partially anonymous. Yet they are also overpopulated with names, crowded with collated attributions to family, friends, social superiors, and printed sources. One cannot read these texts without stumbling across citations such as "Cousin Mabel's way of making almond milk," "Lady Clement's cheese," or "Dr. Allen's water." Even in an era when writing was broadly understood as collaborative, the genre of the recipe book stands out as a peculiarly collective production. Some manuscripts were compiled over the course of hundreds of years, with multiple generations of writers weighing in with opinions, styles, and hands. Often the original compiler backtracked

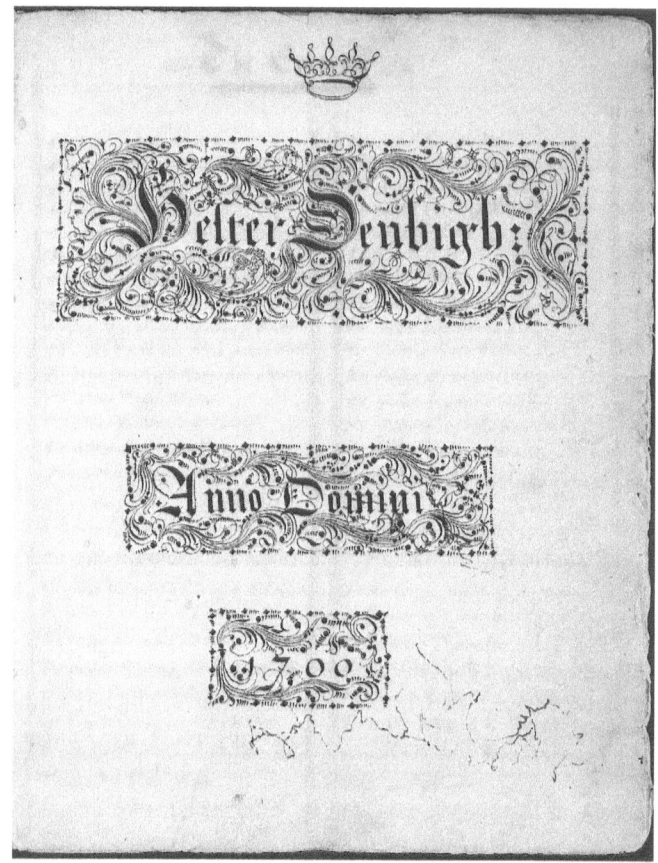

Figure 2. Ornate title page for Hester Denbigh's *Cookery and Medical Receipts*, MssCol 3318, vol. 11. Whitney Cookery Collection. Manuscripts and Archives Division, New York Public Library. Astor, Lenox and Tilden Foundations.

through the collection multiple times amending information. While it is possible in a few instances to trace the precise historical networks registered in a collection, this task is mostly futile (and it's impossible to generalize on the basis of the few collections that we can pin down). I had hoped that these sources would enable me to make claims about what a particular class of people did, made, and ate, or how particular social networks developed through recipe exchange. For instance, I thought I had found a bedrock attributional certainty when I discovered a collection in which the compiler identified her maiden name and married name in the margin: "This I make. E. O. Elizabeth Okeover now Adderly."[20] How much clearer could this be? Given that E. O. also marked other recipes in the collection, it seemed that we could reconstruct *this* recipe community with certainty. But even this declaration (found so rarely in books) proved evasive: the Elizabeth Okeover Adderly who signed her name was not necessarily the Elizabeth Okeoever marked elsewhere in the collection; there were, in fact, two Elizabeth Okeoevers in the family tree (possibly three) who lived far apart, had different connections, and occupied different social stations. Given the lack of extrinsic evidence about the collection and its inconclusive handwriting, we cannot definitively determine the social coordinates of its compilers. While a few scholars have successfully mapped female scribal communities by using recipes, this work can be done for only a fraction of the material. Rather than make faulty guesses about a recipe's provenance or build a sociological argument on such a shaky foundation, I was forced to rethink the questions that I was asking of my printed sources. The new questions I developed moved away from empirically answerable problems, as I sought to make the recipe's elusive collaborative nature the subject of analysis (see Chapter 5). The fact that these books were produced *across* individuals, I realized, *was* the real story: it structured the type of "ownership," "knowledge," and "writing" that recipes embodied.

Manuscript sources also allowed me to glimpse a world of formerly undetected (and largely still unknowable) female writers existing in the early modern world, with recipes sometimes serving as the only trace of their existence. Compilers, scribes, and writers used a mundane form of writing in practical ways—to learn how to create properly textured marzipan, or to display ways to conserve quinces so that they would last a full year. Through this writing, they also asserted particular forms of identity, created durable legacies, opposed or continued family traditions, debated ways of thinking about hospitality, established modes of taste, and tested ways to be a *maker* in their worlds.[21] I have just scratched the surface of what these materials can tell us about reading practices, conceptions of writing, the gendering of medical care, or the social networks forming around food. While I demonstrate that recipe collections register a vibrant world of exchange and contemplation that enfolded writing and practice, more research needs to be done to convert my foray into theorizing kitchen work into multiple textured accounts of specific collections as they traveled and collated knowledge.

Finally, manuscript sources prompted me to think about the formal characteristics that distinguish recipes from other food writing such as memoirs, travelogues, culinary novels, literary banqueting scenes, dietaries, or household manuals. "Receipts," as I have mentioned, implied a contractual relationship between writer and reader, as the reader was enjoined to complete a directive—to "take" and "receive" information mentally and practically (to receive and conceive). The Latin imperative "recipe," which formed the basis for the symbol preceding medical recipes in the medieval and early modern periods—the Rx—served as a visual reminder of this call to action. As "conditional documents," Pennell has argued, recipes create a contract by being pushy, demanding, and imperious in tone.[22] "Draw a large cauldron filled with water," they might order; "take a hog and cut off his head." The use of the second person, a structure not universally shared in recipes in other languages, gave the recipe reader the power to respond to, or refuse, a seemingly authoritative directive. When a recipe reader compiled her own collection, she claimed this commanding voice. "Mix it together if you think good," one recipe tentatively suggests, acknowledging the reader's prerogative in invoking her own judgment over and beyond the speaking agent's.[23] The "transactive" reader often idealized in humanist philosophy as a moral agent wielding practical knowledge is literalized in recipe engagement in instructive ways—as the subject who must "take" a command as well as a material. Make the cream. Censure the recipe. Scribble your judgment in the margin. Pass the recipe to others who will continue the process of acting and accreting words. The recipe's special syntactical form thus correlated with it historical use, as early modern artifacts actively exchanged among men and women, scientific reformers and servants, midwives and artisans. Readers corrected amounts and scribbled sometimes passionate commentary: Elizabeth Godfrey dismissively cancelled a recipe for candied angelica: "this is the worst way to doe them." Lettice Pudsey scrawled beside her pickled cucumber recipe: "This Receipt is good for nothing."[24] Then, as today, people copied recipes in letters, pasted them into books, stole them from sources, presented them as gifts, and lovingly handed them down to daughters or sons. Both the recipe syntax and its mobility contributed to its commemorative and epistemological functions.

Unlike more imaginative forms of food writing, recipes did not strive for lexical variety but instead were deliberately and perhaps comfortingly formulaic. They took the form of a title centered above a brief block of prose language, with no introductory list of ingredients and often only vague amounts. (*The Good Huswifes Jewell* unhelpfully advises the reader to add "all kind of spices" to boiled rabbit, a practice that altered as more precision entered recipes in the next hundred years.)[25] Early recipes repeated conventional commands such as "take," "mix," "stir," "boil," "bake" (and unfamiliar ones such as "smyte," "hack," "anoint," and "smear"). They were repetitive: hundreds of similar recipes marched in lockstep one after another. "How to Make Orange Water" was followed by a string of only slightly varying recipes, each entitled "Another Way." Mary Doggett's collection, we might note, astonishes by following a recipe for cowslip wine with alternatives labeled, in elegant calligraphic hand, "To make Ditto" (Figure 3).[26] While there were exceptions (which I discuss in this book), the early modern recipe presented as fairly impersonal, unforthcoming, and spare.

Yet recipes sometimes strayed from their otherwise uniform and formulaic language to allow a glimpse of the creativity and selectivity of users. Jane Newton likened her sack concoction to rippling water: "some doe fancy to heap the possett with whi[p]ped silbub froth and sett it on like waves"; Mrs. Knight imaginatively conceived one dish as "pigeons transmogrified"; and John Murrell urged readers to beat sugar candy "small like sparks of diamonds."[27] This unusually colorful language conjured up natural motions, twinkling gems and myste-

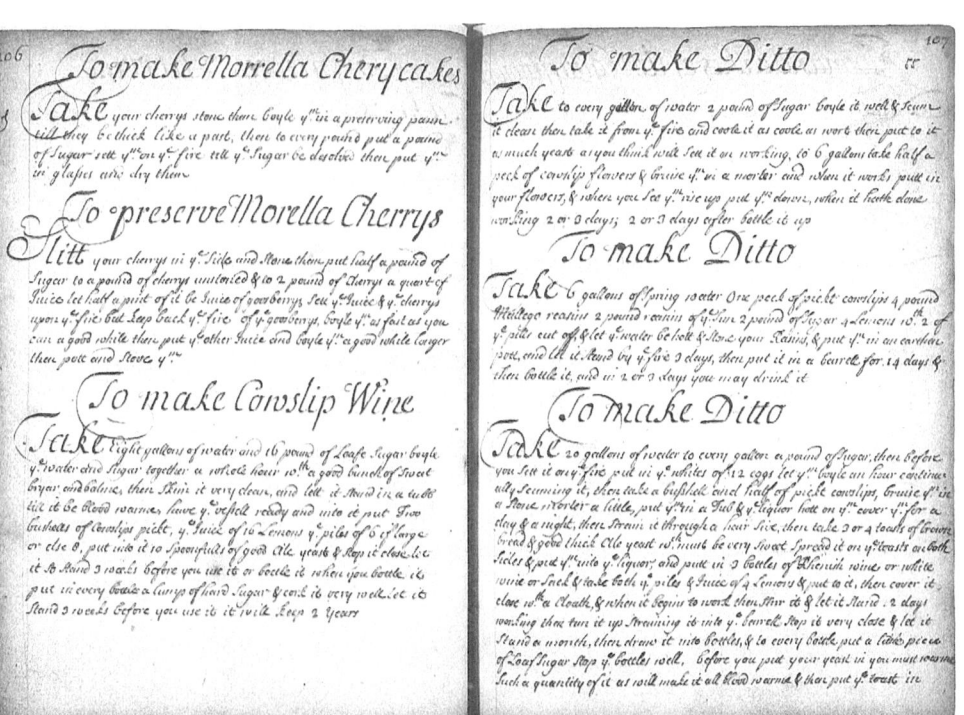

FIGURE 3. "To make Ditto," in Mary Doggett's *Book of Receipts*, 1682, British Library, Add MS 27466, 106–7. Reproduced by permission of the British Library.

rious conversions in which essences utterly metamorphosed. We hear in Mary Granville's claims for her medical panacea a rapturous sense of the spiritual nature of the mission of preserving bodies and worlds: "this pretious water doth marvelously helpe the cough, the Rheume the desease of the Spleene, and many other deseases scarce to be believed; This water was administered, to a person sicke of the palsie for the space of 46 daies, and hee was by the mightie helpe of god, and this miraculous water, throughly healed of his desease, also this helpeth the falling sicknes, and preserveth the body from putrifying, soe that by all these wee may learne that this is as it were a divine water from heaven, and sent from God to serve vnto all ages."[28] While this recipe writer carved out a divine mission for the household worker, other writers took the opportunity of their recipe collections to issue threats to descendants, craft political satire (such as the sly recipe "How to Make a Presbyterian"), mock family members, practice translations, and/or tease out puns in their own names. Mary Cruso, wife of a minister, copied poems and moralisms in her collection that called for the return of the exiled king, parodied French politics, rehearsed sermons, and offered life advice. She marked one pithy saying—"A mans best fortune or his worst a wife / That makes an happy or a wretched Life"—with this note: "*probatum est* Prov. 12:4."[29] By using an erudite Latin phrase often used to indicate the "proven" nature of medical and culinary experiments ("*probatum est*"—"it is proved"), was Mary showing off her knowledge of *sententiae*, Latin, and the Bible alongside her expertise on gingerbread and milk water? Did her role as practitioner of food making, writing, and versifying "prove" her worth as a good wife, or did it challenge the very way the saying typically functioned in the culture (as written *for* a man who determines the value of "his" wife)? What forms of "making" and "knowing" did such a recipe entry register? Hidden within the technical genre of the recipe are detours and idiosyncrasies that catch the eye. I comment on these unusually "voiced" recipes not to track the exceptional personalities behind texts, but to identify what was discursively remarkable within the typical practices and languages they displayed. It was the recipe's almost banal existence that gave it the power and currency it had.

Serve It Forth

The first two chapters of this book analyze printed sources. Chapter 1, "Taste Acts," maps the printed recipe book's social negotiations over the sweep of almost two hundred years. By focusing on ways that the apparatuses of printed books generated particular locales (the closet, kitchen, nation) to configure reading in relation to status and to female labor, I argue that English recipes produced a new concept of domestic "use" out of the ingredients of active reading, manual labor, intellection, and prestige. These locales, along with the notions of expertise and use they entailed, changed as recipes moved away from a concern with social mobility to consolidate a national community that ideally could fuse socially differentiated audiences. The irony of this ideological shift is that the actual labors of the household became more class differentiated, as they segregated the tasks of mistresses and servants that had, for a while, united within the conception of the "good wife." As it outlines the striking taste communities negotiated in printed recipe books, Chapter 1 creates the broad social narrative that frames the concerns discussed in the remaining chapters, each of which investigates the recipe as a site of intellectual exchange, mastery, and reflection.

Chapter 2 argues that the history of recipe publication is also the story of the emergence and decline of culinary "think-pieces" or domestic "conceits." The chapter emerged out of my curiosity about the fact that early recipe publishers insisted that the benefits they offered readers were precisely those of entwined social and intellectual "pleasures." The housewife was both to take pleasure in the act of knowing/making and to "pleasure" others in performing her skills for others. The recipe book thus notably differs from some critically noted discourses in the period, where female artistry and enjoyment were seen as morally and socially suspect. Noting that recipes were called "conceits," a term that also designated poems, artistic devises, and mental formulations, this chapter outlines the ways that food play, like poetic conceit making, functioned as a form of mental apprehension and exercise. What did it mean to invite women to craft "conceits," such as foods that pretended to be naturally growing plants and flowers? Or edible family coats of arms? What were the representational and intellectual stakes of a cuisine that was, as one writer noted, "wrought with no small curiosity"?

The next three chapters foreground ways that *manuscript* recipe collections structured and participated in the intellectual life of households. Chapter 3 examines domestic practice as a complex site of literacy formation and investigation. Given that we now recognize that the domestic arts included writing on surfaces other than paper, how do recipes enable us to reconsider the ways that we conceive of literacy? Did recipes teach women skills that allowed them to write on paper and to perfect particular socially meaningful scripts? Or was "writing" itself conceived in a much more expansive way—as a set of material and expressive marks etched onto food, household objects, walls, plate ware, and paper? This chapter argues that the "handiwork" undertaken by the household maker fused medium and content; recipes created channels of textual circulation whose meaning was inextricably linked to the work they describe. We need only look at the overlap between the handwriting in recipes and the tasty edible alphabetic letters women sculpted to see the stakes of these fascinating connections. What was at stake in some recipe work was nothing short of the processing of material representation itself.

Chapter 4, "Temporalities: Preservation, Seasoning, and Memorialization," takes up the philosophical concerns about death and preservation that a shared culinary and medical practice prompted. In a world without refrigeration or canning, one of the central tasks of domestic life was the preservation of foodstuffs; yet the word "preservation" was also equally or more frequently mentioned in recipes as the goal of medical care. This goal, I argued, then became explicitly linked to the material practice of recipe writing, which was said to preserve family and individual traditions over time. In what ways, I ask, did recipe writers translate the ever-present specter of mortality in the kitchen into the commemorative functions of recipe writing? How did they see their texts, like their labors, as positioning substances in and out of time? Using Shakespeare's play *All's Well That Ends Well* as a way to understand the meanings of "seasoning" (a discourse that surfaces in recipe practice and writing), I attend to the ways that household writing in the seventeenth century registered what poets elsewhere in the culture were vividly portraying as a human battle against time, mortality, and decay.

The final chapter examines connections between the recipe genre and the rise of experimental science in the seventeenth century, with particular focus on how recipe compilers collaboratively defined and authenticated "knowledge." Because recipes involved the circulation of methods for testing procedures and operations, they allow us to document the existence of an informal community of experimenters on the home front. While members of the Royal Society were busy conducting experiments at Gresham Hall, countless unknown women were testing chemical and medical processes and then contemplating the problem of documenting their modes of verification to their scribal communities. Through attributions to recipe donors, source citations, records of personal experience, and imported testimonies, recipe writers took part in epistemological debates that extended into, and resembled, those conducted by virtuosi who have figured prominently in histories of science. With elite women enfranchised within the scope of domestic labor and "ladies" conceptually fused into the roles of "housewives," women had access to a special conceptual site and media for engaging intellectual questions lodged in literate making, preservation, and hands-on knowledge.

The recipe archive harbors riches. It unfolds to our view the intellectual and creative dimensions of daily labors in a past world, yielding to us past recipes for thought laced within practice.

CHAPTER 1

Taste Acts

> I another's Appetite may whet;
> May teach him when to buy, when Season's past,
> What's stale, what's choice, what plentiful, what wast,
> And lead him thro the various Maze of Taste.
> —William King, *The Art of Cookery*

I am acutely aware of how preliminary components set the scene for the remainder of a book, in part because my subject matter in this chapter is the *front matter* of published recipe books. In order to track the changing social stakes of early modern recipe books, I focus on the way that their preliminaries introduced readers to domestic work by generating particular scenes and locales for reading. It is through these apparatuses that recipe books staged what Priscilla Ferguson, in her history of modern French cuisine, calls "taste acts," the process by which culinary subcultures, taste communities, and reading publics are shaped. She writes: "Whereas food calls for eaters, a culinary culture contends with a different sort of consumer, the reader-diners whose consumption of texts rivals their ingestion of food. Reading and evaluating, like eating and cooking, are so many 'taste acts' by which individuals 'perform' their connections to a taste community. That participation in turn—the culinary practices, norms, and values that derive from and support the cuisine in question—sets us in a culinary culture."[1] In positing that food-texts mediate and translate the human activity of eating into a cultural field, Ferguson views *consumption* as a performance implicated in social, textual, and economic protocols. Taking this view of consumption as my cue, I see the early modern recipe book as constituting an understudied representational framework, one that rendered food practices and shifting notions of taste culturally legible in the early modern period.

What was taste in the domain of early modern recipes? Introducing cookery recipes as part of his estate guide, Gervase Markham contended that a housewife should have a sound judgment rooted in sensory expertise. She must possess qualities of character, he observed, chiefly, "a quick eye, a curious nose, a perfect taste, and a ready eare."[2] Markham's fellow recipe writers, by contrast, argued expressly for the cultural capital afforded by recipe knowledge; they recommended that the domestic lady develop a flair for social discrimination that could be demonstrated by serving precisely the right sauces and pies. For most early recipe writers in England, "perfect taste" was less a personal attribute and more a technical expertise that could be used to mobilize social identity. Almost two hundred years later, novelist and recipe writer Eliza Haywood observed that a "woman of *fine taste*" was defined in part by how *little* she knew of the menial tasks of British housewifery. Voltaire, Haywood's contemporary, differentiated current conceptions of taste from earlier incarnations such as Markham's, when he reminded readers that the sense by which the flavor of food was distinguished had become the figurative basis for the apprehension of beauty.[3] The early English recipe book, we discover, marked evolving and contested meanings of taste that configured and reconfigured sensation, status, and aesthetics.

In this chapter, I trace English printed recipe books from their appearance in the 1570s through the eighteenth century, focusing in particular on how their preliminary material used spatially imagined scenes to assert, test, and contest values for the taste communities they crafted out of reading publics.[4] In asking consumers to define appetitive practices within a framework that would later be categorized as "cuisine" or "gastronomy," recipe books performed what sociologist Pierre Bourdieu describes as the work of discrimination and distinction. Because Bourdieu's theories have thoroughly informed cultural studies, it's standard to interpret cultural practices as establishing and negotiating social boundaries. "Taste," Bourdieu has famously written, "classifies, and it classifies the classifier."[5] It's worth returning to his terms to remember the culinary roots of the trope that began to define aesthetics and acts of mental judgment in the Enlightenment. Pre-modern recipes certainly participated in acts of social classification long before taste took on its modern meaning as a refined mental sensibility tied to social hierarchies. In earlier textual and social operations taste was, strikingly, the product of an active practice that women orchestrated—something tied to physical sensation, social judgment, and sweaty labor.

While it's not possible to provide a comprehensive study of the social struggles that recipes engaged during this vast sweep of time, I identify one key conceptual shift that occurred with regard to recipe publication and taste: while early recipe books fantasized about opening an elite closet to female readers, later texts turned to the nationalized kitchen as the primary site of recipe literacy.[6] In the first ninety years of their publication (1570–1660), English recipe books, I argue, marketed a female closet newly accessible in print, a space that was a bookish marker of elite standing and one that entailed a particular conception of manual, cognitive, and somatic *use*. In the 1650s and through the eighteenth century, representations of recipe work shifted to the kitchen, where professional chefs and female housekeepers vied to define the relationship of food to nation building, gender, and class-stratified labor. This transformation in the textual scene of recipe consumption altered the meaning and scope of domestic knowledge, as readers shifted from ladies/housewives to chefs to servants. It also dramatically recalibrated reading and labor. My story concludes at the historical moment when newly aestheticized conceptions of taste filtered into recipe discourse.

Thinking about the recipe book as activating consumption within particular *spaces* allows us to track the evolving relationship between reading and domestic practice. We see that particular recipe producers alternately related and disassociated labor, reading, gender, and privilege as they shifted from broadcasting a culture of prestige to embracing culinary nationalism. It's significant for our understanding of domestic intellectual life, I will argue in this book, that recipe producers founded taste communities precisely on the figure of the female practitioner—a fantasy housewife with "perfect taste" who was also a "lady."

The Recipe Closet

John Partridge kick-started the fashion for publishing recipes to a diverse readership when he put forth *The Treasurie of Commodious Conceits, & Hidden Secrets and May Be Called, the Huswives Closet, of Healthfull Provision. Mete and necessarie for the profitable use of all estates both men and women*. Although recommended for people across the social spectrum, Partridge's book was conceptualized around and named for the housewife, the person who was assumed to possess a closet stuffed with information and goods. English publishers did not initially market recipe books to capitalize on any radical innovation in cuisine. Indeed the taste-scape of early recipe books registered only incremental modifications to what was essentially an elite medieval diet. Instead book producers anticipated that a new group of literate consumers would be interested in purchasing recipes about exclusive foods and methods. The first published recipe collections in England thus promised to unleash aristocratic medical and culinary secrets to a wider population; and they marked that release spatially in terms of gender and class. Partridge's text gambled on the existence of a population ready to be educated in stylish gastronomical "taste," in Bourdieu's sense of the term.

What did it mean to locate domestic information within a closet? Defining the early modern term "closet" turns out to be a surprisingly complicated and loaded problem. In the last decade, scholars of gender, literature, and sexuality have identified the closet as a key site around which to anchor claims about the birth of the individual, the historicity of same-sex relations, the division of public and private spheres, and the clash of gendered subjectivities. Because of its particular modern connotations, the closet has particularly been the locus of recent theorizations and histories of early modern male-male eroticism. As a relatively new, secluded, and locked space within the early modern home, the closet (or cabinet) has also intrigued scholars interested in charting emerging conceptions of privacy, sexuality, gender, class, and property.[7] Alice Friedman and Mark Girouard argue that closets first came into being in England in a wave of radical architectural changes that amplified the number and size of places for polite entertainment, while, at the same time, proliferating spaces for intimate exchange. With the creation of hallways and expansion of rooms used for withdrawal, homes began to differentiate public and private areas.[8] While scholars initially interpreted closets as signifying a newly privatized sense of the individual that correlated to this new division of space, they soon recognized that closets were multipurpose sites where people sat, worked, studied, talked, read, transacted business, counted money, prayed, and even slept. The common denominator for all these spaces, Lena Cowen Orlin observes, was that they could be locked.[9] As such, closets routinely housed the valuable consumer goods increasingly available to a wider range of households on the social spectrum: jewels, miniature paintings, money, and—perhaps unexpectedly for a modern audience—foodstuffs such as spices, drugs, and sweetmeats. The closet, with its multiple functions, dispositions, and affects, endowed goods or activities lodged within its confines with prestige.

How did the analogy of the recipe book as a closet shape the meaning of the domestic information newly disseminated in print? This question is significant because Partridge's association between closets and recipes was not idiosyncratic. In fact, the metaphor of the closet not only flourished in recipe writing for the next one hundred years, but also became the most common lens through which this type of technical writing was viewed. Witness the following titles of recipe books: *A Good Huswifes Handmaide for the Kitchin... Verie Meete to Be Adjoned to the Good Huswifes Closet of Provision for Her Houshold* (1594); *Delightes for Ladies, to Adorne Their Persons, Tables, Closets, and Distillatories* (1600); *A Closet for Ladies and Gentlewomen* (1608); *The Ladies Cabinet Opened* (1639); *The Ladies Cabinet Opened and Enlarged* (1654); *The Queens Closet Opened* (1655); *The Closet of the Eminently Learned Sir Kenelme Digbie Kt. Opened* (1669); *The Queen-Like Closet; or, Rich Cabinet* (1675); *The Ladies Delight; or, A Rich Closet of Choice Experiments* (1672); *A Supplement to the Queen-Like Closet* (1674); *The Accomplished Ladies Rich Closet of Rarities* (1687). Given that many of these texts went through multiple reprints, it is no understatement to say that the print market in England was flooded with recipe-filled closets over the course of a century. This primary fantasized scene of recipe knowledge and taste began to be rivaled by other conceptual frameworks only in the 1650s. In the next chapter, I consider ways that the closet trope in recipe writing mobilized a particular conception of domestic pleasure that was implicated in *eros* and art. In this chapter, I argue that Partridge's use of the closet trope created a powerful and enduring conception of a household *maker* whose manual labor was literate, active, and prestigious.

In *The Treasurie*, Partridge essentially invented a domestic incarnation of the "books of secrets" that had been popular throughout Europe in the sixteenth century. Esoteric in nature, books of secrets offered miscellaneous information about remedies, party tricks, invisible ink, foods, chastity tests, and other sundry skills.[10] Yet *The Treasurie* addressed a domestic and female audience that had not previously been acknowledged in the secrets genre. Partridge sought this audience by identifying his recipes as part of the cheap market that his printer Richard Jones cultivated in the late sixteenth century. Jones was known for published accounts of pirate adventures, monstrous births, treason, and juicy news stories, ballads, poems, and popular defenses of women. Having himself previously translated versified stories of martial combat and martyrs, Partridge took a calculated risk in joining Jones to court a novel audience for his refined, yet practical, housewifery book directed to female and male readers.

Despite an increase in books addressed to female readers during these decades, printed advice on domestic labors might have seemed to hail a nonexistent audience.[11] Who would have read such a newfangled thing? Weren't the women who cooked and made homey medicines largely illiterate servants? Would literate women of means truly have cared to know details of boiling, stewing, and dairying? Despite our skepticism about the project, Partridge seems to have discovered—or perhaps invented—a ready and receptive audience. Reprinted in thirteen separate editions spanning eighty years, *The Treasurie of Commodious Conceits* inspired a wave of like-minded texts. Partridge launched another recipe book called *The Widdowes Treasure* (1588); Jones followed with the anonymous *A Good Huswifes Handmaide for the Kitchin* (1594); and writers such as Thomas Dawson, Hugh Plat, John Murrell, and Gervase Markham moved swiftly to capitalize on this market. Gilly Lehmann estimates that by the end of the sixteenth century, 14,500 copies of recipe books were in circulation in twenty-nine editions in England.[12] Although we cannot assess the exact proportions of men, noblemen, noblewomen, and/or housewives who actually read these books with any degree of certainty, it is clear that Partridge defined a new marketing niche that reached a more encompassing and gender-mixed readership.[13] Ownership marks by non-noble women, for instance, show that the address to women was not merely a flight of fantasy. Noble women were interested in honing the prestigious tasks of confectionery and medical care, while gentry women and affluent merchant's wives sought to introduce expensive foods into their social circles. Recipe texts validated the post-Reformation ideal that sought to unify nobility, wealthy farmers, yeomen, country gentry, merchants, and aspiring householders in the quest for hands-on knowledge about the nuts and bolts of running a home. Branded a "good housewife" (a category that stretched to include high-born ladies and farmers' wives), the new reading consumer was to arbitrate taste and demarcate the class categories she was imagined to traverse.[14] Although the stews and confections that recipe books promoted might have seemed familiar to ladies and lords, these concoctions circulated in public in ways that affirmed a woman's responsibility—as a *housewife*—for diet and health care. If women at all ranks had been supervising domestic tasks to more or lesser degrees in post-Reformation England, their responsibilities took on the added mission of defining public culinary tastes and domestic ideals when these texts appeared in print. For my purposes, it is important to underscore that recipes made housewifery a matter of public written record, something subject to debate by an array of readers.

While Renaissance literary and moralist writings freely depicted food-related longings, pleasures, and reveries with great gusto, early recipe collections surprisingly did not revel in the sensual pleasures of the table. They clearly subordinated the sensory pleasures of food to its medicinal, practical, and social functions. Recipe books would not organize taste communities around preferences for particular styles of food, in fact, until after the 1650s. Instead these early books championed the novelty, exclusivity, profitability, and propriety of foods and goods available to consumers. Thomas Dawson's *Good Huswifes Jewell* proclaimed on its title page that it delivered "most excellent and rare Devises for Conceites in *Cookerie*"; John Murrell's *A New Booke of Cookerie* promised innovative techniques for creating splendor at the table. If recipes offered readers a way to demonstrate good taste, they understood that term to pertain to technical methods and skills that could be obtained through reading.

The closet that Partridge unlocked in print initially materialized as a gentleman's study, the working space of a library. *The Treasurie of Commodious Conceits* opens with a woodcut frontispiece where an elegantly dressed man dutifully copies domestic "secrets" from printed texts and manuscripts (Figure 4). The writer is pictured as the epitome of high fashion, decked as he is with hat, ruff collar, cape, doublet with ornate cuffs, button-studded pantaloons, and accessorizing florets that match hose to prominently displayed shoes. He consults textual sources as he pens the manuscript that presumably has converted into the book that the reader consumes, a commodity that grants access to what is clearly an elite, interior, and literate space. It smacks of textuality and exclusivity.

The Treasurie's subsequent prefatory materials consolidated the frontispiece's identification of expertise in cooking and medical care with an elite knowledge vested in literate practice. In a rhymed envoy (a well-known literary form in which an author sends out a personified book to the public), Partridge framed the book as the object of the reader's gaze: "Goe forth my little booke / That all on thee may looke." Through a thirty-two-line patterned rhyme scheme, Partridge imagined the book's reception by harsh critics in terms conventional for a literary work (A2v). Having promised to stand loyally by the vulnerable book as it ventures on a courageous mission, the author then included a dedicatory letter where he presented himself as a hero disseminating knowledge in the face of foolhardy resistance. Given that dedicatory epistles were typically reserved for Bibles, classical literature, devotionals, and works of religious and political controversy in the sixteenth century and would not become attached to popular pamphlets until later, the author's decision to use the epistle and envoy aired a measure of ambition.[15] In repeatedly signaling

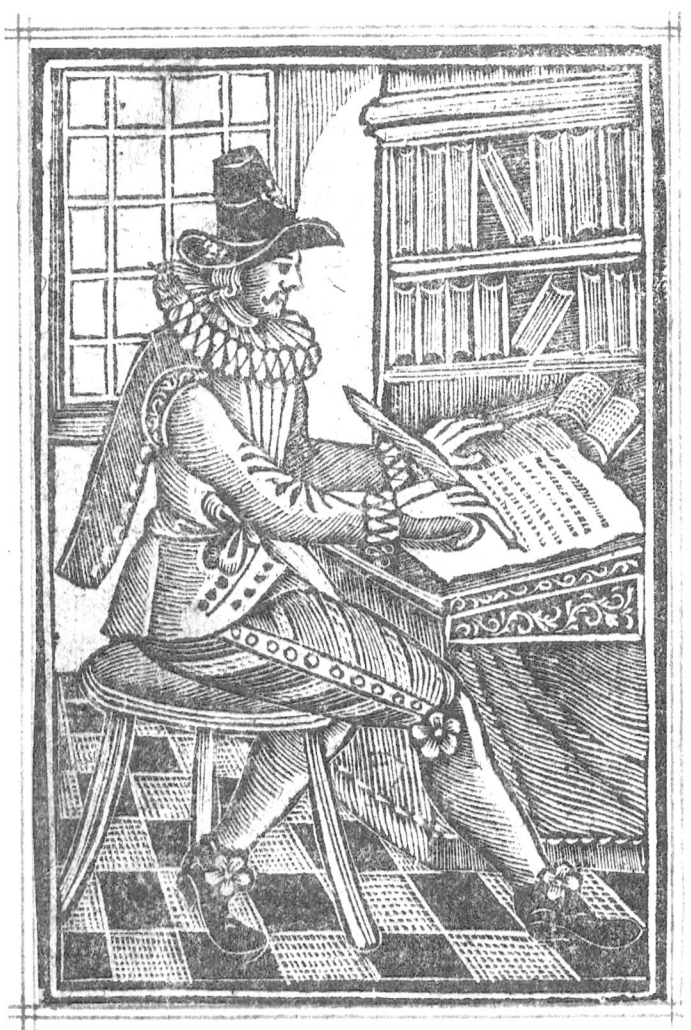

FIGURE 4. Frontispiece to John Partridge's *The Treasurie of Commodious Conceits & Hidden Secrets* (London, 1573). Reproduced by permission of the Huntington Library.

that his "little" form differed from "great workes," Partridge evoked markers of both popular print and learned genres.

After revising book conventions to accommodate a non-noble patron and general reading public, *The Treasurie* included two commendatory poems that testified to Partridge's standing not as an experimenter but as a *writer*; "Thomas

Curteyse Gentleman in prayse of the Auctor" and "Thomas Blanck Gentleman in the behalf of the Auctor" located recipe writing as a classically renowned art. In a final poetic envoy, the author insisted that the book commodity was part of a polite exchange constituted by service and patronage; for he charged the book to prostrate itself in feudal servitude to a "dear and speciall friend," the mistress who catalyzed the project by begging him to put his knowledge in print.[16] Actual recipes appear only after a fulsome seven pages of preliminary addresses, the cumulative effect of which is to conscript humanistic and literary conventions to shape an artifact whose value rests in widespread consumption. The message is not subtle: knowing the latest foods and medicines, such as how to bake chickens or conserve quinces, place one in the company of well-dressed and well-read (literate) persons. *The Treasurie*'s erudite conventions encoded female domestic knowledge as intimate, secluded, and valuable. Recipes were snugly nestled within the world of letters as part of a bid for social status.

How did the recipe book square housework with what we now recognize as the trappings of literary pretension? The printer's 1584 address, "To all that covet the practices of good Huswyverie as well wives as maydes," addressed this issue by elaborating on the how the newly visible closet generated "use":

> Good Huswives here you have a Jewell for your joy,
> A Closet meete your huswivery to practise and imploy.
> As well the gentles of degree, as eke the meaner sort,
> May practise here to purchase helth, their houshold to co[m]fort. . . .
> Therefore good Huswives once againe, I say to you: repayre,
> Unto this Closet when you neede, & mark what ye find there.
> Which is a mean to make most things, to huswives use pertain
> As al Conserves and Sirops sweet to comfort heart and braine.
> For ba[n]quets to, here may you find, your dishes how to frame:
> As Succad, marmalad, Marchpane to, & ech thing els by name . . .
> Thus to co[n]clude, I wish you mark, the benefits of this booke.
> Both Gentles state, the Farmers wife, & crafts mans huswife Cooke.
> And if we reape commoditie by this my friendes advice.
> Then give him thankes, and thinke not muche, of foure pence for
>   the price. (A1v)

While directly attempting to up his sales, the printer also advised women who aspired to be elite housewives to view the book simultaneously as a precious material good, informational storage unit, and analog for a particular form of labor. The printer signaled these meanings by describing the book as a precious "jewel" that the reader could "have" (for only four pence) as well as a closet (or study) in which the reader could "practice" knowledge. "Repayre / Unto this Closet when you neede," he commanded. The analogy of the book as a space into which the reader could enter and "repayre" might seem to indicate the quaint wish that the reader will be passionately absorbed into the material, but this phrasing glossed the way that the book, and domestic closet, might be imagined. The gesture of "repair," with its most obvious meaning of proceeding or going habitually, was closely connected to acts of restoration and remedy. The word derived both from the Latin *reparare* (to restore or recreate) and *repariare* (to resort).[17] When women dwelled, retreated, and had recourse to their closets, they undertook re-creational and restorative projects. In her diary, Lady Margaret Hoby, who regularly used her cabinet as a devotional space for prayer as well as a study for reading, recorded that she was "busy" in her closet just as she was busy in her in housewifery.[18] When Gervase Markham commanded his housewife to sequence an elaborate banqueting course, he described this ordering as happening *within* a storage closet (1623; 125). The secluded study depicted in the frontispiece of the inaugural edition of Partridge's *Treasurie*, where a male author writes, was utterly transformed in recipe books when appropriated as a usable space open to a gender-inclusive (though female-identified) mobile practice.

Knowledge production also became importantly portable within this conceptually spatial framework: the material book served as a closet without walls. For those not rich enough to have a physical closet in their households, the book allowed a metaphorical home renovation, serving as a textual surrogate that could, like locked spatial closets, confer value. Alsemero, in Middleton and Rowley's *The Changeling*, wittily describes ladies maids' privileged knowledge by calling on this trope. "These women are the Ladies Cabinets, / Things of most pretious trust are lock into 'em," he declares.[19] Ironically, the recipe book would likely have been housed *in* the wife's closet (if she were fortunate enough to possess one) along with valuable spices and the tasty sweetmeats that she learned to make while reading the book. The title metaphor thus presented a set of receding closets within closets.

The Treasurie also defined a *transactive* domestic space in which "use" signaled a cognitive, physical, and exalted act. As a "closet meete" in which the reader was to "practise and imploy" housewifery, the book was the medium through which women could energetically process and test information. In fact, the reader is twice asked to "mark" domestic information and its salutary features: "Repaire / Into this closet when you need, and mark what ye find there"; "I wish ye mark the benefits of this book." While "marking," in early modern parlance, meant noticing or observing, it also signaled the material act of inscribing a mark onto a surface. Indeed, according to the *Oxford English Dictionary*, the graphic meaning of marking likely preceded the cognitive meaning. After reading William Sherman's *Used Books: Marking Readers in Renaissance England*, it is impossible to think of early modern reading as an abstract process. His scholarship, along with that of Heidi Brayman Hackel, Carla Mazzio, and Bradin Cormack, goes far in documenting ways that "marking" served as a rich mental and manual activity, a sign of ubiquitous hands-on use by book consumers who transformed the texts they engaged.[20] Early modern readers seemed to have followed schoolmaster John Brinsley's pedagogical advice for boys to identify material in books that should be "marked out." Brinsley instructed students to use a pen to write in their schoolbooks and an erasable pencil for making ephemeral notes in recreational books; smaller children were advised to make "secret markes" "with some little dint with their naile."[21] Early modern readers took this advice to heart as they tackled all kinds of books by underlining, annotating, drawing manicules (pointing hands), adding checkmarks, cancelling text, and making marks with pins and fingernails (the latter being the most embodied reading).[22] Readers who left traces of their lexical tools for apprehension and memorialization— whether through charcoal, ink, or bodily impression—understood this task as "marking." "Marke this," Lady Clifford wrote performatively in her copy of *The Mirror for Magistrates*.[23] Some people even "read" recipes through the operations of pinning, stitching, and sewing. The person consuming a manuscript attributed to Anne Bayne pinned a scrap of paper to the recipe for red currant cake, which emended the amount of sugar required and specified an exact boiling time.[24] Choosing a durable and time-intensive technique, the reader of Elizabeth Okeover's recipes stitched a piece of protruding paper, inscribed "egg pie," onto the recipe page so as to create an personalized indexical bookmark.[25] In these instances, readers used domestic and artisanal skills to highlight and/or transform information. When the printer of *The Treasurie* urged readers to *mark* information, then, he encouraged an embodied, active, and transformative textual engagement; readers were to take on the labor of the writing compiler earlier envisioned in the library/closet.

As Cormack and Mazzio exhibit in *Book Use, Book Theory, 1500–1700*, many of the typical utilitarian operations of early modern reading constituted modes of thinking and identity formation. They introduce book use by pointing to Geoffrey Whitney's emblem book, which glosses reading with this motto: "First reade, then marke, then practice that is good, / For without use, we drinke but LETHE flood."[26] Use "is positioned as the foundation of practice and experience," they argue, "but also, more surprisingly, of memory and knowledge itself" (3). Readers used physical marks to create memory techniques as well as to single out passages for further meditation and study. While we might expect a reader's mark to trigger and unlock memory retrieval in technical manuals, recipe books also inspired "reflection" explicitly through use. The dictum prefacing Hugh Plat's *Delightes for Ladies* (1602), a text so popular that it went through thirteen editions in fifty years, commanded: "Read, Practice, and Censure." Although these actions seem sequential, Plat's text goes on to show that they were mutually implicated. The reader's ability to censure, or pass judgment on, instruction was part and parcel of active *practice*, testing, and labor, a dynamic form of reading carried out between closet and kitchen (or stillroom). In inviting the reader to "practise here," *The Treasurie* further fused the physical and temporal moment of reading into the domestic work it recommended. The reader's spatialized engagement with the artifact ("here") implicated "marking" within the motions of housework. Entering into her closet to alter, test, and memorize its resources, the housewife inhabited a space that endowed prestige on domestic book "use" and labor.[27]

Historians of reading practices have recently analyzed book use to support claims about the physical and social elements of early modern knowledge production. By highlighting reading's physical dimension and assumed practical application, they have turned away from modern depictions of reading as purely abstract. The activities of "marking" and "noting" ubiquitously recommended and conceptualized by humanist pedagogues and thinkers involved imprinting the mind through action. Knowledge was conjured forth through embodied exercise. Household prescriptive reading strikingly demonstrates the inversion of this relationship: recipe work, which we assume to concern itself with practical doing, entailed forms of thinking, an intellectual *praxis* that *The Treasurie* identified squarely by reference to the domestic closet. Extending the cognitive-manual interface that scholars have appreciated as part of early modern humanistic reading to recipe books allows us to see the intellectual contours and social valuation of a previously unrecognized domestic literate culture.

After *The Treasurie* burst onto the publishing scene, numerous recipe books echoed its claim to release elite household knowledge to active readers. When

Partridge promised "to teach all manner of person & degrees to know perfectly the maner to make diverse and sundry sorts of fine conceits," the "gentels of degree and eke the meaner sort," he put the secrets vested in the sanctum of the closet up for sale, available to any literate person with four pence to spare. Partridge offered the "manner" (or means) for becoming a different "manner" (or type) of social being (1573; A3v–A4). Following his lead of offering scaled-down noble concoctions and confections amid tips for making cosmetics, dyes, and practical medicines, subsequent inexpensive collections promoted their information as a fashionable luxury commodity subject to the wife's authority and possession: *The Good Huswife's Jewell* (1587); *The Good Hus-wives Treasurie* (1588); *The Good Huswifes Handmaide for the Kitchin* (1594); *The Widdowes Treasure* (1588); *A Daily Exercise for Ladies and Gentlewomen* (1617); *The Ladies Companion* (1653). In *The Good Huswife's Jewell*, Thomas Dawson assured insecure readers that they could learn "the best and newest fashion" for making almond butter and "the order of meats how they *must* be served at the Table" (32). John Murrell professed to provide "the newest and most commendable Fashion for Dressing or Saucing, eyther Flesh, Fish or Fowle," as part of a metropolitan and international cuisine designed to "beautifie and adorne eyther Nobleman or Gentlemans Table."[28] *A Good Huswifes Handmaide for the Kitchin* bragged that it could deliver "principall pointes of Cookerie . . . after sundrie of the best fashions used in England and other Countries, with their apt and proper sawces." Those on the fringes of elite society were offered the chance to absorb the decorum and protocols for dining. Even people who did not have the means to concoct the most extravagant recipes in a given collection might want to buy it to become privy to the lifestyles of the rich and famous. Why not bolster your social self-esteem by learning how "to make . . . Marmelade very comfortable and restorative for any Lord or Lady whatsoever"? Or an excellent confection "given Queene Mary for a New-yeare's gift"? Imagine the satisfaction of knowing how Lady Gray Clements enjoyed her quince jelly (unstrained): how King Edward preferred preserves; or how Henry VIII liked his rabbits sauced (apparently with parsley, butter, pepper, and verjuice).[29] With the newfound popularity of the printing press, the increased affordability of print materials, and the rise of social mobility, affluent merchants and yeomen were able to traffic in the culinary signifiers of affluent living. While recipe books' claims to reach a wide public were certainly exaggerated (few persons of "the meaner sort" could have pursued these leisure activities), they *did* reach a wide group of people who *did* put this information into practice.[30] The paradox of mobility found in courtesy manuals of the day extended to the recipe guide: these genres affirmed and made legible status lines that they also promised to traverse and attenuate. But unlike courtesy manuals, recipes nominated "every good huswife" as the figure who could integrate social estates and arbitrate taste.

The imagined recipe closet was also, we should note, a free and untroubled international zone. With one glaring exception, which I discuss below, English recipe writers until the 1660s were not defensive about the fact that the diet they recommended depended on the importation of foreign ingredients and on international trade ventures. Stage plays, sermons, and conduct books, by contrast, vociferously denounced luxury commodities and foreign peoples flowing into England as making dangerous incursions on national culture and nationally constituted bodies. Stories in print and on the London stage traded in national stereotypes signaled by food preferences—from Welsh cheese, to French kickshaws (*quelquechose*), to Irish liquor.[31] Dietaries of the day sternly warned against the dire health risks of foreign foods and dining customs. Yet early printed recipe books silently embraced and even celebrated the international cuisine of elite households as the marker of social status. They neither mystified nor celebrated the global coordinates of recipe culture but instead promoted the taste community as congealing within a gendered scene of reading, thinking, and working.

Although collections continued to be reprinted, no new recipe texts appeared in print between 1619 and 1650. In part, this hiatus was caused by the fact that King James banned the publication of all medical recipes except the *Pharmacopeia*, the official book of remedies sponsored by the College of Physicians. Given that the fates of culinary and medical recipes were intertwined, this prohibition blocked the dissemination of cookery information (and, according to Elizabeth Spiller, helped to segregate these knowledges in future books[32]). New publications of recipe books also ground to a halt because of the social, political, and economic upheavals of the civil war, which brought with it horrors of privation and hunger as well as the financial ruin of notable families of standing. When recipe collections resumed in print in the commonwealth, they began to cater to a new readership eager to master basic vocational skills; they addressed, for instance, daughters of landed families who found themselves forced to go into service.

In the mid-seventeenth century, the recipe closet was renovated and then largely dispensed with as the master trope for domestic knowledge. Recipe books in the 1650s initially looked much like their predecessors, in that they continued to vest expertise in aristocratic closets. Yet they shifted the scene and meaning of "closet knowledge" in three salient ways: they (1) cited individual practitioners rather than a given class as the source of knowledge, (2) included women as author-compilers, and (3) lodged domestic know-how within partisan political battles. In 1653, the medical recipes of Elizabeth Grey, Countess of Kent, were published posthumously, paired with a companion text on confectionery and preserving entitled *A True Gentlewoman's Delight*. Grey's *A Choice Manuall, or Rare and Select Secrets in Physick and Chirurgery* would have looked familiar to readers who kept abreast of recipe books because it pointed to the refined nature of its tastes and practices; it imparted a "rich cabinet of knowledge" possessed and practiced by a known countess (1661; A3). Rather than portraying the all-purpose space of the closet, the frontispiece depicted the countess's portrait. Two subsequent publications attributed to female practitioners struck out in new directions by subjecting recipe closets to the fierce battles around royalist politics. W.M.'s *The Queens Closet Opened. Incomparable Secrets in Physick, Chirurgery, Preserving, Candying, and Cookery; as They Were Presented to the Queen by the Most Experienced Persons of Our Times* (1655) claimed to put into print the recipes of the exiled queen Henrietta Maria. This collection, as Laura Knoppers has demonstrated, enacted a public relations mission to combat images of excess at the court and to "English" the suspiciously foreign Henrietta Maria by showing her to be a woman of industry rather than a seditious plotter. In her trenchant analysis of this book's production, presentation, and reception, Knoppers argues that it "proved a remarkable means of assimilating the queen into a multigenerational social network distinguished, above all, by its Englishness" (103). Within the same political vein—though cast in the mode of satire—*The Court & Kitchin of Elizabeth, Commonly called Joan Cromwel[l], the Wife of the Late Usurper* claimed to open the recipe collection of the Lord Protector's wife to the public in the interval between his fall and the restoration of Charles II. This book promoted a royalist agenda by mocking the cuisine of Cromwell's court as vulgar, inelegant, and deceptive.[33] Rounded out by Kenelm Digby's posthumously opened and somewhat atypical *Closet* in 1669, this new breed of recipe collection collectively lamented the decline of hospitality and aristocratic housekeeping caused by the civil war. Rather than attempting to make elite taste transferrable, as the first wave of writing had sought to do, post-1650 books aimed to revivify a courtly milieu disappearing in the wake of turbulent social, political, and economic changes. As they conjured up the particular closets of renowned persons, these books were explicitly rooted in worlds of the past.

Mid-seventeenth-century recipe publications also significantly transformed the represented locale of recipe work. They felt no obligation to train readers to understand the literate and prestigious nature of work-practice, because domestic "marking" was now an accepted component of recipe use. Instead they renovated the basic conception of the closet. To buy and use a recipe collection inserted the reader into heated political disputes where housewifery could establish or contest "proper" royal values; it made the consumer a participant in a political conversation that easily extended into other forms of writing—political pamphlets and ideologically charged poems. One's taste in making sauces and baking pies was mobilized to prove the gentility of an *original* individual practitioner and thus to assert allegiance to a particular social network, courtly circle, or form of government. The nature of the taste act, and its imagined locations, had changed.

From Closet to Kitchen

The story of the early modern recipe takes a dramatic turn in the 1660s, when recipe use and authorization moved out of the elite closet altogether and into a kitchen staffed with paid professionals. In this new scenario, recipe writers did not nostalgically cling to an aristocratic lifestyle but instead staked their expertise on the professional experience of compilers who now were to oversee English taste and culinary values. Rather than venerating the status of domestic work, recipes collections placed the kitchen front and center as an *entrepreneurial* site of practice. Though social standing would always be an alluring feature of the recipe world, cookery books began to show less interest in advertising the thrill of exclusivity and instead promoted new ways to imagine recipe use and ownership. Two groups battled for control over the soul and meaning of cuisine in its publicly circulating form: female housekeepers and male chefs.[34] In the heated debate that unfolded in print, they posed new questions to readers: was food preparation and its concomitant role in arbitrating taste best controlled by amateurs or those with formal training? Should cooking be a constituent part of general household management or a specialized vocation? Should cuisine exhibit national values or introduce readers to exotic fashions? Should food practices model conduct for women? While the foods recommended in English guides moved cautiously away from centuries-old traditions, the publishing world became sharply polarized about how people should think about taste communities, with some books clinging to an image of food making as housework (along with medical care and confectionery making) and others classifying it as a cosmopolitan style grasped by individual genius. For the first time, these communities distinguished actual foods as they distinguished readers.

Robert May's *Accomplisht Cook* was a landmark book in this debate. While identifying good taste with royalist political networks, this text newly defined cookery as an *artistic* skill acquired through specialized training. Cuisine-in-print did not obtain value because it opened an elite closet to a wider audience. Instead it was the proprietary knowledge of exceptional individuals who were able to communicate some measure of their extensive training through writing. The extensive prefatory materials to *The Accomplisht Cook* presented May as a monumental *author* worthy of commendatory poems and a formal portrait; it constructed, as Sandra Sherman argues, the first modern celebrity chef.[35] Whereas Partridge had been presented as an erudite textual *compiler*, May visually appears on the page in the monumentalizing portrait form reserved typically as a sign of aristocratic or authorial power (Figure 5). The consumer of May's text was to appreciate individual accomplishment rather than practice-based "use," a message underscored in the poetic command accompanying the portrait:

> What wouldst thou view but in one face
> All hospitalitie, the race
> Of those that for the Gusto stand,
> Whose tables a whole Ark command
> Of Natures plenty, wouldst thou see
> This sight, peruse May's booke, 'tis hee.

Using the high style of encomium found in texts such as Shakespeare's First Folio (which commanded readers to gaze upon the book not the man), this poem hyperbolically invites the reader to view a figure whose face emblemizes "all hospitalitie." The central operation of this verse is compression: as the book collapses into the figure of its author, it offers a "sight" that unifies nature with people of good taste. May embodies the "race" of persons devoted to "gusto" (from the Latin *gustas*, taste), a term whose cultural meaning was only gradually expanding to signify aesthetic appreciation. Rather than instructing the reader to repair into a closet to produce knowledge, as earlier books suggested, *The Accomplisht Cook* urged readers to be struck with wonder at the spectacle of a culinary Noah.

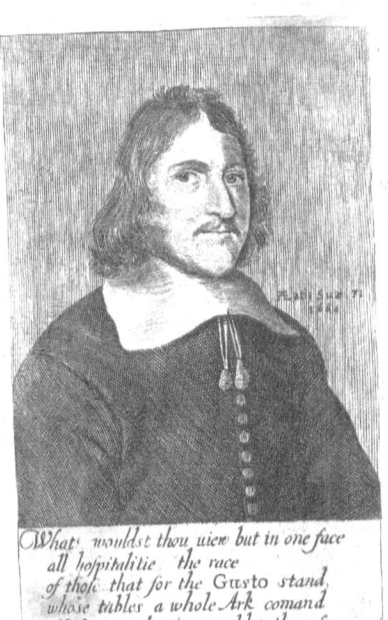

FIGURE 5. Title page to Robert May's *The Accomplisht Cook* (London, 1685). Reproduced by permission of the Folger Shakespeare Library.

The title page, dedication, epistle, and commendatory poems for *The Accomplisht Cook* go on to define a chef as someone possessing a culinary philosophy and authorial monumentality. Lords testify to May's greatness; John Town poetically mourns the fact that Ben Jonson, the only author capable of genuinely singing May's praises, is dead and thus unavailable to offer a blurb. May himself nostalgically laments the demise of old-fashioned noble entertainment while celebrating the vibrant patronage network that has allowed him to develop into a culinary wizard. The publisher then offers something never seen in English recipe books: a biography of the recipe author. This narrative threads the tale of May's training as the son of a cook and apprentice in French and English noble households within two sweeping contexts: a celebration of the golden age of religious belief, hospitality, and charity; and a brief for cookery's role in ancient Rome. As an esteemed tradition of antiquity exercised by "most worthy Artists" (A5, A4), cookery appears as a pedigreed skill, one likened, as one commendatory poem suggests, to academic arts such as mathematics, geometry, architecture, and military fortification. From its place within the grand tradition of the humanistic arts, cooking hardly seems frivolous entertainment, or, for that matter, housework.

After the publication of *The Accomplisht Cook*, numerous books sought to establish cookery as an elevated tradition circulating from and to a vocation of trained men. Influenced by translations of French texts such as *The French Cook*, *The Perfect Cook*, and *A Perfect School of Instruction for Officers of the Mouth*, Joseph Cooper, William Rabisha, Charles Lamb, Charles Carter, and other chef-authors consolidated a brethren of cooks. Celebrating Italian, Spanish, and French cosmopolitanism as the signature mark of pre–civil war noble hospitality, these texts added a royalist patina to previous articulations of taste. One writer, for instance, chalked up his publication to the "blessed restauration of our long-exiled Luminaries" who replenished "the Life of Arts and Sciences."[36] Cookery texts became publicly available as sites where writers could gently protest the protectorate or celebrate the restoration of cavalier housekeeping.

Fully ensconced within this tradition, Rabisha's *The Whole Body of Cookery Dissected, Taught and Fully Manifested, Methodically, Artificially and According to the Best Tradition o[f] the English, French, Italian, Dutch, & c.* (1661) mandated an international, authentic, and newly rationalized cuisine that could not be learned simply by reading. The book opened by calling for nothing less than the complete eradication of all previous culinary knowledge:

> Cooks burn your Books, and vail your empty brains;
> Put off your feigned Aprons: view the strains
> Of this new piece, whose Author doth display
> The bravest dish, and shew the nearest way
> T'inform the lowest Cook how he may dress,
> And make the meanest meat the highest mess:
> To please the Fancie of the daintiest Dame
> And sute her palate that she praise the same.
> Give him return of worth, (besides due wages)
> And recommend his Book to future ages. (A6)

Using heroic couplets, this anonymous commendatory poet introduced would-be cooks to an author whose authentic and brave cookery promised to transform meager food into elegant eating. Women entered the picture as finicky consumers rather than textually engaged housewives. The good taste ("palate") of the "daintiest Dame" is important chiefly because it might catalyze her to render the artist-chef immortal by employing him. This poem follows on the heels of Rabisha's dedication of his book to five elite female patrons and "nourishers of all ingenious Arts and Sciences" (A2). When Rabisha later reassures a "fraternity of Cooks" that his publication will not allow "every kitchen wench" to pretend to a grand art, he classifies cookery as outside the sphere of female domestic labor.[37] Dainty dames do not work, nor do gentlemen amateurs. They nourish and feed through their generous funding.

The Whole Body of Cookery Dissected appealed to a sophisticated reader who might put a premium on the ancient authority of the culinary arts. The opening poem playfully figures Rabisha as a second Jacob, whose exceptional skill promises to turn diners into Esaus willing to sacrifice a birthright for savory stews. "His Broth, Pottages, to the taste and sight," the poet claims of Rabisha, "would Esau-like make some to sell their right." Part of the poem's wit rests on the tension between the formality of the iambic pentameter couplets and the seemingly mundane operations they describe. Sauces, pickles, jellies, leaches, hashes, puddings, and boiled meats jostle against an elevated style and diction: "To Carbonado, and to Hash and Stew, / He all correcteth, by this Art more new: / To Fry and Frigasie, his way's most neat. / How he compounds a thousand sorts of meat!" Rhyming "sallets" with "pallats," and "season" with "reason," the poet jauntily collapses domestic and artistic registers: "To Marinate, to Sowce, and pickle fish / So rich, so high, as any heart could wish." The resulting humor, however, is tempered by an overarching earnest ennobling of cookery; the poem advances cooking as an art requiring "admired reason" and sophistication both on the part of the maker and the consumer.

As they separated housewifery from cooking, recipe writers redefined taste as a marker of social distinction. In *Royal Cookery; or, The Complete Court Cook* (1710), Patrick Lamb (master chef for fifty years under Charles II, James II, William and Mary, and Anne) welcomed readers into his book as guests who needed to be ushered to their proper seats at a lavish banquet. He denounced stingy consumers who condemned and refused to buy recipes. "As a viscious Palate is, by no means, a proper Judge of Tastes," he proclaimed, "so were it a great Pity, One or Two peevish Cynicks should put Good-Eating out of Countenance."[38] Being refined, according to master cook Robert Smith, meant rejecting the menial tasks associated with rural estate management and female cosmetics. In his 1723 *Court Cookery*, Smith mocked recipe books that deigned to present "washes and beautifiers for ladies or making ale for country squires."[39] Charles Carter, chef to the Duke of Argyle, admired ingenious culinary makers as feeders of elite taste. "No Occupation in the World is more oblig'd to Invention," he wrote in *The Complete Practical Cook* (1730), "every year and every ingenious Artist constantly producing New Experiments to gratify the Taste of that Part of Mankind, whose splendid Circumstances make them emulous to excel in the Delicacies of this Mystery."[40] Criticizing recipes by those "tavern bred," Carter offered his full resume to his "brethren" while urging the ideal chef to review international cuisine so as to "chuse, with some Distinction, from all, what might gratify the most elegant and various Tastes." Labeling his text a "treatise" and a "performance," Carter orchestrated a self-conscious taste-act for consumers, one in which tasting (sampling) dishes both delighted the palate (taste sensation) and exhibited good judgment. Distancing food preparation from the utilitarian concerns of medical care and the vulgarities of cosmetics, these writers understood taste to rest on a prepossessed style, elegance, and cosmopolitanism.

Leading the charge against chef-oriented cookery collections was the phenomenon known as Hannah Woolley, a domestic female celebrity who acted as the Martha Stewart of the seventeenth century. In her recipe books, Woolley (also spelled Wolley) reclaimed food preparation as part and parcel of female-managed domesticity. Given her own lack of formal education and social standing, she embodied a rags-to-riches narrative that made domestic expertise the key to social mobility. Having been orphaned as a child, she apprenticed as a servant and married the master of a free school at Newport Pond, where she served as resident nurse to students. When widowed, she enjoyed stints as a housekeeper, overseer of boarders, and cooking teacher before becoming the first female professional domestic writer and the most popular author of recipe books in the latter part of the seventeenth century. Reprinted numerous times, her texts became a significant bookselling trend. They included *The Ladies Directory in Choice Experiments* (1662) and *The Cook's Guide* (1664), together reprinted as *The Ladies Delight, Or, A Rich Closet of Choice Experiments & Curiosities* (1672); *A Guide to Ladies, Gentlewomen and Maids* (1668); *The Queen-Like Closet; or, Rich Cabinet* (1670), which was translated into German; and *A Supplement to the Queen-Like Closet* (1674). Three additional books have been attributed to her, some of which recirculated material from her previous works—*The Accomplisht Ladys Delight in Preserving, Physick, Beautifying and Cookery* (1675); *The Gentlewomans Com-

panion; or, A Guide to the Female Sex (1673; a text Woolley disavowed); and *The Compleat Servant Maid, or the Young Maidens Tutor* (1677).[41] While the texts that bore her name and used her material varied, they all promoted cookery as a constituent element of household management. Domesticity, within the Woolley corpus, was to be informed by the ethos of thrift and exercised so as to signify proper womanhood. Straddling the genres of conduct book, moral guide, and technical manual, Woolley's texts identified food preparation as the requisite knowledge of a "woman," whether lady, housewife, or servant. Unlike male cookery writers, Woolley was less concerned with making judgments about proper palates than with ensuring thrift and propriety in home management.

Woolley eagerly ushered the recipe consumer from the literate closet into the literate and practical kitchen. Although the female figures populating books attributed to Woolley inhabit a range of social stations, they are unified in their belief in, even their *adoration of*, hands-on involvement with work. Addressing "all Ladies and Gentlewomen . . . who love the Art of Preserving and Cookery," *The Ladies Directory* opened with a mannerist frontispiece in which women, situated within the rich material resources of an elite kitchen, figuratively roll up their sleeves and concoct distillations and sweetmeats (Figure 6). Woolley offered this instructional book on confectionery in hopes that women would find "pleasant Employment both for Winter and Summer" (A2–A2v). Her *Queen-Like Closet; or, Rich Cabinet* may appear invested in an earlier figuration of elite knowledge; yet Woolley repurposed the cachet of the inner sanctum, redefining the closet as a space that could be effectively *simulated* and marked as different in its imitation. Playing off the title of the earlier *Queens Closet Opened* (with its endorsement of the proprietary space of a noble person), she offers a "queen-like" closet, the product of a mimetic process to be carried out by, as the title page states, "ingenious persons of the Female sex" (1675). In a prefatory poem, Woolley directly critiqued an earnest reading of her own title by comparing the insubstantiality of a rich cabinet laden with jewels (containing fancy necklaces that "please the Taste, also the Eye") to the functionality of her cloned and simulated closet, which allowed people to fill their bellies (A6v). As the title page image illustrates, the faux royal closet encompassed multiple and proliferating sites in the home, where ladies of means as well as servants busied in preserving, candying, distilling, baking, and roasting (Figure 7). "Cuisine" may be a male ancient art, she implicitly said to rival chefs, but what households needed were ingenious women who knew the intricate byways of the complexly defined house.

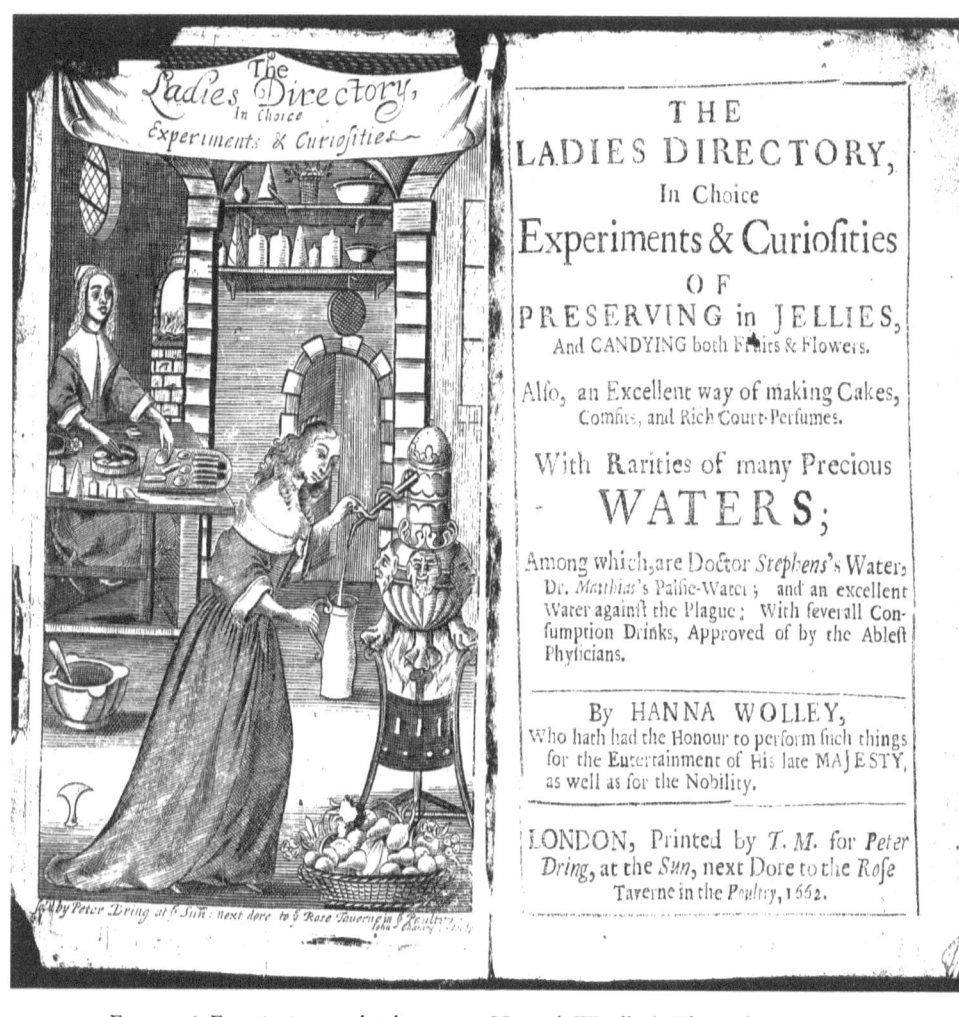

FIGURE 6. Frontispiece and title page to Hannah Woolley's *The Ladies Directory in Choice Experiments & Curiosities* (London, 1662).

Woolley's defense of female kitchen expertise was nothing short of an attempt to change the way that people viewed culinary knowledge and discourse. She sought to reset the scene and meaning of recipe work. As she returned food preparation to its earlier placement alongside medical care, distilling, carving, dairying, and confectionery, Woolley also expanded recipe topics to include manners, deportment, letter writing, handwriting, decorating, arithmetic, money handling, wax working, and moral behavior. Seeking—

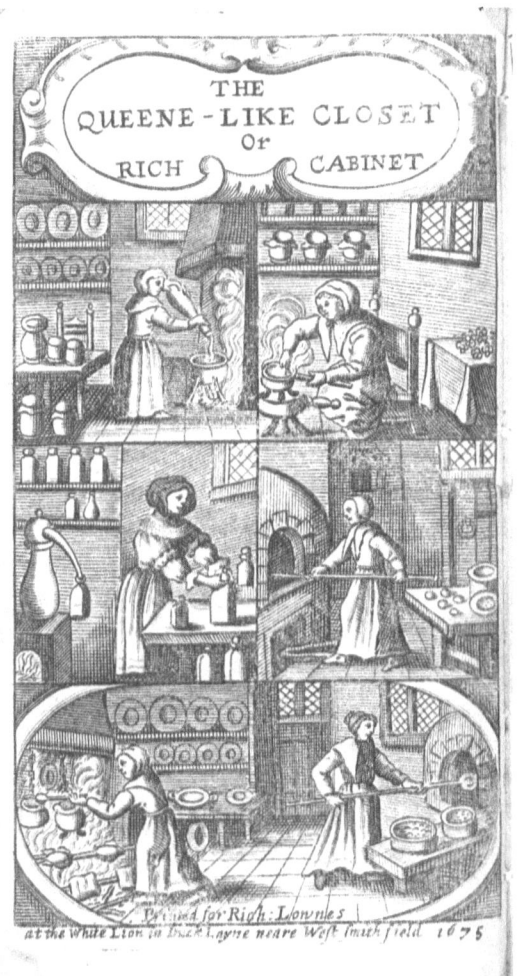

FIGURE 7. Title page to Hannah Woolley's *The Queen-Like Closet; or, Rich Cabinet* (London, 1675). Reproduced by permission of the Folger Shakespeare Library.

pie by pie—to construct the proper lady who possessed useful knowledge, Woolley offered the most explicit brief for budgeting that recipes had yet aired.⁴² Impractical and fanciful recipe books, she wrote, proved obstacles to cooking, "confounders" rather than "instructors," in her terms (*Directory*, A2v). Her works, by contrast, did not, as she said, "[confound] the Brains with multitudes of Words to little or no purpose, or vain Expressions of things which are altogether unknown to the Learned as well as the Ignorant" (*Queen-*

Like Closet, 1675; 181). The grand proclamations and humanist trappings that featured in chefs' recipe books are noticeably absent as Woolley insisted on a nontechnical and practical food discourse readily accessible to readers.[43] For Woolley, imagining the workspace as a library-closet would hinder true domestic skill; experience trumped decorum, erudition, and eloquence.

In championing home management as revealing the *character* of the housewife, Woolley extended a tradition established by Gervase Markham, whose immensely popular *English Housewife* had nevertheless existed as an outlier within status-based "closet" recipe writing earlier in the seventeenth century. *The English Housewife*, published first as a companion text to a guide for male estate owners before emerging in numerous editions as a stand-alone book, was the first text to situate the imagined scenario of recipe work in the nation rather than the closet. The ever prolific Markham experimented with playwriting, translation work, and romance writing, while offering a steady stream of published expertise on horsemanship, sports, military matters, beekeeping, husbandry, veterinary care, land management, gardening, and epistolary writing. In *The English Housewife*, Markham strikingly grafted the imagined nation onto the boundaries of the household and the individual female worker.[44] In a brief section on conduct preceding his recipes, Markham explained that the housewife's labor, habits, and physical appearance should manifest the Christian values of godliness, constancy, and temperance:

> It is meete that our English Hous-wife be a woman of great modesty and temperance as well inwardly as outwardly; . . . outwardly, as in her apparell and dyet, both which she shall proportion according to the competency of her husbands estate & calling, making her circle rather straight then large, for it is a rule if we extend to the uttermost we take away increase, if we goe a hayre breadth beyond we enter into consumption: but if we preserve any part, we build strong forts against the adversaries of fortune, provided that such preservation be honest and conscionable: for as lavish prodigality is brutish, so miserable covetousnesse is hellish. Let therefore the Hus-wifes garments be comely and strong, made as well to preserve the health, as adorne the person, altogether without toyish garnishes, or the glosse of light colours, and as farre from the vanity of new and fantastiqe fashions, as neere to the comely imitations of modest Matrons; let her dyet be wholesome and cleanly, prepared at due howers, and Cookt with care and diligence, let it be rather to satisfie

nature then our affections, and apter to kill hunger then revive new appetites, let it proceed more from the provision of her owne yarde, then the furniture of the markets; and let it be rather esteemed for the familiar acquaintance she hath with it, then for the strangenesse and raritie it bringeth from other Countries. (1623; 3–4)

For Markham, the ideal housewife balanced preservation and expenditure, a negotiation that he figured spatially in terms of a fortressed "straight" circle linked (through the phrase "therefore") to the housewife's physical appearance. As he mapped the appropriate material expenditure for apparel and diet, Markham superimposed the bounded domain of the housewife's *person* onto the borders of the estate and nation. In saying that the English housewife should model a self-sufficient domestic economy that eschews domestic and foreign markets, he suggested that personal inward character extended into and out of moderate and ordinary practice.

In *The English Housewife*, the female worker seems to hold within her obligations and knowledges that are then projected outwardly: "Now we have drawne our *Hous-wife* into these severall knowledges of Cookerie," Markham writes, "in as much as in her is contained all the inward offices of houshold" (1623; 125). As she expresses her "outward and active knowledge" she is to consider civic virtue more than elite standing. Markham thus fantasizes a national taste community that obliterates social distinctions, not because recipe skills could not shuttle across ranks, but because, at a deeper level, practice should emanate from core national virtues. His *English Housewife*, reprinted numerous times throughout the seventeenth century, offers a potent recipe counter-fantasy that would become the norm one hundred years after its initial publication.

Kim Hall has argued that Markham's text was part of a larger project in which recipe books offered women creative powers only by mystifying the foreign origins of domestic products and abetting in the formation of European nationalism.[45] Hall identifies and develops a central contradiction in Markham's recommendation for native foods: his reliance on imported spices and foreign methods was utterly at odds with his stated philosophy. Indeed the culinary Englishness he imagined was, we might say, *theoretical*, in the sense that the domestic worker was to demonstrate her Englishness chiefly by using "native" values as a compass for judging how to process ingredients, including imports. Hall's point is that women were complicit, through domestic practice, in fueling a national consciousness that concealed its colonial investments. In the recipe publishing industry, where status-conscious appeals to culinary pretension ruled the day, Markham's touting of national pride remained a popular anomaly—a well-used utilitarian protest book that echoed advice given in sermons and dietaries. While Markham's text resembles other recipe books of the day in exhorting women to use sugar and imported spices, it was one of the few early seventeenth-century books that might be said to conceal those investments under the veil of Englishness. Almost all other recipe texts exuberantly embraced (rather than attempting to nationalize) the international cuisine they shared. Over the next fifty years, *The English Housewife* joined other texts to form an avid debate, on booksellers' stalls, about conceptions of domesticity and the national contours of the taste communities they endorsed. Only later did English recipe books give concrete substance to Markham's vision by defining actual diet in national terms.

After the mid-seventeenth century, Woolley embraced, popularized, and adapted Markham's utilitarian vision. Woolley echoed Markham's interest in making recipe skill and home management go hand in hand with character development; she also rejected the elite closet as the primary scene of recipe work. Yet she departed from Markham in her enthusiasm for market forces and paid service relations. Woolley recognized how nostalgically quaint Markham's vision of a self-contained domestic universe was in the late seventeenth century (and perhaps in his own day). Instead of abstracting recipe work from commerce, Woolley made market and service relations central to domestic advice. She defined skills for all levels of domestic service, from low servants to nursemaids, from housekeepers to ladies. Her texts unabashedly instructed readers on how to improve their resumes so as to take advantage of critical job opportunities. While, as David Goldstein has argued, Woolley moved between the personae of friend, confidant, and servant in her writing, she also did not shy away from offering extra-textual services for a "competent gratuity."[46] In *The Supplement to the Queen-like Closet*, she explains the limits to what one could learn solely by reading: "I have set down every thing as plain as I can; and I know there are many who have done things very well by my Books only: but you may imagine that if you did learn a little by sight, of my doing, you would do much better; For if my Pen can teach you well, how much better would my Tongue and Hands do? The one to make answer to any Objection or Questions; the other to order or to shape any thing. . . . Be pleased to afford me some of your Mony; And I will repay you with my pains and Skill" (*Supplement*, 61). Explicitly entrepreneurial, Woolley calls attention to the deficit of reading as opposed to embodied apprenticeship ("doing"). While pitting personal give-and-take and embodied teaching against any reading experience, she emphasizes the commercial dimensions of any exchange: "Be pleased to afford me some of your Mony," she urges readers. In *The Ladies Directory*, she directs readers seeking additional instruction to the bookshop where she could be contacted for a fee (A3v–A4). Along with book publishers who indelibly shaped her image as recipe author, Woolley works to prioritize economic relationships rather than abstract notions of taste.[47] In the latter half of the seventeenth century, texts attributed to Woolley shifted the imagined scenario of recipe production from the newly permeable closet to a nation shot through with global and domestic economic concerns. As English national diet emerged from a pan-European cuisine in the mid-seventeenth century, her books recast the locale in which that cuisine was vested as well as the terms through which it was to be valued.

In the eighteenth century, recipe writers such as Ann Cook, Sarah Harrison, Eliza Haywood, Elizabeth Moxon, Ann Peckham, Elizabeth Raffald, and Eliza Smith elaborated and consolidated Woolley's template for domestic culture. Yet they subsumed the qualities of professional female expertise, economic savvy, and frugality under the banner of "Englishness." Following male writers who had generated culinary cults of personality around individual figures, these works outpaced, outsold, and eventually pushed out chef-authored texts addressed to fraternities of cooks. Housekeepers, that is, won the battle to control culinary taste in England.[48] Criticizing pretentious rhetoric and suspect French methods, their texts ironically recoded the dishes using imported spices from Asia as quintessentially "English" products resistant to French incursions. They nationalized a modified medieval diet by calling it the cuisine of dear old England newly attuned to budgeting. Assuring ladies that one could produce elegance that exhibited "frugality and good Conduct" (A2v), Sarah Harrison downplayed costly recipes and advised housewives to economize by using pears, apples, and figs as occasional sweeteners. Ann Peckham, represented in *The Complete English Cook, or Prudent Housewife* (1771) as "one of the most noted Cooks in the County of York," promoted an elegant English fare "not stuff'd with a nauseous hodge-podge of French kickshaws" (3). "Our Cook," Martha Bradley declared, "will be able to shew that an English Girl, properly instructed at first, can equal the best French Gentleman in everything but Expence."[49] Eighteenth-century cookbook writers (the genre into which the recipe book evolved) offered shopping tips, weighed the relative costs of ingredients, and promoted goods available in their own shops.[50]

A key feature of the new cookbook was its embrace of the plain style of language that had increasingly gained value with the rise of empirical methods in the century earlier and that was a hallmark of new aesthetic styles generally. National cuisine, for recipe writers, was only in part a matter of eating; it was also a mode of communication (and, as we shall see in Chapter 5, a means for verifying truth claims). In *A House-Keeper's Pocket-Book . . . with Plain and Easy Instructions* (1733), Sarah Harrison accuses fashionable writers of being unfamiliar with genuine work and true kitchen-speak; she sees the conjoining of frugality, experience, and "plain and easy instructions" as an ethical and social imperative. Entrepreneur, caterer, shop owner, and famed housekeeper Elizabeth Raffald introduced her *Experienced English House-keeper* by mocking esoteric and rhetorically complex accounts of cookery. "I can faithfully assure my Friends," she states of her instructions, "that they are truly wrote from my own Experience, and not borrowed from any other Author, nor glossed over with hard Names or Words of high Stile, but wrote in my own plain Language."[51] Raffald guarantees that her text, which persisted in twenty editions published across three cities (Manchester, London, and Dublin), is the product of a "frugal Hand," stylistically and practically.

It is appropriate that the most popular book of cookery in America and England for over one hundred years bore the promise of *facility* in its title. Hannah Glasse essentially characterized *The Art of Cookery Made Plain and Easy; Which Far Exceeds Any Thing of the Kind Ever Yet Published* as a translation. She sought to convert unnecessarily technical and expensive arts for an aspiring and burgeoning middle class. First published in London in 1747 anonymously, but with the assurance that the author bore the status of "a lady," this influential text appeared in over twenty editions in the next hundred years. Insisting on the practicality of English fare, Glasse, who eventually was outed as the text's author, consolidated values pioneered by previous female cookbook writers and prepared the way for Victorian domestic gurus such as Catharine Beecher and Isabella Beeton. As the illegitimate daughter of a prosperous gentleman, Glasse presented herself as someone straddling the line between fancy living and austerity. Tapping the market of upwardly mobile city folks who had little idea about how to run a prosperous household, Glasse directed her cookery book to "young and Ignorant" yet literate servants in a middle-class kitchen.

In *The Art of Cookery*, Glasse made representational style a centerpiece of her culinary system. In keeping with her avoidance of "high polite Stile," her preface did not outline a theory or history of food. Instead she offered concrete examples of her two central subjects: how to avoid culinary jargon and how to simplify recipes. "When I bid [my readers] lard a Fowl," Glasse stated, "if I should bid them lay them with large Lardoons, they would not know what I meant. But when I say they must lard with little pieces of bacon, they know what I mean. So in many other Things in Cookery, the great Cooks have such a high Way of expressing themselves that the poor Girls are at a loss to know what they mean. And in all Receipt Books yet printed there are such an odd Jumble of Things as would quite spoil a good Dish; and indeed some Things so extravagant, that it would be almost a Shame to make Use of them" (A1). For Glasse, omitting rhetorical ornamentation was an integral part of culinary streamlining. Grammatically linking stylistic and culinary simplicity by transitioning from confusing wording to confusing cooking, she imagined readers as "poor Girls" desperately seeking clarity. She thus used her preface to offer step-by-step instructions for how to make a rich sauce that could rival a French *cullis* at a fraction of the expense. "If Gentlemen will have French Cooks, they must pay for French Tricks," she concludes (ii). Acknowledging that cost-cutting measures were certain to be scorned by elite chefs and their noble employers, Glasse professed a desire only to deserve the "good Opinion of [her] own Sex" (ii). Gender cemented her taxonomy of taste. Everyone is, at heart, a "poor Girl" who seeks lucidity in a world of facades.

As we see, the figure of the "good housewife," which had formerly conjoined gendered labor, reading, and status, was strikingly reimagined in the new recipe environment. In collections such as *The British Housewife* and *The Complete English Cook*, the housewife transforms into an ideal distributed across the work, body, and positions of servants. Bradley's 1760 *British Housewife* opens with an image (Figure 8) that marked the distance recipe scenarios had traveled since Partridge's *Treasurie*, which, we remember, visually presented the author in a library (Figure 4). Bradley's frontispiece instead pictures three female servants wearing kerchiefs and aprons, busily working within a space filled with expensive plate ware and utensils; they spear chickens, crank spits, and shape pies. As the accompanying motto commends thrift and experience, it urges the reader to distinguish the domestic positions sharing these ideals: "Behold ye fair united in this book; frugal housewife and experienced cook." As the title indicates, the working non-noble culinary expert models the *fairness*—aesthetic and ethical—that exemplifies the nation. The unified housewife and cook do not, however, replicate the idealized housewife imagined in earlier recipe books; for domestic labor, now specialized into particular domestic roles, has separated from knowledge production and consumption. The image opening Catharine Brooks's *Complete English Cook* (1767) similarly

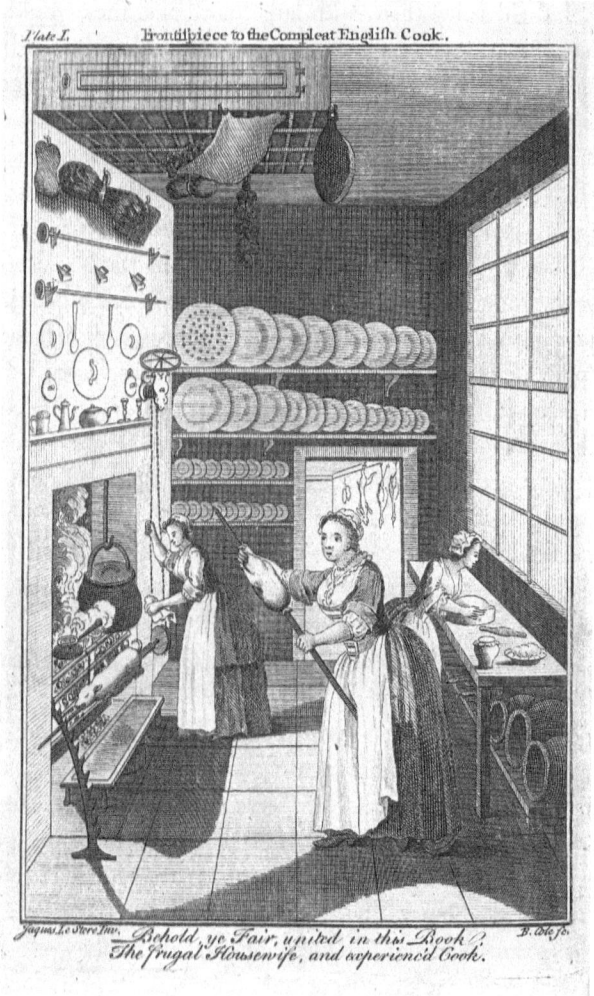

FIGURE 8. Frontispiece to Martha Bradley's *The British Housewife* (London, 1760). Reproduced by permission of the Beinecke Rare Book and Manuscript Library, Yale University.

detaches the working kitchen from the scene of reading. In this frontispiece, two female servants spit animals for the chimney fireplace and cut pies, while a male servant delivers newly killed poultry and rabbits. The attached motto, drawn from Proverbs 31:27, repeats the verse that post-Reformation conduct writers had earlier used to announce the signature characteristic of all women:

"She looketh well to the ways of her Houshold, and Eateth not the Bread of Idleness." In this context, however, the verse does not hail women from all social stations to act the role of "good housewife." Instead the pronoun "she" points to an absent mistress, or, we might say, that the figure has converted into an ideal made manifest explicitly through other delegated laboring household bodies. The chief domestic female authority exists somewhere off the page as the purveyor of a decidedly non-aristocratic English taste, diet, and cuisine implemented by unnamed workers.

Eighteenth-century texts thus represented recipe literacy in ways that constructed a hierarchy of work practices in the home. The frontispiece to William Henderson's *The Housekeeper's Instructor* (1790), for instance, depicts a "lady," as she is identified in the caption, who carries a book into the working space of the kitchen. She consults the printed book (that the reader now holds) to instruct and perhaps to oversee a female servant (Figure 9). Possession of printed instruction marks authority over the practitioner rather than serving as the tool promising social mobility. The image also shows a man using a printed carving manual to instruct a male servant. In Henderson's text, reading plays a central role in domestic management, but the privileged reader (and possessor of the valuable book) must "translate" for the laboring practitioner. Hannah Glasse also maintained that the lady of the house was a mediating recipe consumer and editor. In the 1775 edition of *The Art of Cookery*, an affluent lady is pictured consulting her newly purchased recipe book so as to select and copy individual recipes for her servants.[52] The scene of recipe reading and writing is not within the secluded working closet but instead lies just outside the kitchen space in a formal parlor. While ladies reserve a role within the recipe community of book buyers and readers, they centrally function as finicky judges of taste removed from practice. The recipe reader inhabits a supervisory role within a fantasy in which national cuisine is authorized by hands-on but class-divided female labors. The actual cost of Glasse's recipe book made it a significant investment for a servant (equal to a week's pay for a kitchen maid). It is no wonder that the employer safeguards the manual and acts as an intermediary for the reading servant.[53] This division of labor constructs, as it were, a new definition of book "use" in relation to physical practice.

Other guides—such as Eliza Haywood's *A New Present for a Servant Maid* (1771), *Town and Country Cook; or Young Woman's Best Guide* (1780), Mary Holland's *The Complete British Cook* (1800), and Ann Peckham's *The Complete English Cook*—reattach reading to labor but remove the household mistress

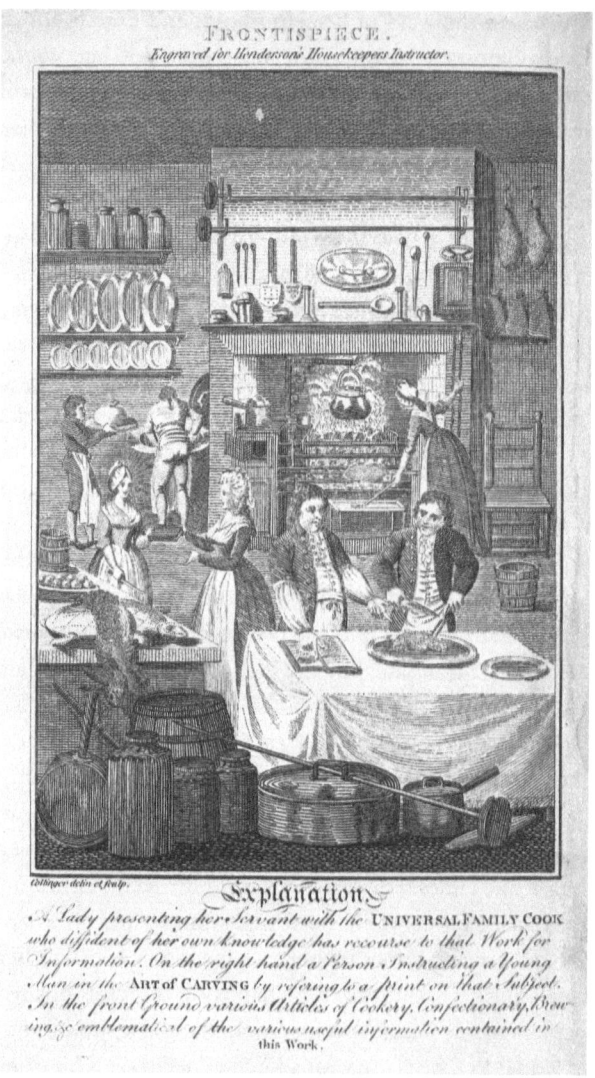

FIGURE 9. Frontispiece to William Henderson's *The Housekeeper's Instructor* (London, 1790). Reproduced by permission of the British Library.

entirely from the economy of work, reading, and domestic judgment. Following the lead set by *The Compleat Servant-Maid* published in the century before, these texts are written directly to literate servants. Haywood's frontispiece recasts the reading experience by presenting a worker who stands ready to cook with pan in hand while studying a book. Just to make sure that the reader grasps the specificity of this reflexive moment, the book that the servant peruses is identified specifically as "Haywood's New Present" (Figure 10). In Holland's guide, a servant turns a spit and sets a pot on an open fire, next to an opened book of recipes. And *Town & Country Cook* opens with an engraving in which a housekeeper delivers a single page handwritten recipe to the male and female workers who populate a lively kitchen scene (one in which cats and dogs compete with the humans for control over foodstuffs). The culmination of these images comes in *The Complete English Cook*, which addressed the recipe fashion of exempting elite women of taste not only from the

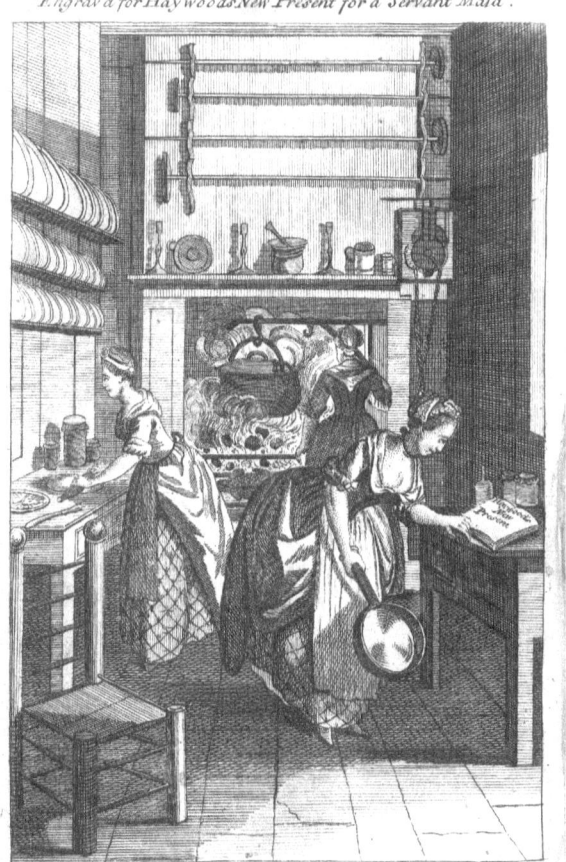

FIGURE 10. Frontispiece to Eliza Haywood's *A New Present for a Servant Maid* (London, 1771). Reproduced by permission of the Huntington Library.

kitchen, but also from the literate culture that made up the recipe community. According to Peckham, a literate servant could precisely relieve a lady of trivial manual responsibilities and improve culinary pedagogy: "Such mistresses as think it a burden to be continually dangling after their maids in the kitchen," she wrote, "may be exempted in a great measure from that trouble, by putting these rules into the hands of their servants; for special care is taken to make everything easy and intelligible to the meanest understanding. And it is certain, that the direction, which may be read with coolness and deliberation at a leisure hour, all more easily be retained in the memory, than those that are given in the hurry of business from the mouth of the most respectable mistress" (4). The lady bustling about instructing her servants was not a figure of ideal womanhood but an inefficient teacher. Giving the servant the (proper) recipe book enables better education while freeing the mistress for worthier endeavors. Only a plain style of writing could enable the sorting and differentiation of labor in the home. If the lady meddles in the kitchen, she is, according to Peckham, at risk of self-identifying as having the "mean understanding" and lower intellectual capacity that recipes authors saw in their target audiences.[54] Peckham imagines that experienced housekeepers might enjoy reading published recipes not because they learn new tricks but because they might take "satisfaction of seeing their own methods approv'd by one who is generally allow'd to be a competent judge."[55]

In these texts, reading is disaggregated from the more capacious definition of "use" that had formerly staked status on experiential methods. "Every Servant who can but read will be capable of making a tollerable good Cook," Glasse writes (i). In *English Housewifery*, Elizabeth Moxon sees recipe books as "*necessary for Mistresses of Families, higher and lower Women*" (title page). Servants were invited to bypass apprenticeship and engage directly from books; housekeepers could read technical books as a leisure activity confirming pre-existing knowledge; and ladies are left out of the equation altogether. Peckham's portrayal of herself as "almost worn out in the service of the kitchen" highlights the fatigue (rather than the intellectual pleasure or cultural capital) that the domestic knowledge-practitioner experiences, a position any elite woman would naturally want to avoid. This is precisely the view that Ann Cook mocked in a scathing poetic rebuttal to Glasse in *Professed Cookery* (1735), where the aptly named Cook excoriated "a Lady" (Glasse's pseudonym) for thinking that "the Author and sov'reign Cook" could convey "so much art, that each ignorant Maid / By reading it, is Mistress of the Trade; / Shall know to do the Art of Cook'ry well, / Examines not for Judgment, Taste or Smell."[56]

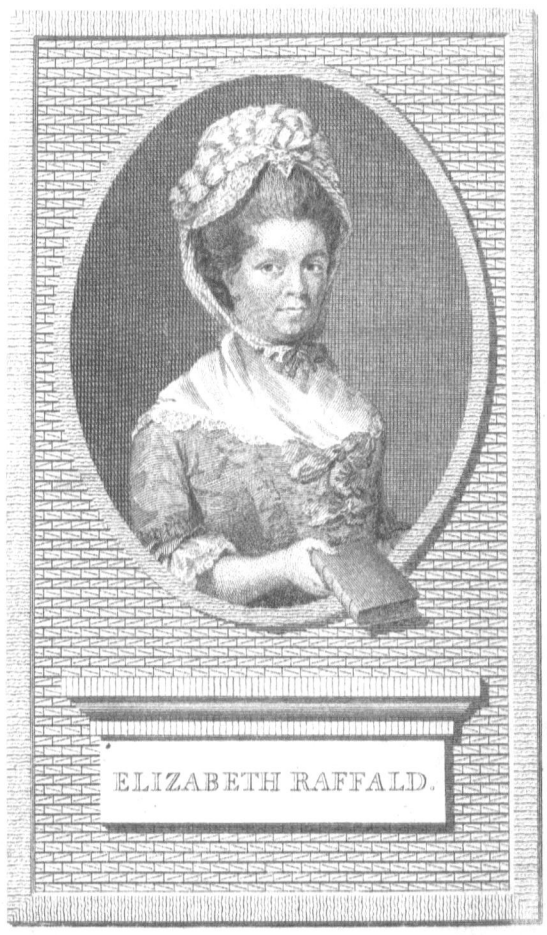

FIGURE 11. Frontispiece to Elizabeth Raffald's *The Experienced English Housekeeper* (Manchester, 1784). Reproduced by permission of the British Library.

How could servants enact the sophisticated operations required in reading and recipe wisdom? Doesn't this make the servant a purveyor of taste?

Despite Cook's mockery, servants able to obtain and read recipe books responded to the allure of social mobility. Elizabeth Raffald, for instance, rose from servant to authoritative housekeeper for noble families as well as celebrity author. She visually marked and sought to reduplicate her own rise by portraying herself as housekeeper (in simple apron and bonnet) reaching out from within the elevated posture of the oval portrait, to hand her book directly to her reader (Figure 11). As Janet Theophano notes of this "personal and intimate gesture," Raffald's unnervingly steady gaze seems to break the "constraining frame of sturdy brick that encircles her likeness."[57] The portrait, punctuated by the intrusive hand-off, erases the elite lady from book commerce. The prestige of a literate recipe culture embodied in the idealized "good housewife" eroded as servants and housekeepers began to publish and purchase newly affordable cookbooks and thus to manage imagined and material reading taste communities.[58] Eschewing overwrought rhetorical exercises, they further devalued the "literate" characteristics that made the first recipe books appealing to consumers.

The British Housewife, The Complete English Cook, The Experienced English Housekeeper: the nation/commonwealth saturated the imaginary locale of eighteenth-century recipe writing. These texts are strikingly aware that the national dimensions of their taste acts were implicated in global relations. As Sandra Sherman argues, the community produced in eighteenth-century recipe books was explicitly an artifact of a recognizably international market, with "community" signaling both the cohesion of readers aligning as "English" and the material book trade circulating information.[59] Martha Bradley thus finds it appropriate to laud the truly British nature of culinary methods that depended precisely on global imports. Cayenne pepper, she notes, is "imported . . . from the Negroes of our Plantations. The fruit is common in Africa, they have been accustomed to eat it there, shewed our People the way in America, and they have taught us."[60] Thus was the "British" cook overtly the product of international trade and the slave system. Manuscript recipe collections also newly acknowledged the international commercial system underlying even seemingly native products, regardless of whether these texts embraced or rejected a national definition of taste. Witness Katharine Palmer's intriguing entry, "A Poetical Receipt to Make a Sack Posset, 1699," which begins:

> From fam'd Barbardoes only Western Main
> Fetch Sugar half a pound, fetch Sack from Spain
> A pint and from the Eastern India Coast
> Nutmeg the glory of our Northern Tost.[61]

To prepare a traditional English drink, the reader is required to traverse the globe as well as to stir, boil, and mix. Palmer poetically materializes—without denouncing or celebrating—the Atlantic, Mediterranean, and European trading routes that invisibly supported the production of English taste, even going so far as imply that the cook herself had to globe-trot to concoct foods and drinks. Even as they recoded traditional dishes in national terms and defended a national cuisine, recipe texts acknowledged imperial and commercial international networks.

Whereas recipe producers of the early seventeenth century had toiled to install working literate housewives/ladies as arbiters of taste and whereas they envisioned recipe culture as a means of proving gentility, eighteenth-century recipe writers reconceptualized domesticity so that the leisured lady's status depended on her removal from the nitty-gritty details of work. (This campaign was so successful that it has obscured our ability to recognize the labors of elite women in earlier eras—to imagine, that is, that a countess would genuinely *know* a cheese recipe.) When women were instructed to head to the drawing room and delegate housekeepers, professionals, and servants as administrators of a national cuisine, the housewife no longer served as a vital switch-point for the textual and social operations that aggregated within taste acts. The axes of classification—the way that taste was imagined to classify the classifier—shifted. We have ample evidence of broader historical changes in conditions of labor and ideologies of gender. Tradesmen's daughters, for instance, began attending boarding schools that emphasized leisure arts rather than domestic skills. Meanwhile, writers felt free to smirk at housewifery: in the *Spectator*, Joseph Addison mocked sewing, embroidery, and the making of sweetmeats as "drudgery"; and, in *Humphrey Clinker*, Tobias Smollett satirized interest in housework as quaintly old-fashioned.[62] Eliza Haywood went so far as to declare that a woman of *fine taste* could show only so much interest in domestic knowledge and practice. This is where the story of recipe books opens onto the history of manners, of the construction of a middle-class cult of domestic womanhood, and of the civilizing process.[63] Upper-echelon ladies began to oversee a sphere that scholars lament as increasingly devalued economically and overinvested emotionally, a domestic domain cordoned off from the critically noted (but contested) public sphere.[64] Printed recipe books do not alter significantly this familiar story, which scholars endorse while contesting its particularities; instead the recipe archive helps us to recognize the role that the literate domain played in this story; for targeted readers morphed from social climber, to professional chef, to prudential British housekeeper, to aspiring servant.

Coda: Debating Recipe Taste in the Restoration and Enlightenment

> Sorry, Charlie. StarKist don't want tuna with good taste, StarKist wants tuna that tastes good.
> —Television commercial, 1980s

In 1764, Voltaire defined "taste" as "the sense by which we distinguish the flavor of our food," a feature, he noted in his dictionary, that has "produced, in all known languages, the metaphor expressed by the word 'taste'—a feeling of beauty and defects in all the arts. It is a quick perception, like that of the tongue and palate, and in the same manner anticipates consideration. Like the mere sense, it is sensitive and luxuriant in respect to the good and rejects the bad spontaneously. . . . As a physical bad taste consists in being pleased only with high seasoning and curious dishes, so a bad taste is pleased only with studied ornament, and feels not the pure beauty of nature."[65] Voltaire reminded readers of the culinary trope founding emerging conceptions of aesthetic taste. As he analogized the judgment of beauty to the physical sensations of tasting, he assumed that the sign of a universal bad taste was appreciation for "high seasoning and curious dishes," precisely those foods that had been the foundation of fashionable dining centuries earlier. More important is the fact that Voltaire defined taste as a spontaneous sensation rooted in nature that bridged aesthetic and culinary experience.

As eighteenth-century recipe books reconfigured gender, status, and domestic labor, they began to register aestheticized definitions of taste circulating in writings throughout the culture. After Eliza Smith accused fancy recipe books of peddling "impracticable" and "whimsical" dishes (a common charge), she went a step further, for instance, and grounded her judgment in a conception of inherent bad taste. Some dishes, she wrote, were "unpalatable, unless to depraved Palates" (the "palate," or roof of the mouth, was the conventional seat of taste; A4v, A4r). Smith did not just indict "capricious Appetite" as a facet of an immoderate or intemperate Epicureanism, a long-standing moral charge; she converted identifiable food preferences into essential personality traits. Similarly, when Charles Carter acknowledged recipe readers who "have not the highest Taste of elegant Eating," his possessive verb ("have") implied a conception of internal (in)capacity.[66] The title page to Charlotte Cartwright's *The Lady's Best Companion; or, Complete Treasure for the Fair Sex* (1799), by contrast, poetically identified "taste" as both a style and personal quality:

> If in the modern Taste you'd learn to cook,
> Study the perfect Method in our Book;
> Then the best Table you may serve with ease,
> And the nice Appetite exactly please.

While first defining taste as a mode "in" which one cooks, this passage concludes by referring to the "nice" (or refined) "appetite" of the diner. Modern techniques, it seemed, catered to an ideal reader's *habitus*, a preexisting discriminatory palate that could be attached to the perception of beauty. Perhaps it is not surprising that cookbooks in the mid-eighteenth century, as Jean Flandrin notes, were recategorized in bookshops under art rather than medicine.[67]

As they grappled with *taste*—as physical perception and habit of mind—recipe writers moved closer to writings where cuisine was heralded explicitly as an art. In his satiric poem *The Art of Cookery*, to take one example, William King elaborated ways that food making was prone to routine artistic flaws of the day, including deceptions of appearance, extravagance, contortions of scale, redundancy, disregard for natural essences, and outlandish combinations. King opens his poem by asking his reader to imagine certain dishes as grotesque portraiture:

> Were a Picture drawn
> With Cynthia's Face, but with a Neck like Brawn;
> With Wings of Turkey, and with Feet of Calf,
> Though drawn by *Kneller*, it would make you laugh!
> Such is (good Sir) the Figure of a Feast,
> By some rich Farmer's Wife and Sister drest.
> Which, were it not for Plenty and for Steam,
> Might be resembled to a sick Man's Dream,
> Where all Ideas hudling run so fast,
> That Syllibubs come first, and Soups the last.
> Not but that Cooks and Poets still were free,
> To use their Pow'r in nice Variety;
> Hence Mac'rel seem delightful to the Eyes,

> Tho dress'd with incoherent Gooseberries.
> Crabs, Salmon, Lobsters are with Fennel spread,
> Who never touch'd that Herb till they were dead. (E3v–E4)

The speaker mocks reversals in the order of serving as well as hybrid, excessive, and artificial dishes. In his argument for artistic decorum, King pointed to meals that failed to respect natural correspondences; seafood, for instance, should be served with herbs associated with their living state. True cookery, in this poem, rests not simply in emulating one's social betters, affirming political allegiance, or displaying national virtue, but in its regard for a naturalized (even mimetic) aesthetics. When King figured its violation as a grotesque female portrait pieced from diverse animal and human elements, he points backward to satiric renditions of the blazoned woman as a body literally composed from jewels, cosmological elements, flowers, and food. Extending arguments familiar in poetic treatises to the realm of gastronomy, King insisted that cookery concerns judgment, proper ordering, and balance: "When Art and Nature join th' Effect will be / Some nice Ragout, or charming Fricasee," he declared. Believing such to be the goal, he urged cooks to steep themselves in classical theories of art and subject themselves to critical review. The ideal meal should be an artistic masterpiece:

> Tables shou'd be like Pictures to the sight,
> Some dishes cast in shade, some spread in light,
> Some at a distance brighten, some near hand,
> Where ease may all their delicace command:
> Some shou'd be mov'd when broken, others last
> Through the whole treat, incentive to the taste.

Visual presentation should manifest intrinsic culinary properties while catalyzing a desire for flavor: the artful arrangement of texture and lighting was to draw out the reader's natural taste, which signifies, here and elsewhere, a mental compulsion, process of discrimination, and sign of self-regulation.[68]

"All of the major Enlightenment philosophers of taste were involved," Denise Gigante writes, "in the civilizing process of sublimating the tasteful essence of selfhood from its own matter and motions, appetites and aversions, passions and physical sensibilities."[69] According to Gigante, writers as different as Shaftesbury, Hume, Addison, Burke, Johnson, and Godwin sought to extricate taste from its connection with lower-bodily appetitive cravings so as to reclaim it as the basis for a refined civic sensibility. Defining the relationship of physical taste to its aesthetic and social operations is indeed a question that has preoccupied thinkers for centuries. "How might it have happened," Immanuel Kant mused, "that the modern languages particularly have chosen to name the aesthetic faculty of judgment with an expression (*gustus*, *sapor*) which merely refers to a certain sense-organ (inside the mouth) and that the discrimination as well as the choice of palatable things is determined by it?"[70] Just as food flavors, freed from the demands of humoral dietetics, became significant entities in their own right, taste was culturally emptied of physical meaning (referring, as Kant notes, "merely" to a sense organ) and made to serve as a signifier primarily for aesthetic judgment. As part of the civilizing process, taste began to be abstracted into a faculty of discernment whose connection to appetite and sensation was suppressed or fraught. Recipe books seem at a far remove from this lofty cultural project, yet, as we have seen, they also struggled to manage, perhaps within a more practical realm, the circuitry between decorum, privilege, and taste sensations. In one sense, it seems unremarkable that the recipe books we have considered in this chapter labored to construct discerning readers and refined palates, but in the eighteenth century they were also silently pulling against the current of an aesthetics predicated on transcendence of the physical realm. By virtue of their subject matter, which invited recognition, to some degree, of sense organs and eating, recipes departed somewhat from the civilizing impulse that Gigante describes. In this sense, recipes constituted a discursive field of conversation and knowledge that joined and differently configured the debates about sense and sensibility carried out in more recognizably "literate" domains.

    I close with attention to one striking moment on the title page of Ann Shackleford's 1767 *The Modern Art of Cookery Improved*, where literary and recipe conversations about gastronomy and aesthetics intersected. In choosing an epigraph from a classic literary epic, John Milton's *Paradise Lost*, this book introduced readers (perhaps unwittingly) to the vexed problems surrounding taste that philosophers and poets of the day addressed. While the other prefatory materials to Shackleford's book conventionally praised novelty, use value, and prudence, the title page cited, without commentary or explanation, Milton's Eve in the midst of preparing dinner for the angel Raphael in the bountiful world of Eden:

> She turns, on hospitable thoughts intent
> What choice to choose for delicacy best,

> What order, so contriv'd as not to mix
> Tastes, not well join'd, inelegant, but bring
> Taste after taste upheld with kindliest change.[71]

Commentators on the poem, stretching back to Leigh Hunt in the early nineteenth century, have been fascinated by the fact that Milton decides to have a resplendent angel arrive in Eden exactly at dinnertime, or rather, that Adam and Eve's first response to a heavenly visit is to render the visitor a dinner guest.[72] In choosing this occasion, Milton required himself to address not only the sensibility and corporeality of angels but also prelapsarian domestic and culinary life. Eve's "hospitable" thoughts in this moment, phrased ambiguously so as to suggest that they are both *about* hospitality and a thought process modeled on a welcomed opening of options, demonstrate that she values "delicacy" over the indiscriminate mixing of flavors. Her goal is to "bring" (or produce) variety and multiplicity in generous provision, but she does not assimilate the flavors she assembles from the garden's fruits; instead she maintains distinct "kinds." Milton elaborates this process by tapping into the roots of *kinship* (of a kind) and *kindness* (generosity), so as to saturate the passage with the weightiness, ethics, and obligations of hospitality. Eve's gastronomical concern for multiple and distinct flavors reflects the aesthetics of modern cuisine even as it refers to current deliberations about the relationship of aesthetics to physical eating.

As critics have long understood, food and eating not only form the core and climactic scene of *Paradise Lost* but also saturate its themes and idioms. The epic repeatedly defines communal relations and tests individual virtue by constituting what Michael Schoenfeldt teasingly calls a "Garden of Eating."[73] For Schoenfeldt, food choices in the poem serve to try moral principles, particularly the ability to calibrate temperance. For David Goldstein, Milton creates a "gastro-theology" to establish the ethics of commensality.[74] For Gigante, Milton deploys an "alimentary cosmology" that complicates the relation of physiology to judgment and paves the way for Enlightenment and Romantic constructions of taste (2). While some critics argue that Eve's preparation of food for the divine guest models a natural and sin-free female aesthetic operative in Eden, others point to Adam's misguided praise for Eve as "exact of taste" when she offers him the forbidden fruit and thus read Eve's desire for a culinary "effect" ("taste after taste") as suspiciously "contriv'd" and "aloof from the divine plan." In this latter view, Eve's concern with taste is a sign of her winding and circuitous overgoing of natural and moral order.[75] Although they disagree about the moral encoding of the scene, critics appreciate Milton's striking decision to represent the meeting of divine and human as a staging of a culinary aesthetics.

The publisher of *The Modern Art of Cookery Improved* perhaps cited this passage simply to establish an erudite frame of reference that might endow his recipes with the patina of authority. Readers even with a passing familiarity of the epic, however, might have wondered if this literary moment was somewhat wrenched out of context when recruited to serve as the introduction to a cookbook. In *Paradise Lost*, Edenic "food" is technically uncooked (meaning not heated); hence Milton's joke: "No fear lest Dinner cool" (book 5; 396). This passage can apply to recipe work, of course, because Eve does "act" on nature to transform gathered vegetation into a meal: she must collect fruit, strew herbs, and press grapes in this her primal act of biblical housewifery. The publisher of Shackleford's text may have seen Milton's text as transparently approving Eve's attempts to manufacture a variety of tastes at the dining table. Regardless of our speculations about the intentions behind this citation, it is safe to say that *The Modern Art of Cookery* conscripts and recodes Eve's ambiguous moral and aesthetic cookery so that she models a housewifery that the recipe book endorses. Eve's interest in taste is made to illustrate, that is, the economy, prudence, health, and pleasure that the preface recommends.

But surely it was remarkable for any text to point to Eve as not only a female role model but particularly a *culinary* model. In an epic in which the climactic moment of humanity's fall centers on a woman's misguided act of eating, food emerges as of paramount importance but also as a particularly vexed issue. As Lord Byron later quipped, "since Eve ate apples, much depends on dinner."[76] Referring to Eve's famously problematic relationship to dinner hardly seems a way to urge women to hunger for culinary expertise. Might mistresses and servants in the eighteenth century imagine themselves as taking on the rehabilitated role of "daughters of Eve" not as sinners (as the phrase often suggested), but as aesthetically sensitive chefs? Were they to imitate a primal shaping of "tastes" as a moral and artistic act? In asking readers to identify with this culinary Eve, *The Modern Art of Cookery* ushered the recipe book reader into a dialogue about taste that was taking place in elevated and literate communities in the culture. While labor had been delegated to workers, recipe readers were still to appreciate the intellectual problems that an Edenic kitchen inspired.

We have only scratched the surface of the social struggles and debates that the recipe archive reveals as it makes visible vibrant textual communities in early modern England. Within these communities, women were recruited to join in ideologically charged debates about the nature and stakes of the social identities they took on in relation to domestic work and domestic writing. As we will see in the next chapter, recipe books had not forgotten the role that pleasure played in the taste acts they performed; it was not only, as we might expect, the *gusto* of the table but rather the desires surrounding creative wit that they heralded as the ultimate reward for the recipe book consumer.

CHAPTER 2

Pleasure: Kitchen Conceits in Print

Let your conceits be nimble and ready.
—*A Gentlewomans Companion*

I will now give you some Directions for several sorts of Work, which may pleasure you in your Chambers and Closets.
—Hannah Woolley, *A Supplement to the Queen-Like Closet*

You must begin at the Kitchin. There, the *Art* of *Poetry* was learnd, and found out, or no where: and the same day, with the *Art* of *Cookery*.
—The Cook, in Ben Jonson's *Neptune's Triumph for the Returne of Albion*, 1623

A shopper at St. Paul's in late sixteenth-century London might have discovered this array of books on display: William Phiston's *The Welspring of Wittie Conceites*; Thomas Blague's *A Schole of Wise Conceytes*; Anthony Munday's *A Banquet of Daintie Conceits*; Robert Hitchcock's *The Quintesence of Wit Being a Corrant Comfort of Conceites, Maximies, and Poleticke Devises*; Bonaventure Des Périers's *The Mirrour of Mirth and Pleasant Conceits Containing Many Proper and Pleasaunt Inventions*; numerous "merry conceited" plays; and John Partridge's *The Treasurie of Commodious Conceites, and Hidden Secrets*. Nestled among handbooks of maxims, lyrics, popular figures, translated sayings, dramatic works, and verses were the first printed recipes, indistinguishable from recreational and literary titles in their designation as "conceits."

And yet no one seemed to have accused any book publishers of false advertising. How was an early modern recipe a conceit? If we think about a *food* conceit, the answer is obvious; in fact, the term might appear to be redundant, because the word "conceit" could mean a sugary trifle or fanciful sweetmeat. When George Gascoigne complained that "daintie fare" has led to "excesse on Princes bordes, / And every dish, was chargde with new conceits, / To please the taste, of uncontented mindes," he meant to condemn frivolous and luxurious banqueting dishes.[1] Yet publishers and authors did not merely have this narrow meaning in mind when they titled their recipe texts, for it's clear that they classified the full creative and intellectual enterprise of domestic making under this rubric.

For those versed in Renaissance poetry and poetics, "conceits" signified abstract ideas conceived in the mind as well as particularly ingenious and witty modes of expression. When Philip Sidney famously defended poetry by celebrating the Neoplatonic "foreconceit" as driving imaginative writing, he used the term to indicate a mental foundational idea that was then figured or bodied forth. "The Poet onely," Sidney wrote when praising the exceptionality of ideation in poetic making, "bringeth his owne stuffe, and dooth not learne a conceite out of a matter, but maketh matter for a conceit."[2] Fulke Greville deployed the more generic meaning of "idea" when he described painting as "the eloquence of dumbe conceipt," with ideal conception imagined as deficient until the moment of expression.[3] Often the term was used to refer to some combination of these meanings, when, for instance, it named mental facility, intellection, or the general faculty of apprehension. When Falstaff insults Poins in *Henry IV, Part 2* by complaining that "his wit's as thicke as Tewksbury mustard, there's no more conceit in him than is in a mallet," he suggests that knowing how to wield conceits—displaying that you "have" them within you—was a serious early modern cognitive skill (2.4.243). Poets of the day paradoxically debated ways to shape conceits (thoughts) into conceits (language). Edmund Spenser's "sweete conceited Sonets" were praised for their rhetorical turns of phrase, named after *concetti*, or Italian pictorial conventions. Positioned at the meeting point of the mental and material, the conceit posed a key conceptual problem for poets and philosophers contemplating the relationship of cerebral labor to material craft. Domestic creations in the form of recipes might be seen as crafty tricks (another meaning of "conceits"), but they also engaged the critical philosophical problem of yoking the abstract to the concrete, precisely the issue that poets identified as a central conundrum of intellectual wit.

Readers of *The Treasurie of Commodious Conceits* quickly discovered that the guide did not offer eloquent literary devises or pithy sayings but *recipes*, formulas for making "sundry sorts of new conceits, aswel of meats, conserves, and Marmalades, as also of sweet and pleasant Waters, of wonderful Odors, Operations & Vertues." In the prefatory matter, the reader was nevertheless schooled to think of these formulas as recreational. Partridge, on the pretense of modesty for his "little" enterprise, grouped his book with learned works that "pleasure every one" (A2v). Dedicatory poems singled out the reader's "pleasure" and "delight" as central aims of the book. Partridge sent his book out, he professed in an introductory poem, precisely so that his mistress could "pleasure" her friends. Subsequent recipe books flooded the print market, offering "prettie conceits" (Plat); "conceits in cookerie" (Dawson); "conceits in sugar-workes" (Murrell); and medical conceits (*Handmaide*).[4] John White's 1651 book of secrets, a genre overlapping with, but distinct from, recipe books, chimed "receits" with "conceits" in its title, as if signaling their ready interchangeability; it presented *A Rich Cabinet, with Variety of Inventions; unlock'd and opened, for the recreation of ingenious spirits at their vacant houres Being receits and conceits of severall natures.* White's terms are worth noting: the variety of "receits" and "conceits," yoked by their lexical similarity, provided newly disclosed modes of "recreation" for persons who possessed cleverness and leisure time. We might note that etymologically the word "conceit" emerged from "conceive" only by analogy with "deceive"/ "deceit" and "receive"/ "receit."[5] White's text reminded the reader of their shared lexical past, even as he evoked the conceptual meaning (the "conceit") harbored within the "receipt" as a term. He offered diverse "inventions" to be received and conceived.

Given ubiquitous sermonizing in the period about how housewifery should function as a moral prophylactic against female idleness and wayward fancy, we might expect early recipe books to stress the spiritual benefits of household labors for consumers. Yet much like the "merrie conceited comedies" and poetic inventions sold alongside recipes on booksellers' stalls, the first wave of English recipe books were introduced as technologies of pleasure—that is, as consequential and highly *intellectual* modes of (re)creation. A glaring contradiction snaps into focus: Puritan-influenced sermons and conduct books posited the household as the chief site for inculcating moral and national values just as "delight-centered" recipe books proliferated in the book market.

This chapter argues that we should read early recipe books in England by looking past the early modern ideological framework of female recreation as a sign of trivialization. Such reconsideration will enable us to see that recipes constructed a notion of domestic pleasure centered on the intellectual wit of food making. In the previous chapter, we saw that class-conscious readers were eager to master the leisure skills offered by early published recipe books. We are now in a position to think about the intellectual component of even recreational food work, its necessary investment in transforming natural substances into human artifacts. The artificial element of this conversion was especially evident in a period when people valued foods that smoothly compounded ingredients rather than those that accented natural flavors. The transmutationalist gastronomy that Renaissance England inherited from the medieval period conceived of nature primarily as material to be manipulated, disguised, and reconstituted.[6] Edible conceits, foods that served as forms of performance art, not only exaggerated the basic values of the cuisine but also interrogated and explored its fundamental categories: nature, art, representation, form, essence. Foods served as think-pieces for a print and domestic audience interested in probing ways that nature related to its artistic end products.

One strand of my argument concerns the historical parameters of foods-as-conceits. Between 1570 and 1650, recipe books emphasized the delights that readers might take in managing food, contemplating its uses and meanings, and reveling in its transformative potential. After midcentury, as artful concoctions (increasingly deemed "frivolous") declined in popularity, recipes began to promote a culinary knowledge based on frugality and efficiency. Both the underlying conception of food and the packaging of recipes as recreational wit disappeared in the late seventeenth century. While Hugh Plat marketed his 1602 *Delightes for Ladies* "to all true Lovers of Art, and knowledge," Ann Peckham saw her 1771 recipes as transforming a reader into *The Complete English Cook; or Prudent Housewife*. No one could have mistaken Peckham's guide, that is, for a poetic or rhetorical manual. Pleasure and wit as categories either dropped out of culinary discourse after 1650 or were redefined and conscripted to promote the values of frugality, nationality, propriety, and rationality. Yet the intellectual questions driving culinary conceits did not vanish from the domestic scene or from recipe culture in the eighteenth century. Questions about the domestic worker's role in negotiating and probing the relationship between nature and (food) culture, I argue in the conclusion to this chapter, surfaced in the front matter of published recipe books, where histories and mythologies of cookery became the subject of explicit discussion.

My chief interest in using the recipe archive to explore food conceits (and recipes-as-conceits) is to recover a history of the culinary arts that recognizes the serious intellectual and creative dimension of domestic work. As documents, recipes enable us to filter past modern understandings of domesticity so as to acknowledge its alien early modern incarnations. What we find is that household culture and life could provide an enclave in the social world where women indulged in intellectual inquiries protected, in part, by their designation as simultaneously work and "play."[7]

The Joy of Cooking

Recipes have long been associated with pleasure in ways hardly concerned with specific dishes that promoted food-wit. In Plato's *Gorgias*, Socrates disparages rhetoric by comparing it to cookery (*opsopoiike*), seeing both as insubstantial experiences whose failure to rise to the level of "art" (*techne*) registers precisely in their ability to produce a superficial form of satisfaction:

> *Socrates.* Will you ask me, what sort of an art is cookery?
> *Polus.* What sort of an art is cookery?
> *Socrates.* Not an art at all, Polus.
> *Polus.* What then?
> *Socrates.* I should say an experience.
> *Polus.* In what? I wish that you would explain to me.
> *Socrates.* An experience in producing a sort of delight and gratification, Polus.
> *Polus.* Then are cooking and rhetoric the same?
> *Socrates.* No, they are only different parts of the same profession.[8]

For Socrates, rhetoricians and cooks offer analogously inconsequential forms of experience. Food preparation pretends to the truth of medicine just as rhetoric pretends to the truth of philosophy. Cookery produces only a fleeting by-product called "delight," a response more like "charm" than the "pure happiness" that Joseph Conrad later claimed cookbooks unleashed.[9] The "delight and gratification" that Socrates disparaged, however, were precisely the responses that early English recipe books championed as indicators of the recipe's social, economic, and intellectual value. Given the use of the word "conceit" in culinary and poetic discourse, late sixteenth-century commentators might have agreed with Socrates about the connection between rhetoric and cookery, but they would have rejected his devaluation of these arts. Many humanist proponents argued that rhetoric enabled precisely the philosophical density and truth that Socrates opposed to cookery. As classical rhetoricians had acknowledged, delight could be a component of the "art" that defined recipe work. The etymological connection of sweetness (the Latin *suavis*) with persuasion (*suadere*) is only one manifestation of the link humanists assumed as they advised writers to create palatable sweet truths.[10]

While people from different cultures and different eras have long appreciated recipes as sources of enjoyment, the pleasures that the first recipe books promised to women in late sixteenth-century England were distinctive. It's worth thinking in this regard about similarities and differences between early modern recipes and modern cookbooks.[11] In offering a preview of the array of flavors, smells, and colors that the kitchen might provide, modern recipes often anticipate and translate into writing the sensory stimulation of tasting, beholding, smelling, touching, and swallowing. Reading about food production catalyzes the cookbook reader to approximate and to "conceit" (or to conceive of) aromas, flavors, and textures (e.g., sweet, salty, bitter, sour, smooth, or crunchy), to delight in *anticipatory sensation*. Social dimensions might filter into an awaited meal, whether as a candlelit moment soundtracked with clinking cocktail glasses or a ritualized public display of decorum. Early published recipes were remarkably uninterested, by contrast, in prompting the reader to imagine food's sensory pleasures or concrete dimensions as the primary joys they offered.

What then of the recipe's investment in what we might identify as the *transportive fantasies* offered in modern recipe writing? Recipes are often said to prompt readerly fascination with exoticism or nostalgia, as they invite consumers to imagine a world other than it is through the vehicle of food. Modern cookbooks promise a release from the strictures of everyday life, whether by jettisoning readers into exotic landscapes (e.g., through culinary tourism) or into the past (e.g., conjuring forth the smell of biscuits in grandmother's kitchen). Curling up with a cookbook filled with glossy pictures of gleaming oiled eggplants served on a rustic wooden table against the backdrop of a Tuscan hillside, the reader can be transported imaginatively elsewhere. Conversely, cookbooks that promise a return to the simpler days of yore (where one used only local products from a nearby farm), offer nostalgic time travel. As we saw in the previous chapter, early modern fantasies about recipes often revolved around the release they offered from a fixed social hierarchy; they promised the ability to traverse a class-based landscape by traveling into the closets of the elite. Until the mid-seventeenth century, however, English recipe books did not exoticize food in any explicit way; in fact, they largely ignored both the heated xenophobia in food dietaries and the lush literary exoticization of cuisine.

Finally, modern cookbooks engage the logic of what we might call a *substitutive aesthetics*, or the fetishizing of the recipe-as-art. If we return to the glossy image of eggplants served on a Tuscan patio, we notice that it trades on a desire for exoticism precisely by creating what Roland Barthes terms "openly dreamlike cookery" or what has been dubbed "food porn."[12] High-definition pictures surrogate the gratifications of eating into the aesthetics of looking. Angle of view, lighting, and arrangement transform the image into an object of desire in its own right. Although early printed books were not illustrated until the appearance of basic line drawings in the 1650s, early texts used graphic design work to aestheticize the book object rather than to represent food itself.[13] Plat's *Delightes for Ladies*, *A Closet for Ladies*, and Murrell's *A Delightful Daily Exercise* exist as lovingly designed printed objects, complete with decorative printer's lace borders (made up of geometric or floral intersecting patterns) as well as historiated capitals (Figure 12). In Partridge's *Treasurie of Commodious Conceits*, design clearly trumped functionality, as we see in the five-page table of contents, which simply lists all recipes in the miscellaneous order in which they appear in the text, with no sectional groupings or alphabetical index (Figure 13). Asterisks and pilcrow marks, which in other books of the day served as lexical aids, serve as ornamental designs to enhance the visual appeal of the page. The apprehension of beauty within the act reading stood in for, or lent itself to, the creativity of making in the kitchen and eating at the table.

Some early English recipe books theorized the pleasures they offered by pointing not simply to their visual appeal but also to the reader's exercise of prerogative over and beyond the directives encoded in the book. *The Ladies Cabinet Enlarged and Opened*, for instance, methodically ordered its material within a format that writer M.B. celebrated as creating "readier use" for the reader.[14] Yet "use" becomes, as the text reveals, a synonym for pleasure. Using the text's indexical aids, M.B. promised, the reader can "quickly view the particulars of [one's] Treasury, and know where to find them at pleasure." In case this notion of readerly satisfaction remained too general, M.B. then elaborated the book's tripartite organizational structure: the portion of the book devoted to "stately" medicine was flanked by "the more delightful" sections on preserves and cookery, the latter two serving as "palaces of pleasure" surrounding a central mansion. "Here [when reading about cookery and preserves] you may sport," the reader was instructed. "There [in the section on physic] you may rest. These are for pomp, the other for safety." The true "sport" of the

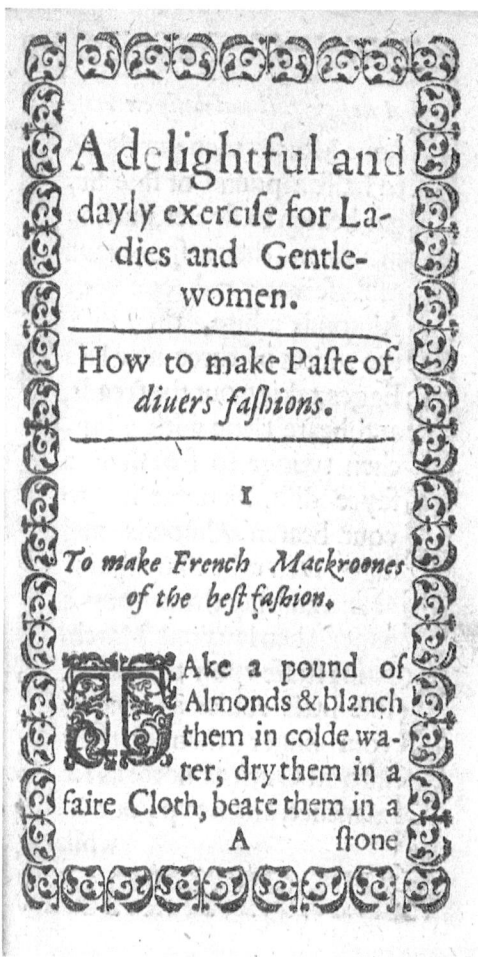

FIGURE 12. Sample page from John Murrell's *A Delightfull Daily Exercise for Ladies and Gentlewomen* (London, 1621), A12. Reproduced by permission of the Huntington Library.

recipe ("sport" being a word that carried erotic undertones in other writings) lay in the apprehension of *all* recipe knowledge, M.B. explained, regardless of its content: "But lest I should be thought tedious to little purpose, or any way to endeavour to by[p]asse your affections, or abridg your freedom, I shall thus leave you at liberty as Lovers in Gardens, to follow your own fancies. Take what you like, and delight in your choice, and leave what you list to him, whose labour is not lost if any thing please." Wandering through the book like "Lovers in gardens," readers could convert order into a leisurely labor that cultivated imagination and feeling. Defining *use* as bibliographical and intellectual freedom, the recipe book traded on the trope of the book-as-garden, a figure common in poetic anthologies such as *The Arbor of Amorous Devices, The Garden of the Muses*, and *Britton's Bowre of Delights*. Such collections invited gentlemen readers to pluck out verses to suit their desires and needs. "Thou which delight'st to view this goodly plot," a prefatory poem to one garden anthology

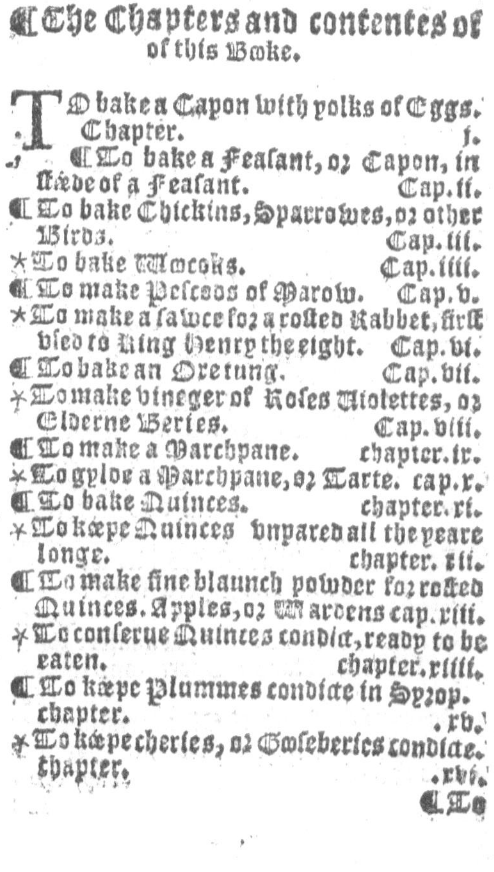
¶ The Chapters and contentes of
of this Boke.

TO bake a Capon with yolks of Egges.
Chapter. i.
¶ To bake a Feasant, or Capon, in
stede of a Feasant. Cap. ii.
¶ To bake Chickins, Sparrowes, or other
Birds. Cap. iii.
To bake Wodcoks. Cap. iiii.
¶ To make Pescods of Marow. Cap. v.
To make a sawce for a rosted Rabbet, first
used to King Henry the eight. Cap. vi.
¶ To bake an Oretung. Cap. vii.
To make vineger of Roses Violettes, or
Elderne Beries. Cap. viii.
¶ To make a Marchpane. chapter. ix.
To gylde a Marchpane, or Tarte. cap. x.
¶ To bake Quinces. chapter. xi.
To kepe Quinces unpared all the yeare
longe. chapter. xii.
¶ To make fine blaunch powder for rosted
Quinces. Apples, or Wardens cap. xiii.
To conserue Quinces condict, ready to be
eaten. chapter. xiiii.
¶ To kepe Plummes condicte in Syrop.
chapter. xv.
To kepe cheries, or Gooseberies condicte.
chapter. xvi.
¶ To

FIGURE 13. Table of contents for John Partridge's *The Treasurie of Commodious Conceits* (London, 1573), sig. Avi. Reproduced by permission of the Huntington Library.

stated, "Here take such flowres as best shal serve thy use."[15] It's remarkable that the recipes in *The Ladies Cabinet* could be slotted so easily into the role of posies, poem-flowers to be picked at will by female readers as they navigated textual gardens. Clearly there was an imaginative and rhetorical crossover between the recipe and the conceit, if only in the pleasurable utility that they saw the reading experience as delivering. Like a lover meandering through a lush bower, the reader could take whatever caught her eye, flip the pages, "sport," and choose recipes that excited her "fancy" and liberated her "affections."[16]

But then there was the food itself, or more specifically, the issue of how food practice served as imaginative play. Most early English conceit making described in recipes turned on the ability to create pliable food substances that could be used to fashion referential and nonreferential designs. Readers could create a versatile food medium by manipulating one or more of six main ingredients: (1) isinglass, a firm semitransparent gelatin made from the air bladders of freshwater fishes; (2) marzipan, made of almonds mixed with sugar and rosewater; (3) gum tragacanth, a tasteless, water-soluble mixture derived from the resin from an eastern Mediterranean shrub; (4) gum arabic, the resin of the acacia tree; (5) sugar plate, made of boiled sugar syrup poured into molds; and (6) coarse pastry crusts. From these supple substances, readers modeled banqueting dishes, such as marzipan tarts, clear cakes, wafers (stamped with iron wafer irons), "Genoa pastes" (thick translucent jellies made from fruit pulp), quiddanies (hardened quince syrups stamped with designs), and jumbals (dough twisted into pretzel-like "knots"). Jumbals, by far the most popular sweetmeat, appeared in almost every manuscript and printed recipe collection in the early modern period regardless of the writer's social station or food preferences. While these sweetmeats could be served alone, they were commonly grouped on a centerpiece platter, decorated with comfits (spiced seeds), lozenges (almonds candied in rosewater), suckets (hard candies made of roots, spices, or citrus fruit peels, served "wet" in syrup or "dry"), leaches (stiff creams), candied flowers, and dyed jellies.

Labor-intensive sugar work often required sequential stages of blanching, crushing, straining, and rolling mixtures that were then dried using a heat source (fire, oven, or tripod) and molded into shapes or imprinted with designs. One of Plat's sugar paste recipes, to give some idea of the scope of the endeavor, involves four pages of detailed instructions. If the housewife or lady had ample resources and access to markets, she could purchase pewter or wooden molds to form ornamentation on pastes or crusts. Murrell's *A Daily Exercise for Ladies and Gentlewomen* mentions that readers could avail themselves of one-stop shopping by buying the molds mentioned in the recipes at the printer's shop where the book was sold (A12). Budget-conscious women who elected to make molds at home out of relatively cheaply plaster of paris could find information about how to do so in some recipe collections.

Banqueting dishes cultivated pleasures that combined artistic ambitions with the luxury of expenditure. Readers were to heighten the visual appeal of foods by experimenting with ways to make rainbows of precisely graded color-dyes. As *The Ladies Cabinet Enlarged* theorized of reading practice ("Take what you like, and delight in your choice"), individual recipes emphasized the creative freedom that readers could exercise through culinary design work. Strings of confectionary recipes concluded with variations on the same popular phrase: "print it in what fashion you please," "print it as you please," "put it in whatever shape you please," and "print it with your moulds." While these phrases were meant to signal the reader's prerogative in selecting patterns or shapes, they also encouraged domestic practitioners to *identify* what pleased them and thus to imagine domestic knowledge as a technology of pleasure.

In order to understand the illusionistic play and interpretive potential of recipe dishes, we should consider their connection to medieval and Renaissance court entertainments. Chef Robert May's 1660 collection of published recipes, in fact, related lavish noble spectacles to scaled-down printed conceits, for he opened the book by including a description of a surreal food spectacle in a work otherwise concerned with advice about preparing standard puddings and boiled meats.[17] "Triumphs and Trophies in Cookery, to Be Used at Festival Times" offers instructions, as critics have noticed, for how to replicate a sumptuous noble interlude by molding paste into a theatrical stage set complete with backdrop and props. In this "triumph," a word derived from the Italian term for the sculptural components of banquet, or *trionfi di tavola*, the reader is to devise a ship with gunpowder-laden cannons, a deer, and a castle decorated with battlements and drawbridges. Eggshells are to be filled with scented "sweet water" made from distilled flowers. The reader is to oversee the baking of a huge coarse pastry pie that can house live frogs and birds. Rather than providing details about how to make these component parts, the "recipe" focuses on scripting the action of the spectacle. Ladies in attendance, it dictates, are to begin the festivities by plucking an arrow out of the sugar-paste stag. To the "admiration of the beholders," the faux animal will release delectable claret wine "as blood running out of a wound."[18] The participants will next stage a mock war in which the ship and castle fire at each other. To cover the odor from the discharged gunpowder, the diners will be instructed to throw perfumed water from the eggshells at each other. After this carefully orchestrated and refined food fight—when "all danger" is past—huge pies will be cut open to release hopping frogs and flying birds. The fluttering of the birds' wings will put out the candles and leave everyone in the dark, which "will cause much delight and pleasure to the whole company." After the candles are relit, musicians will play while the diners narrate the events aloud and relive the spectacle. The desired response, as is repeated three times, is to produce "delights" for the audience.

"Triumphs and Trophies in Cookery" reads like a compressed Renaissance masque. Like the masque, a spectacle popular in the early Stuart court, this dining entertainment is concerned with producing wonder among spectators through scenic machinery, investing participants as stakeholders within the illusion, and celebrating artifice through extravagant contrivances. In the masque proper, courtiers performed roles and then collapsed the distinction between stage space and real world by stepping out to dance with audience members. Unlike the food festival described May's recipe book, however, the masque relied on a formally crafted script that included characters, disguises, and versified language. It was also, as many critics have explored, explicitly ideological, in that it typically staged threats to the social, natural, political, and economic order that were (perhaps incompletely) contained by the power of the monarch. Compared to the grandeur of spiraling stage sets and moving seas routinely devised by Inigo Jones for masques, the "Triumphs" illusions may seem unambitious or underwhelming, but the "Triumphs" had the added challenge of producing a visual spectacle made entirely of food.

The opening imperatives of "Triumphs"—"Make," "binde," "place," "stick," "bake," "cut"—align it grammatically with the hundreds of recipes presented in May's manual; and the recipe title observes that this script is "to be used." Yet the writing awkwardly shifts into present tense ("out skips some Frogs, which makes the Ladies to skip and shreek"), future tense (the birds "will put out the candles") and past tense ("These were formerly the delights of the Nobility"). As such, the account strains against the recipe format, unstably moving between prescription and description. When is a masque also a recipe? the text asks. Are these two forms compatible? In nostalgically mourning the demise of luxurious festivities, the narrator seems to admit that the reader will not, in all probability, enact the "recipe" at all. "These were formerly the delights of the Nobility," he laments, "before good Housekeeping had left England" (A8). In this way, the text marks the demise of the golden age of pre–civil war hospitality; it is a recipe aware it that will not, sadly, be made.

The fact that this spectacle appears in the prefatory matter of a cookery book rather than within the body of the text might seem to mark its exceptional status, yet "Triumphs and Trophies in Cookery" is nevertheless formally presented as a *recipe*. Scholars tend to point to May's "recipe" as historical evidence for what actually happened at court banquets,[19] or to dismiss it as nostalgic fantasy clearly out of place in a cookery advice book. Yet each of these approaches overlooks two important stories that May's text helps us to tell. First, May's recipe/account can provide a means of understanding the interpretative possibilities of *printed* recipe conceits that had only recently declined in popularity in England. Second, May's text actively converts food conceits from one frame of reference into another, as it disseminates food conceits to a new print audience. *Reading* about frivolity offers pleasures and puzzles in their own right; it has its own poetics.

In May's "Triumphs," food work involves a playful inquiry into the nature of representation and the "real," particularly as those terms relate to food practices. It asks readers to imagine an edible war on a grand scale, much like the architectural food designs and interactive sculptures presented as "sotelties" at noble feasts, where the medium and content productively clashed. In a commendatory poem prefacing *The Accomplisht Cook*, James Parry precisely points to this alignment by praising May as a master confectioner able to create simulacra of cities and military fortifications out of ephemeral materials. He is the artful Cook

> Who can in Paste erect, of finest flour,
> A compleat Fort, a Castle, or a Tower.
> A City Custard doth so subtly winde,
> That should Truth seek, shee'd scarce all corners finde:
> Plat-forme of Sconces that might Souldiers teach
> To fortifie by Works as well as Preach. (B1; 1660)

Parry teasingly lauds the ingenuity of culinary structures so realistic that they can serve as working models for military strategists; that is, May's culinary inventions are said to join the world of the real by modeling that world for viewers. Yet these creations are also firmly positioned within the ranks of an "art" that eludes "Truth," a figure defeated by the intricate mazes of the confectionary landscape ("should Truth seek, shee'd scarce all corners finde"). The product is "compleat," realistic enough to train soldiers, and yet also visibly a subtle piece of artifice. Ben Jonson's *The Staple of News* uses similar terms to praise the cook's ability to devise artificial worlds based on an expansive knowledge of astronomy, military strategy, chemistry, engineering, philosophy, and architecture, as Lickfinger exclaims:

> A *Master-Cooke*! Why, he's the *man* o' men,
> For a *Professor*! he designes, he drawes,
> He paints, he carves, he builds, he fortifies,
> Makes *Citadels* of curious fowle and fish . . .
> He raiseth *Ramparts* of immortall *crust*;
> And teacheth all the *Tacticks*, at one dinner:
> What *Rankes*, what *Files*, to put his dishes in;
> The whole *Art Military* . . .
> And so to fit his relishes, and sauces,
> He has *Nature* in a pot, 'boue all the *Chymists*,
> Or airy brethren of the *Rosie-crosse*.
> He is an *Architect*, an *Inginer*,
> A *Souldiour*, a *Physician*, a *Philosopher*,
> A generall *Mathematician*. (3.2.1631)

Jonson's poet-cook is a master of intellectual knowledge because he is a grand maker of simulated worlds. Putting "*Nature* in a pot" means making artifacts that only seem to be trivialized as curiosities but, in fact, serve as intellectual and imaginative triumphs. Indeed they transcend the intellectual efforts of chemists or secret esoteric societies (Rosicrucianism).

In a masque that he devised specifically for the 1624 court, Jonson celebrated the culinary arts by having a Cook take the stage with a Poet to declare their affinities. In *Neptune's Triumph*, the Cook declares, "you shall see I am a *Poet* no lesse than *Cooke* . . . Ile fit you with a dish out of the Kitchin / Such as I thinke will take the present palates, / A metaphoricall dish!" (A4v). In the masque, the Cook attempts to supplement the visual deficiencies of poetry by creating props and scenery that can be enjoyed by the palate: "I would have had your Ile brought floting in, now, / In a brave broth, and of a sprightly greene / Just to the colour of the Sea," he proclaims, after seeing the forlornly bare nature of the represented island. The Cook also supplies the missing antimasque by creating a metaphorical "Olla Pordrida," a miscellaneous stew of satirized occupations and people who emerge from a pot to dance. Jonson's masque strikingly rejects Plato's denunciation of cookery as a shadow of art: the masque asserts the correspondences between poetic rhetoric, material substance, and the truth of art. "A Good *Poet* differs nothing at all from a *Master-Cooke*," the Cook declares, "Eithers Art is the wisedome of the Mind."[20]

Although these hyperbolic food worlds might seem only the whim of fantastical writers, they had a referent in actual medieval and Renaissance feasts, where lavishly "realistic" *sotelties* or *entremets* were presented amid a sensory-rich world of music, dancing, perfumed scents, and costly objects.[21] Edible sculptures of animals, monarchs, ships, cities, and battle scenes punctuated courses of eating at these events. The earliest extant manuscript recipe book in England, *The Forme of Cury* (penned by master cooks serving under Richard II), documents the existence of individual "surprize" dishes that could be served as such banquets, including peacocks whose feathers were restored and capons stuffed with other easily recognizable flesh. Deliberately confusing essences and forms, veal would masquerade as duck or pudding would impersonate a chicken. Such spectacles might take place on a grand scale: at a feast in England in 1454, twenty-eight live musicians secreted within a large coarse pastry played music before dramatically breaking from their pastry-encrusted symphony shell—to great applause, we might imagine. The pageant in May's cookery book partakes of conventions from both masque and court feast. Although it does not rely on verse or speech, it makes an effort to script confectionary tableaux into a chronological sequence. The pie, for instance, punctuates the event with a finale, as flying birds extinguish the candles and plunge the audience into the dark.

The Accomplisht Cook's recipe for a sea-land battle in pastry-scape is framed by two highly representational moments: the feigned wounding of a deer and the surprise revelation of live creatures secreted in a pie. It is specifically on the meaning of these symbolically rich moments that I focus my interest. The thrill generated by these bookended disclosures stems from the instability of the category of "food," a term that usually marks the conversion of natural live creatures into processed human artifacts. Food becomes food precisely at the pivotal moment when the organic transforms into a dead object: pigs to ham, sheep to mutton, apples to pies, quinces to jelly. The bleeding deer and animated pie in May's spectacle tap into a long-standing cultural fascination with the "raw/cooked" axis that anthropologist Lévi-Strauss named as a critical fault line in culture. In myth, Lévi-Strauss argues, cooking straddles the line between the two as it marks a transition from nature into culture.[22] Surprising diners with pies housing live creatures is designed to evoke a sheer sense of marvel about the quandary of definitively separating "food" from an animate natural world. This dilemma is precisely the one registered in the nursery rhyme, "Sing a song of six pence, a pocket full of rye," where vocal blackbirds emerge from a pie. In transforming food so as to cite its prior live sources, "Triumphs" reverses the teleology of cooking and exposes the artful processes that underwrite a cuisine invested in the disguise of nature. The wit of the pie, that is, is to make strikingly visible the logics and processes that delineate "food" and "culture." In the spectacle, viewers act as agents who can "liberate" nature from culture and enact the dream of restoring nature to itself.

The opening gambit of presenting a *pastry* deer stabbed with an arrow further complicates the issues surrounding the live blackbird pie; for the deer is portrayed not as *food* but as a wounded animal that has been only partially denatured as it is injured in the hunt. When the guests remove the arrow, the shocker is that the deer bleeds (and so simulates being alive), but the second-order revelation is that the blood is actually consumable wine. The liveness of the deer is merely a ruse. Made out of coarse pastry, the deer's "naturalness" rests solely in its outward form; its "essence" turns out to be a processed beverage—offered freely to guests—that has only pretended to be a bodily fluid. Much like the conceit underwriting the eggs, which turn out to contain perfume rather than yolks, the deer tableau trades on the semblance of a natural form that gives way to a fully and unfamiliar artificial reality. Together, the pie and deer represent counterfeit foods whose "virtuality" blurs the natural and the artificial.

The deer aims to prompt spectators into "admiration" partly on the grounds that they witness a nonliving creature bleeding and partly by the fact that blood was a substance whose *convertibility* was precisely the subject of fierce religious controversy. Diners in the "Triumphs" are to deconstruct elements of the Christian sacrament of the Eucharist as they release the stag's blood and find that it has been transubstantiated into drinkable wine. As such, the spectators experience the grammar of the Eucharist in a festive register. The ritual of blood-turned-to-wine is subsequently symbolically reversed, when diners witness the seeming resurrection of "dead" and cooked animals. The wit of the scene turns on the staging of transubstantiation and resurrection in a culinary mimetic form. While the "Triumphs" does not directly comment on vexed debates surrounding the Eucharist, it appropriates the power of a religious food transformation to generate a secular "consumption" to admire.

After reflecting on the seemingly reversible processes of wounding and revivification, diners might nibble on the stage set and consume the stage on which they had acted. Yet the final conversion takes place only when they revivify the events by making them into stories designed to outlive any time-bound experience. The end result of the pageant is a narrative that reproduces itself endlessly, freed from its material incarnation. The banquet itself was a form, as Julia Lupton brilliantly analyzes, whose positioning as the final act in the sequence of the meal enabled it to "curat[e] moments of digestive reflection" and usher in a self-consciousness about the procedures and processes by which hospitality occurs. For Lupton, this aligns dessert with the phenomenologically oriented work of theater.[23] May's "Triumphs" makes the punctuating awareness of the banquet evident by calling attention to its transformation into narrative. When the dramatic spectacle is then included as part of a printed collection and marked as the product of a *past* age, it anticipates its ability to escape temporal bounds and to be reincarnated by future readers. In modeling the story that the event asks participants to produce, that is, the recipe refuses its designation as a moribund historical practice and flaunts its status as a technology of proliferation. It becomes a recipe for narrative, newly available to print consumers who might not be privileged enough to be physical witnesses to equivalent spectacular feasts.

While it's tempting to dismiss "Triumphs" as a throwback to archaic courtly entertainments, it fits, I argue, the logic of ingenuous foods that had been fashionable in cheaply published recipe books in the eighty years prior to its publication. While May explicitly addresses his work to professional chefs, previous recipe books trading in food conceits had charged women with the task of orchestrating banqueting dishes and puzzles for diners. In fact, in these recipe books women striving to be ideal housewives and/or proper gentlewomen were authorized to assume the power that Jonson and others invested in professional culinary artists. Thomas Nashe makes this clear when he pens a debate about the merits of country and urban life that holds up the perfect country gentlewoman as pious model, emblem of chastity, biblical scholar, linguist, musician, poet, painter, and, perhaps surprisingly, master of food conceits. Nashe writes:

> Sometimes againe she goeth into the Dairy, and converseth with the dairy-maide, and in a familiar manner of discourse (so curteous she is and loving to the meanest) learnes of her the mystery of her Art. Sometimes againe into the Pastry, where she takes much delight, and there either in raising of a Marchpane like unto a Pyramides, or in ye pourtrayting out a Pheasant, Cocke, or Partridge, she doth a while recreate her selfe: Sometimes she walkes into the open ayre, to see that no wrong be done to the seedes of her huswifery, her Hempe and Flaxe which is growing without.[24]

It is not a problem for this "Diana," as the countryman later terms her, to create faux confectionary pyramids out of marzipan or to create food portraits of fowl as she makes her domestic rounds, communes with the servants, and goes "into" the space called "the Pastry." Indeed these microbursts of domestic artistry enable her to embody perfection and "recreate her selfe" (both to entertain and produce herself). If we imagine that Renaissance audiences saw the housewife's food artistry as involving the revered attributes that Parry and Jonson attributed to the male cook, the housewife's "recreation" made her a home philosopher and poet, someone skilled in producing the "metaphoricall dish." "The *trompe l'oeil* dimension of cooking and confectionery," I have argued previously, "playfully invited people into a world of fantasy that could confuse critical categories operative in early modern life, namely by putting quotation marks around the "'real.'"[25] Part of the joy that recipe books offered makers and readers stemmed from the wit involved in scrutinizing the categories and abstract ideas structuring food making. Recipes that instructed the housewife to create *representational* arts introduced the philosophical conundrums seen in exaggerated form in the "Triumphs."

In the late Middle Ages and early Renaissance, artful elements of dining experiences began to be segregated into a distinct event called the "banquet," a word derived from *banket* or *banchetto*, the bench or board on which foods were displayed. The word signified not only a feast but a course of wines and candied spices served after the main meal while dishes were cleared or "voided." Gradually the banquet, formerly known as the "void," began to be served in houses built precisely for this purpose. Patricia Fumerton has written about how banqueting revealed a fragmentary aristocratic identity based on an aesthetics of culinary detachment, the airy nothingness of the banquet serving as a correlate for the profound emptiness of an aristocratic self in flux.[26] While this argument brilliantly captures the function of banquet practices, it fails to account for the appeal of scaled-down banqueting conceits in printed books marketed not only to a new breed of noblewoman but also to the wives of gentry, merchants, and yeomanry.[27] As printed cookbooks offered ways for women far from centers of power to create elite kitchen art, they morphed "sotelties" into the imaginative possibilities of print. Rather than being an anomaly or a mournful reference to a lost world of courtly feasting, May's "Triumphs" constitutes a belated version of a widespread phenomenon saturating the print industry in England from the onset of the published recipe collection. May's pageant-recipe simply makes visible conversations about art and nature occurring in and through printed recipes.

How did individual edible conceits signify when dishes were not integrated into elaborately scripted spectacles? *The Accomplisht Cook* points toward an answer, because it includes a few recipes that activate the inquiries raised by the "Triumphs." May's "To Make an Extraordinary Pie, or a Bride Pie, of Severall Compounds, Being Several Distinct Pies on One Bottom," is, as the title suggests, an intricate concoction designed for a special occasion. It involves baking several different pastries, composed of meats, oysters, fowl, custards, and fruit, which are merged into a single geometrically elaborate dish (Figure 14). May mentions a detail that gives the dish a surprise element: "it being baked and cold, take out the flour in the bottom, and put in live birds, or a snake, which will seem strange to the beholders, [when you] cut up the Pie at the table. This is onely for a Wedding to pass away time" (219). The dilemma of live food, which "Triumphs" sees as a characteristic of spectacles of the past, nevertheless survives in a recipe designed to create a diversion or "to pass away time." But even when not dreaming up fabulous concoctions for

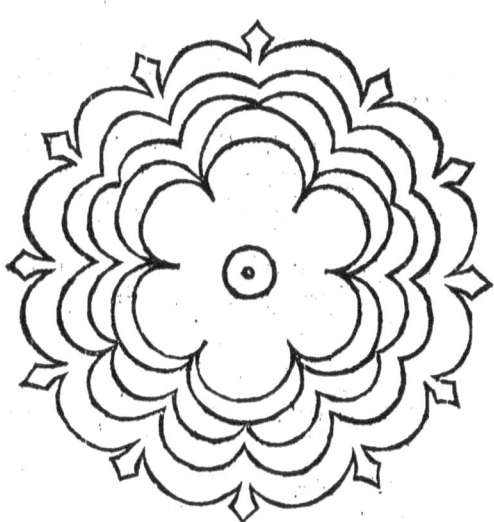

FIGURE 14. "Bride Pie," in Robert May's *The Accomplisht Cook* (London, 1660), 218. Photograph by Wendy Wall, from the collection of the Folger Shakespeare Library.

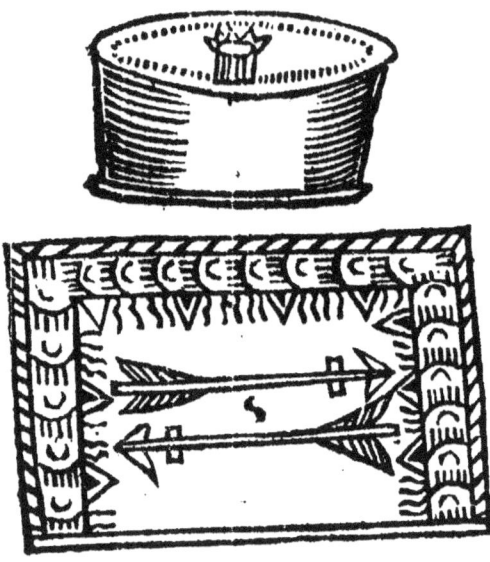

FIGURE 15. "Red Deer Pie," in Robert May's *The Accomplisht Cook* (London, 1660), 173. Photograph by Wendy Wall, from the collection of the Folger Shakespeare Library.

a wedding, readers can create less explicit and more modest food conceits. In a recipe for red deer pie, for instance, May has readers imprint the pastry crust with two hunter's arrows, in opposed directions (Figure 15). Unlike pies that boast geometric and floral shapes, this design references the deer's status as a live creature threatened by human weapons. The red deer baked in a seasoned egg custard subtly hearkens back to the critical moment when the animal converted, with some labor and violence, into food.

Renaissance food conceits often exemplify what food philosopher Lisa Heldke calls "thoughtful practice," praxis that entails self-critical reflection or theorization.[28] Recipe books promising delights for ladies promoted thoughtful practices by recommending foods that investigated their relationship to natural sources. In *A Daily Exercise for Ladies and Gentlewomen*, for instance, John Murrell offers instructions for molding sugar paste into the form of plants and animals, including snakes, frogs, and snails. In order to create cherries or strawberries, the reader should take the additional step of using double molds to construct a three-dimensional form whose similitude will be enhanced by "stems" made of dried birchen twigs sealed with dyer's fat. "They will be as they grew upon staulks," Murrell promises (F2r). His recipes for manufactured roses, primroses, marigolds, gillyflowers, and cowslips similarly aim for realistic representations of flowers in prepicked states. Among the many signs of evidence that recipe readers took these recommendations to heart is a manuscript collection by Ann Goodenough, which includes entries such as "how to Candy Violetts or any other Flowers and keepe them that they will looke as fresh as when they are first gathered."[29] In devising what one recipe describes as candied roses that look "as naturally as if they grew upon the Tree," household makers aspired to fabricate artistic products with natural appearances.[30] Such decoctions playfully pressed the boundary between organic and artificial material, even as they made readers vividly aware of their distinctiveness. In having a diner seem to pick a violet or pear from a faux vine, recipes referenced the linear process of cookery, offering a false return to nature, which, the diner discovered, was already saturated with layers of artifice. Such recipes encouraged sophisticated food wit and food play.

The artistic and intellectual impulse in this type of food work has been contextualized by Jayne Elisabeth Archer, who surveys ways that literary and recipe domains intersected. In teasing out deep structural connections between the making of mental and material worlds in the household, Archer uncovers the symbolic and poetic potential of the recipe form. She focuses specifically on how tropes of housewifery, particularly distillation and healing, figured in both celebratory and satirical conceptions of early modern female authorship. Archer identifies a passage in Thomas Wright's 1693 comedy *The Female Virtuoso* that wonderfully encapsulates this representational power. In this play satirizing emergent empirical culture, a character named Mrs. Lovewitt attempts to distill plays in a limbeck so as to extract their pure literary qualities for commercial profit. "I have made an exact Collection of all the Plays that ever came out," she states, "which I design to put into my Limbeck; and then extract all the Quintessence of Wit that is in them."[31] Mrs. Lovewit's plan to mechanically boil imaginative works down so as to extract their core quality, "the quintessence of wit," is held up to ridicule. Nevertheless Archer shows how this passage capitalizes on the transformative power of distillation and recipe work broadly to envision female poetic making. Housewifery did not merely provide a vocabulary for describing women's intellectual work, however; it also was the site in which practitioners might investigate categories central to acts of representation. Mrs. Lovewit's quest to identify a substance called "wit" was only laughable in its literality. In confectionery, as in distillation, recipe work involved precisely these cognitive quandaries.

It was the difficulty of separating art and nature that some recipes adopted as their subject. *The Ladies Cabinet Enlarged*, a book marketed specifically to "Industrious improvers of Nature by Art," offers a recipe in which readers are to crush violets to form a coloring and flavoring agent for a paste that was then shaped to look like a real violet.[32] The writer brags that this violet is not comprised of "painted colors," but instead retains its own "color and taste." In creating a natural dye, the recipe presents an artificially *reconstituted* yet natural flower. Certainly it produces something that does not fit our modern classifications: part dessert, part home decoration, part preserved food, and part medicine. But it also posed a brainteaser to its contemporary audience: if a violet is dissolved and then reconstituted into a violet-shaped paste, is it (still) a real violet? Or a representation? Or is it something else altogether? Does this violet retain its *essence* while sacrificing its *show*, as Shakespeare's speaker intimates of the distilled rose in Sonnet 5? "But flowers distilled, though they with winter meet," the speaker argues to his beloved, "Lose but their show; their substance still lives sweet."[33] Although Shakespeare's sonnet aligns the reconfigured rose with the immortalizing power of poetry, his flower, like homey violet paste, ponders the relation of essences to forms, copies to originals, technologies of artifice to nature. If we have doubts about whether such considerations could have been activated by the making of something as mundane as a candied flower, we need only consider the fact that recipe collections offered a range of flower recipes, each with strikingly different effects. A home confectioner might attempt a domestically processed flower that appears as "rock candy" shimmering with "sparks of diamonds" (entities that revel in their synthetic status). Or she might craft a candied flower whose leaves, stems, and stalks bear, as one recipe terms it, their "true form." She might use ground flowers to paint imitation versions of an original, as the violet paste recipe dictates, or she might stamp a tart with an image that "cites" its ingredients (for instance, a rosewater-scented marzipan printed with the image of a rose).[34] With these options for made flowers on display, the recipe worker entered a world where the question of food's relationship to nature and art was at issue.

As confectioners tested ways to position nature in relation to their kitchen artifice, they stumbled onto the hermeneutical and ontological issues that vexed poets and philosophers of the period.[35] Critical tomes have been written on the subject of Renaissance literature's pronounced self-consciousness, its interest in theorizing its own representational status and interrogating the nature of artifice. In one critically noted instance in Shakespeare's *Winter's Tale*,

Perdita, for example, engages in a lively disagreement with Polixenes, her beloved, about whether carnations and streaked gillyflowers should be allowed in proper gardens. Perdita declaims against grafted plants as inauthentic bastards and perversions of nature: "There is an art which in their piedness shares / With great creating nature," she complains (4.4.89–90). Polixenes defends hybridization by arguing that nature itself can be mobilized to improve other elements of nature:

> . . . So over that art
> Which you say adds to nature, is an art
> That nature makes. You see, sweet maid, we marry
> A gentler scion to the wildest stock,
> And make conceive a bark of baser kind
> By bud of nobler race. This is an art
> Which does mend nature—change it rather; but
> The art itself is nature. (4.4.92–97)

Critics have long pointed to this passage as crystallizing an ongoing debate among Renaissance writers about the proper relationship of art to nature. For Polixenes, the terms "art" and "nature" are simply too reductive to account for a synthetic substance artificially compounded from natural elements. Perdita disagrees. The play thus stages a debate about the ethical boundaries of artifice and the proper social status of "the natural," a discussion carried out, we might note with special regard to this passage, in gardening manuals as well as literary works.[36] When the recipe reader chose among radically different options for naturalizing artificial flowers or counterfeiting natural ones, she inadvertently engaged a consequential topic of the day. Did one want to be an "industrious improver of Nature by Art" or were those very terms untenable? If one altered nature, did one hubristically convert, as Polixenes argues, "base" substances into "nobler" ones?

One of the most famous scenes in all English Renaissance literature designates the trompe l'oeil artistry seen in domestic confectionery as an immoral sleight of hand. In Edmund Spenser's epic romance *The Faerie Queene*, the knight representing the virtue of temperance concludes his quest to conquer the witch Acrasia by landing on her home turf, the exquisitely sensual Bower of Bliss. As almost all readers notice, Spenser innovates the Homeric myth of Circe by having Acrasia serve as the maker of a gorgeous garden whose aesthetic beauty shares features with the poet's own invention. Unlike other tempting environments in fairyland, Acrasia's bower is a verdant artistic construction, complete with lyrical sounds, gorgeous sculptures, and lush greenery. While its luxuriant flowers and vegetation appear to be nature at its finest, the questing Guyon discovers that they are part of the ruses and deceptions of the garden. He comes across a lush vine bending down under the weight of purple, green, and red grapes, for instance, with some made of "burnisht gold, / So made by art, to beautifie the rest."[37] Nestled among the real grapes, in other words, are artificial ones that invisibly enhance the authentic grapes. Guyon similarly discovers an ivy of dyed green gold used to ornament a fountain; it confounds spectators who "surely deeme it to be yvie trew" (2.12.61.5). The culprit in this pleasure garden is artifice masking as nature. Tellingly, with regard to the recipe world, the narrator mentions that when Guyon destroys the bower, he tears down all the structures it housed:

> Their Groves he feld their gardins did deface,
> Their arbers spoyle, their Cabinets suppresse,
> Their banket houses burne, their buildings race,
> And of the fairest late, now made the fowlest place. (2.12.83.6–9)

Late in the episode, the reader discovers that Acrasia's wanton groves harbored banqueting houses, the Renaissance buildings designed precisely to house the culinary artifices recommended to housewives in English recipe books. The bower also included "cabinets," the central metaphor that recipe collections of the day used to describe their printed forms. Acrasia, it seems, serves up a sensual art specifically associated with the trickery of domestic sugar works. The evident moral coding presented (that women should not orchestrate such delights) is complicated by the epic's status as a lush representational practice much like the banqueting dishes it condemns. Rather than settling the issue, the poem opens the debate about how to experience an explicitly artificial nature through the reading of epic. While candied and preserved flower recipes seem a far cry from the intricately structured world of Spenser's remarkable poetic allegory, both take up basic metaphysical questions about the mechanics of representation and its central categories.

Hugh Plat's poetic preface to his recipe collection, *Delightes for Ladies*, serves as the period's most elaborate manifesto on the representational complexity and power of cookery. Seeking to forge a heroic domestic how-to genre, Plat championed the housewife's ingenuity in using "sweet compoundes of arte" to rival and resurrect a natural world that has been reconfigured beyond recognition. His book, he grandly proclaims, could teach readers to perform almost miraculous and mystical domestic tasks:

> Of marmalade and paste of Genua,
> Of musked sugar I intend to wright,
> Of leache, of sucket, and Quidinea,
> Affording to each Ladie, her delight.
> I teach both fruits and flowers to preserve,
> And candie them, so Nutmegs, cloves, and mace:
> To make both marchpaine, paste, and sugred plate,
> And cast the same in formes of sweetest grace.
> Each bird and foule, so moulded from the life,
> And after cast in sweet compounds of arte,
> As if the flesh and forme which Nature gave,
> Did still remaine in every lim and part. (A2v–A3)

In the trompe l'oeil of the kitchen, the housewife might reproduce a chicken's natural "flesh and forme," as if a real bird's animate quality figured somehow in the creation of dessert. While Plat probably meant that an actual animal would have been used to create a cast-work mold, (which then could be used to fashion marzipan), his ambiguous use of the word "remain" suggested a lingering vitality within the sugar imitation. The effect is echoed by his use of the word "lim," which referred both to a technique of drawing and painting (to "limn") and to a body part (a "limb"). The cook's "compoundes of art" rivaled and seemingly (re)produced the organic world it imitated. In fact, one of the delights that Plat imagined ladies to take was that of managing the tension between nature and art, live and dead creatures, organic entities and the thing that we call food. "Are wee not more delighted with seeing Birds, Fruites, and Beasts *painted* than wee are with Naturalls?" John Donne queried.[38] In trompe l'oeil cuisine, it was not merely the tricky nature of representation that afforded pleasure, but also its inscription within a physically consumable form that estranged "food" itself. Purposefully confusing the category of animation, these artful confections provide a way of thinking through the ecology of food, delving into the type of reflective practice that Julian Yates identifies as part of the metaphysics of early modern "kitchening."[39]

Plat's preface and the "Triumphs" indicate that recipes could focus broad questions about food artifice by referencing "liveness" on the table. Yet some culinary concoctions additionally raised the question of food genres. Among its candies, pastes, cordial waters, and conserves, *A Closet for Ladies and Gentlewomen* presented "all kinde of Birds and Beasts to stand on their legges in cast work" (38), edible forms created by boiling seasoned Barbary sugar to form a moldable paste (47). Birds and beasts commonly eaten at the table reappeared in these dynamic and lifelike postures, which, like the sugar-shaped cherries on the vine, reminded diners of the previous unprocessed natural status of the organic world. Yet, these concoctions also called attention to the particular form in which animals could be served. Yes, fowl were typically present at dinner, the recipe acknowledged, but not usually in *this* incarnation; they usually lay prone ready to carved or chopped. While the conceit drew its wit from the deceptive nature of exterior form, it specifically alluded to the "warner," a medieval term for a food that masqueraded as another type of edible. One of the most popular recipes in the seventeenth century of this ilk was for marzipan "collops" (bacon) and eggs, made by devising natural dyes to simulate streaky slabs of meat and sunny yolks. These modest banqueting dishes relied on an insubstantial ingredient, as sugar was conceptualized, to counterfeit "substantial" food. The wit of the conceit turned less on the elusive quality of the dish's natural origins or the vexed artifice of food preparation than on the fun of having one genre of eating impersonate another. A luxury dessert slummed as a lowly foodstuff; sweet counterfeited as savory. In Plat's "A Most Delicate and Stiffe Sugar Past Whereof to Cast Rabbets, Pigeons, or Any Other Little Birde or Beast," the reader could shape isinglass to resemble a capon, pig, or blackbird (B3v), but she could then give her creation a savory appearance by dredging it in a bread crust mixture. "A banquet may be presented in the forme of a supper," Plat proclaimed, as if unveiling a magic trick (B4). The diner's surprise was the discovery of insubstantial sugar rather than roasted flesh. As taste was divorced from the food's visual appearance, the issue at stake was the reliability of categories of dining—did one eat a supper or a banquet?

When Philip Stubbes listed the moral threats that foods posed, he interestingly singled out for special condemnation edibles that abandoned their natural form. In *The Anatomie of Abuses*, Stubbes predictably denounced *variety* in foods as leading to gluttony, a sin starring prominently in medieval Christian representations. Yet, in a strangely materialistic reading, Stubbes charged Adam with displaying the vice of gluttony when eating forbidden fruit in Eden; he read Satan's temptation of Christ in the wilderness in the same vein. When turning to modern sources of corruption, Stubbes declaimed against lavish foods as inciting lust, excess, and bodily distemper, but he less expectedly objected that "dainty" fare had a representational *structure* that could confuse the distinction between essences and forms: "true Hospitality consisteth not in many dishes," he wrote, "nor in sundry sortes of meates (the substance whereof is changed almost into accidentes thorow their curious Cookeries)."[40] The language Stubbes used surely had Eucharistic significance, chiefly as it raised the question of whether bread and wine lost their "substance" or merely changed in terms of their "accidents" (that is, their apprehensible concrete features); these were the very terms that theologians used in arguing about the communion. In food conceits, the question was not whether one substance converted into another, of course, but rather how an essence was "almost" but not quite identical to its appearance. It was a problem familiar to audiences who attended London playhouses.

Culinary conceits could and were mobilized into domestic performance art for spectator-diners. The "thoughtful" nature of the practice, in these cases, emerged in the moment of consumption. Yet independent of the dining event, the recipe as a written text raised intellectual questions specifically for its *user-reader*. Let's consider two recipes whose wit rested as much in the reader's consumption of text as in the creation of spectacles for others. In prescribing an "out-landish" roasted leg of mutton, Gervase Markham instructed housewives to prepare a sweet, spiced, egg-and-cream-based pudding, dye it vibrant colors, and encase it in the skin of a sheep's leg. "Serve it up as a legge of Mutton with this pudding, for indeed it is no other," Markham declared (1623; 81–82). A reader might have scratched her head at this assurance: the mutton *minus* the meat is no other than what it "is"? And what would that be? Food substantially that is and is not? Something embedded within—but also miraculously enduring out of—nature, a term that, in its semiotic and ontological registers, was held up for inspection? How could mutton be a simile for itself? We might gloss the knotty issues raised by Markham's mutton recipe by looking to the moment in Shakespeare's *Tempest* when Ariel has spirits display a banquet table laden with exotic foods to the hungry Italians shipwrecked on a seemingly bare island. For a moment, Gonzalo and the other noblemen marvel at the contrast between airy spirits and the material abundance they create. But, as they quickly discover, the food turns out to be a mirage, part of the world of illusion used to produce a moral condemnation that leads to political change. In his outlandish mutton recipe, Markham teaches readers to act as domestic magicians, who, in the act of reading the recipe, grapple with the conundrums raised by illusion making.

In *Delightes for Ladies*, Plat similarly presented a recipe whose full wittiness was appreciated chiefly by the cook. In a "Paste Made of Fish," he advised: "Incorporate the bodie of saltfish, Stockfish, Ling, or any fresh fish that is not full of bones, with crums of bread, flower, Isinglasse, &c. and with proper spices agreeing with the nature of everie severall fish, and of that paste molde off the shapes & forms of little fishes: as of the Roch, Dace, Perch, &c. and so by arte you may make many little fishes out of one great and naturall fish" (F5–5v). The diner eating this meatloaf-like fish mixture might have recognized that the small fish shapes referred to their material, much like "baby carrots" purchased in supermarkets today consist of ground carrots pressed into smaller forms of themselves. Yet only the cook would fully appreciate that isinglass (derived from a fish bladder) was the bonding agent used to create the pliable fish mixture. The proliferation of fish categories in this recipe boggles the mind: a large fish donates the taste, a small fish materializes the form, and a fish-product is the magic that generates the texture and structure. Slyly alluding, perhaps, to Christ's miraculous multiplication of fish and loaves, Plat marveled at the expansion of "naturall" fish by "arte." The reader was not invited to savor the tastiness of the dish (Plat did not even bother to describe its cooking method). Instead Plat dwelled on the culinary "pun" created by stylizing fish in different media. The proof of the pudding might rest in the eating, but the wit of the dish seemed to lie, in this instance, in the reading.

When the reader put recipes into practice, she generated fundamentally ambiguous signifiers for eaters to interpret. In *Treasurie of Commodious Conceites*, to take one fascinating example, Partridge instructs the reader to stencil words or images onto a marzipan tart. "Take and cut your leaf of gold," he begins,

> as it lieth upon the book, into square pieces like Dice, & with a Conies tails end moisted a little, take the gold up by the one corner, lay it on the place being first made moist, and with another tail of a Cony dry press the gold down close. And if ye will have the form of an Hart, or the name of Jesus, or any other thing whatsoever: cut the same through a piece of paper, and lay the Paper upon your Marchpane, or Tart: then make the void place of the Paper . . . moist with Rosewater, lay on your gold, press it down, take off your Paper, and there remaineth behind in gold the Print cut in the said paper. (1584; A7)

If the reader so desires, Partridge states casually, she can print something decorative onto the tart—the image of a "hart" (a deer or, perhaps, a valentine shape) or "the name of Jesus, or any other thing whatsoever." While Partridge's recipe is relatively unusual in specifying a religious theme for a sugar work, other texts in the period refer to food conceits that depict manger scenes, saint's lives, the Lamb of God, the Virgin Mary, angels, and the holy infant. If the confectioner did stamp the name of Jesus onto the tart, she would have created a word-oriented version of these religious "sotelties."[41] Would the "name of Jesus" create a talismanic deity-wafer, a luxury Eucharist good with God incarnated into edible signifier? Did this recipe literalize the eating of God by having the wafer imprinted with a *name?* Or did it parody the literalization of that trope? It's hard to answer this question because early modern people thoroughly absorbed the Eucharistic concept of consuming and incorporating God as a means of achieving spiritual union and salvation. Spirituality and ingestion were so closely associated in the culture that it was not heretical in the least for George Herbert to depict God as offering himself to the poetic speaker as "meat" to be consumed in a game of flirtatious courtship ("Love III"). Herbert's "The Banquet" also specifically compares Holy Communion to a secular course of sweetmeats and drinks, which God inhabits as a means of physically touching the physical realm. "Having rais'd me to look up," the speaker states, "In a cup / Sweetly he doth meet my taste."[42]

Recipes that advocated for women to create domestic versions of religious iconography did, however, take a risk. In Ben Jonson's *Bartholomew Fayre,* Puritan Busy condemns Joan Trash's gingerbread as "thy basket of popery, thy nest of Images."[43] While the play undercuts Busy's objection, it points to the close association that culinary icons could have with Catholicism. So too, when José de Acosta denounced Native American religious practice as idolatry, he compared the natives' crafting of bread shaped as feet or hands to familiar simulacra in English "marchpane."[44] While iconoclasts burned crucifixes and smashed statues, home confectioners manufactured religious images in the kitchen. In a comedy called *The Citye Match*, one character makes this association (albeit in a different register) when he jokes that his wife's scalding of preserved quinces turns them into "acts and Monuments in sweet-meats," that is, edible versions of Protestant martyrs burned at the stake.[45]

While some recipe books invited housewives and ladies to orchestrate kitchen practices that simulated, enacted, and/or mimicked sacred rites, others directed readers to consider the status of luxury commodities in the culture. Collections abound with recipes concerning ways to shape sugar plate and marzipan into extravagant household objects such as keys, plate ware, household utensils, cards, gloves, saucers, jewelry, beads, chains, shoes, slippers, knives, and family crests.[46] Many of these consumer goods—including embroidered gloves, jewelry, and expensive plate ware—proliferated in homes of the middling sort at the end of the sixteenth century and early seventeenth century.[47] What did it mean to re-present goods typically used to exhibit social standing in the expensive yet ephemeral form of sugar? These culinary representations present the same hermeneutical quandaries surrounding the wafer imprinted with the name of Jesus: did the reproduction of goods in the banquet *reduplicate* conspicuous consumption? Or did the translation of durable goods into ephemeral foodstuffs mock its pretensions, showing that, like the flesh, all earthly things wither away? While we have no extant archive that allows us to resolve this issue, we can consider the violence involved in consuming labor-intensive simulacra of saucers, dishes, and bowls. "At the end of the banquet thei may breake all, and eate the platters, dishes, glasses, Cuppes, and all things," Partridge writes, "for this paste is very delicate and flavorous" (1573; A4r). As Fumerton has astutely analyzed, we have textual traces of the excessive militancy and zeal with which sugar works were eaten, razed, and destroyed (132–33). While Fumerton sees this destructiveness as emanating from the perceived analogy between human and culinary ephemerality, we might also see it an exposure of the hollow or transient nature of social display. Food conceits could investigate not just the nature of the "real," as we have seen, but also the use value of material practices.

The interpretive possibilities of sugar simulacra further expands when we consider those recommended by the ever-practical Markham, who, as we've seen, published his *English Housewife* to offset what he saw as the trivialization of domestic labor. Because diet should be "rather to satisfy nature than our affections, and apter to kill hunger than revive new appetites," housewives should not look for "strangeness and raritie" of cuisine, Markham advised (1623; 4). He championed a homegrown self-sufficiency that seemed precisely at odds with the cerebral and coy games of banqueting recipes. Markham's terms are worth considering, especially his sense that "nature" battles "affections" within the moral framework of eating. Affections, the "action or result of affecting the mind in some way," seems a mental detour from the basic task of eliminating physical hunger.[48] Strange foods that "affect" the psyche also were problematic in that they stimulated rather than satisfied appetite and thus perpetuated restless desire. In identifying appetite as a suspect sexual and bodily desire, Markham drew on the very classical and medieval topoi that he later contradicted when he presented "Banqueting stuffe and conceited dishes, with other pretty and curious secrets, necessary for the understanding of our English Houswife" (111). "Albeit they are not of general use, yet [in] their true times they are so needful for adornation," he wrote, "that whosoever is ignorant therein is lame, and but the half part of the compleat Hous-wife" (111). What Markham formerly condemned as extravagant becomes "necessary" for the production of the housewife who could only boast of comprehensive knowledge and skills if she were able to create ornamental feasts. Markham then listed forty-three conceits as part of this "needful" "adornation," including printed quince pastes, dyed jellies, ornamental gingerbread, jumbals, and artificial cinnamon sticks. He argued for arranging banqueting dishes so that they would "not onely appear delicate to the eye, but invite the appetite with the much varietie thereof" (1623; 125). It proved difficult for Markham to ignore the social demands of dainty fare or the appeal of stimulating the appetite.

Markham did, however, offer two recipes that strikingly recast the material and social meaning of conceit making. In "The Making of Strange Sallats," he urged the housewife to use pickled and preserved flowers and vegetables "for better curiositie, and the finer adorning of the table" (1623; 62). His reader was to arrange roses into the shape of a large flower, creating stalks and leaves from vegetables and herbs. Markham explained that it was best if this dish reflected stages of natural development: some leaves should resemble buds, while others should be fully opened. In offering a salad designed both "for shew and use," he forged a compromise between competing value systems (63); that is, he identified foods that substantially fed the body while also exciting curiosity and wonder.

Markham also recommended ornamental "Sallats for Shew Onely," which were composed of boiled vegetables arranged into "many shapes and proportions, as some into knots, some in the manner of Scutchions and Armes, some like Birds, and some like wild Beasts, according to the Art and cunning of the Workman" (1623; 63). In appealing to the "cunning" artistry of the housewife-turned-workman as she fashioned simulations of family crests and live creatures, Markham embraced the playful wit that fueled the wasteful practices he elsewhere decried. When recipe writers advocated the making of edible sugar-cast family crests, they potentially posed the interpretative complexities that surrounded culinary religious icons and valuable goods. Such patently false simulacra of the family coat of arms might hint at the counterfeit nature of a primary marker of gentility. We might remember that this was an era when social climbers eagerly sought to purchase family coats of arms so as to inhabit a prestigious family lineage. The dessert family crest, or escutcheon, was part of a status game coextensive with elite banqueting, both dependent on expenditure. But lodging the sign of family lineage in a consumable form that might be smashed and eaten at the end of the meal subjects that symbol to the insubstantiality so clearly visible in "the void." At the least, we see that the evanescent family crest of the banquet clashed with its function of creating longevity. In staging this representational problem through the inexpensive material of carrots, Markham cast a potentially critical light on the expenditure routinely practiced in domestic conceit making. What form of cultural capital might decorative *vegetables* offer? While displaying inventiveness, did Markham's ornamental salad mock the elaborate confectionaries of the "void," even as he hastened to show that the good English housewife was skilled enough to imitate elite practices she might find suspect? Did the wholesomeness or the cheapness of the carrot offset the frivolity of its "show"?

John Murrell asked this question in different form in his recipe for "fond pudding," small fried meatloaves made of mutton, veal, or lamb, which were mixed with beef suet, spinach, parsley, marigolds, endive, thyme, savory, nutmeg, sugar, dates, currants, breadcrumbs, egg yolks, rosewater, and verjuice. "Work them up like Birds, Beasts, Fishes, Peares, or what you will," Murrell directed.[49] As in Markham's "out-landish" mutton dish, Murrell signaled the silliness of the pudding through its name. And like Markham's heraldic carrots, Murrell's pudding offered a substantial "soteltie" that could satisfy hunger while also stimulating curiosity. The meatloaf bird, pear, fish, or beast might deflate as well as express the pretensions aired in costly conceit-making enterprises. With no extrinsic evidence about their reception, we are only able to identify the interpretive possibilities of these utilitarian forms of conspicuous consumption. Read alongside other early modern writings, we see that these forms pressure the meaning of "use" and "show." They reveal a degree of self-reflexivity that we might not expect to find in technical writing. Delights for ladies, it seems, involved knotty interpretive quandaries.

Sanctioning women to undertake creative artistry in the household had clear social stakes. As I have argued elsewhere, the permission that recipe books offered female domestic makers flew in the face of widespread pronouncements that women must prioritize their roles as stewards of precious family and national resources. In inviting housewives to design sumptuous commodities to be devoured at the table, recipes voiced a conservative preacher's worst nightmare. Through culinary games of wit, practical sustenance was subordinated, or awkwardly yoked to, the thrill of social performance. William Harrison expressed horror at "outlandish" feasts popular in merchants' households, which included "jellies of all colours, mixed with a variety in the representation of sundry flowers, herbs, trees, forms of beasts, fish, fowls, and fruits, and thereunto marchpane wrought with no small curiosity, tarts of divers hues, and sundry denominations, conserves of old fruits, foreign and home-bred, suckets, codinacs, marmalades, marchpane, sugar-bread, gingerbread, florentines, wild fowls, venison of all sorts, and sundry outlandish confections."[50] Recipes for elaborate creations also countered ubiquitous early modern warnings that women were especially prone to the snares of artifice, a concern most heatedly aired in denunciations of women's cosmetics.[51] In fact, the "painted lady" who might dabble with mysterious chemicals in her closet was a conventional figure for waywardness in Renaissance plays. Witness Hamlet's seemingly illogical digression when holding Yorick's skull in the graveyard: his mind wanders from mortality to the dangers of female makeup as the ultimate emblem of human vanity.[52] Early recipe books that taught women to take pleasure in using "cunning" artistry to devise false realities flew in the face of these strictures. As such, recipes pointed to a spectacular contradiction in Renaissance ideologies of gender and domesticity. While we have begun to appreciate the fact that domesticity offered a site for testing gender constraints, we have not yet fully considered the representational and intellectual stakes of their involvement in producing a cuisine "wrought with no small curiosity."

As late sixteenth- and early seventeenth-century recipe books reached people who would never attend noble feasts, they subjected banqueting conceits to new frameworks of analysis. Rather than displaying the empty status of aristocratic identity, as Fumerton argues of banqueting, printed recipes spoke to a wider reading public. Certainly the conceit's premium on malleability made it a perfect expression for a metamorphic worldview. With the increased affordability of printed materials, the rise of social mobility, and a slight decline in the price of cane sugar, affluent merchants and yeomen could use marzipan to signify a world that could be molded at will. A carrot need not be confined to its natural shape but could miraculously transform into a family crest. A chicken might take the form of venison or be poised to fly from the table. These concoctions articulated an ideology of utterly reconstructable essences and identities, even as they held up terms such as "nature," "matter," "substance," and "representation" for investigation. Unlike May's "Triumphs," conceits in early seventeenth-century recipe books were not nostalgic but future looking; that is, they circulated a decidedly new way for non-noble people to engage in intellectual games through culinary aesthetics. In fact, when May branded the artifice of the feast as archaic, he erased the history of confectionery that had been popular in the English print world.

Ingenious desserts fell out of favor over the course of the seventeenth century in England as French-led preferences for "naturalist" foods reshaped food tastes.[53] The more naturalist ethos of European cuisine rendered highly artificial sugar designs a relic of the past. Fewer and fewer "outlandish" marzipan and pastes appeared in recipe collections, though extravagant culinary spectacles remained popular in court celebrations. Jean-Louis Flandrin argues that cuisine was affected by neoclassical seventeenth-century art and architecture, which rejected the twisting exuberance and shocking contrasts characteristic of baroque and rococo styles.[54] Thus affected, recipe books began to advise readers to value delicacy and refinement over and above abundance and variety. Confectionery was not to produce intellectual vexation but to accentuate cultivated textures and tastes. In *The Compleat City and Country Cook: Or, Accomplish'd Housewife* (1736), Charles Carter condemned cookery that worked to "disguise Nature and lose it in Art."[55]

Rather than concentrating on the surprises possible in malleable foodstuffs, ladies began to be schooled on how to *refine* the textures and colors of leaches, jellies, creams, and puddings. Dairy dishes, which had come into fashion in the sixteenth century but which had formerly been stigmatized as lower class or rustic, became one of the chief remaining culinary sites for displaying "natural" domestic artistry. Creams served in transparent sculpted glasses took center stage on the table. In the eighteenth century, Hannah Glasse spruced up the humble syllabub (a drink of wine mixed with cream) by dying it in rich colors. Like Markham's carrot salad or Murrell's fond pudding, Glasse turned a modest drink into an unexpected thing of beauty. "Jellies," as gelatins were called, rose in status and began to be prominently stacked in geometric pyramids dyed in "ribbons" of luminous colors. Glasse was a tad apologetic for the superfluity of her "ribband jelly": "You may add Orange-flower water, or Wine and Sugar, and Lemon, if you please but this is all fancy," she explains (1747; 145). While women continued to make sweetmeats and preserves, the lady of the house no longer oversaw the design of culinary brainteasers, the stuff of mere "fancy."

The modern concept of "dessert" as a final course of sweetmeats cordoned off from savory foods truly emerged only in the eighteenth century, though the term had been used earlier. Only then did sweet dishes that had been served alongside savory dishes throughout the meal become singled as a distinctive and culminating finale, pleasures in their own right. Foods masqueraded as other foods only in the service of economy: one could make "artificial red deer" or "artificial venison" by marinating mutton or cheaper meats to create the semblance of luxury dishes. Food designed to shock and surprise fell out of fashion.

As aesthetic culinary concerns turned to table layout, late seventeenth- and early eighteenth-century recipe books began to include engravings and copper-plated diagrams to illustrate the placement and shape of dishes in relation to each other. The reason for this shift undoubtedly had to do with an increase in the affordability of producing print engravings as well as the emergence of a readership interested in illustrations within technical books. Charles Carter's *The Complete City and Country Cook; or, Accomplish'd Housewife* opened with a title page pointing out to readers that the text had "forty-nine large copper plates, directing the regular placing [of] the various Dishes on the Table." These plates use oval figures to show eager readers the proper arrangement of items on the table. Although concoctions from older recipe books continued to be popular, they were newly positioned to conform to new standards for appropriate placing. Recipe books as different as Elizabeth Moxon's *English Housewifery*, John Farley's *The London Art of Cookery*, and Martha Bradley's *The British Housewife* relied on illustrative techniques: from simple line-drawn diagrams that correspond by numbers to lists of foods (Moxon); to models showing the relative size, shape, and position of dishes (Farley); to more elaborate representational and graphic images that indicate the visual appearance of foods or their substance (Bradley) (Figure 16). John Nott spends three pages describing protocols for positioning a dessert course, complete with visual model and "explication" of design rationale (2–3). Stimulating the diner's eye no longer required a sleight of hand or a prerogative to choose "what form you please"; instead it turned on the correct display of tastes, forms, color combinations, and contrasts.[56]

After the 1650s, recipe books emphasized the rationalization of recipe knowledge rather than its witty pleasures. Following Woolley, who opened *The Cook's Guide* with a ten-page "Alphabetical Table of the Heads contained in this Booke," writers such as Elizabeth Raffald, Eliza Smith, and Martha Bradley included indices, headers, demarcated chapters, and tables of contents to make their texts easily readable. Hannah Glasse's *Art of Cookery, Made Plain and Easy* contained elaborate orienting mechanisms in the name of utility, including a twenty-two-page table of contents. As her title suggests, Glasse staked the value of her book on the ease with which cookery could be learned.[57] The world of economy had little truck with the marvels of food conceits.

When recipe books did emphasize the reader's pleasure, they tended to posit a finicky female diner enjoying fine fare, or they retrofitted the term to

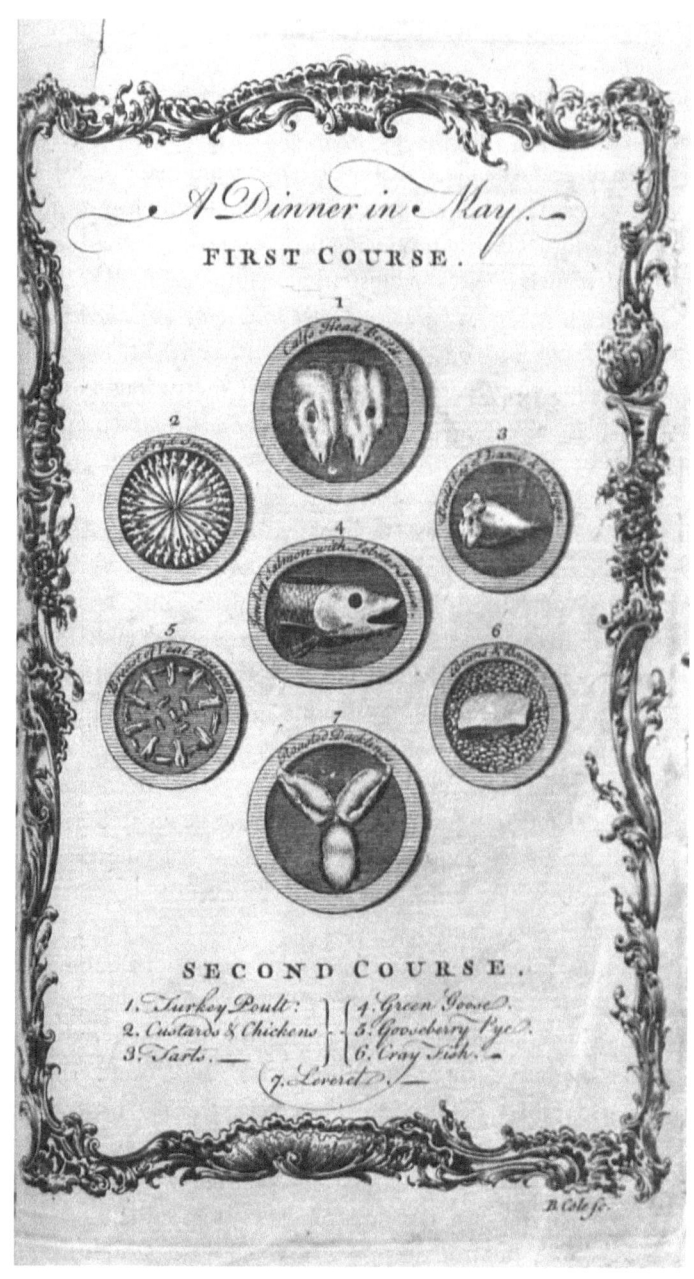

FIGURE 16. Martha Bradley's table arrangement for "A Dinner in May," in *The British Housewife* (London, 1760), 456v. Reproduced by permission of the British Library.

accommodate a new utilitarian ethos. John Town introduced May's *Accomplisht Cook* with the claim that cookery could work "both toe please, and tickle / To the pretty Ladies palate with delight." He located "delight" in the domain that earlier recipe books had avoided: the experience of sensory consumption. In *The House-Keeper's Pocket-Book*, Sarah Harrison thought of pleasure in terms of consumption. "A few good Ingredients make the best Dishes, and a crowd of rich Things, are apter to satiate than to please the Palates of those who have the nicest Taste," she argued, opposing the superfluity of satiation to a more wholesome pleasing simplicity (ix). In her account, the palate took precedence over profusion and variety.

As civil war uprooted English life and culinary tastes across Europe underwent dramatic change, the language and practice of pleasure in the English cookbook changed. The kitchen and dining room abandoned their identification with cunning artistry and became the proving ground, as we saw in the previous chapter, for national identification and virtue. What could be more pleasurable, modern recipe books asked, than ordered and refined eating?

Coda: Art and Nature in the Eighteenth-Century Recipe Book

> Conceit is false taste; and very widely different from no taste at all.
> —William Shenstone, 1768[58]

Although the underlying structure of recipes as conceits fell out of popularity, the recipe world did not lose its intellectual focus. Eighteenth-century recipe books simply shifted the medium through which they engaged metaphysical problems: they grappled with these issues through the front matter of their books rather than through the food practices they recommended. Recipe writers and publishers raised the problem of how to relate nature to the culinary arts through verbal and visual prefatory materials that delved into the histories and mythologies of cuisine. If cookery was an "art" divorced from entertainment and defined as critical "work," it needed, writers implied, to be positioned in relation to civilized life as a whole. Although writers of literary, philosophical, and religious texts had long regarded food as an index of civilization, recipe producers had not been interested in raising these issues in relation to the domestic world of making until the late seventeenth and eighteenth centuries. One way that cookery books addressed this topic was by recourse to "fall" narratives.

John Nott's 1723 *The Cook's and Confectioner's Dictionary; or, The Accomplish'd Housewife's Companion* is a case in point. The text opens with an engraved frontispiece by John Pine featuring a landscape populated by animals and allegorical figures (Figure 17). A classical figure with rays emanating from his head (possibly Apollo) is seated on a cloud. He floats in the sky presiding over—and indexically pointing to—a pastoral scene below where semiclothed women repose in a natural setting. Harbored under the shade of a tree beside a lake, these women are surrounded by the live and dead animals that will presumably be converted into food in the recipes that follow. Deer, cattle, geese, rabbits and other animals flock beside the stream, as if drawn to the two lounging female figures, who casually pet foxes and receive fish that seem to have leapt voluntarily into their hands. These classical figures, one draped with a crown of grains like Ceres, appear to represent abundance and ease.

Pine's image draws on a long-standing utopian tradition in which the natural world exists in harmony with human consumption. This ideal had one source in the medieval legend of the mythical land of plenty and ease called Cockaigne, which appeared in variations in German, Dutch, Italian, French, and English. In Cockaigne, cooked foods fall from the skies, and foodstuffs serve as the architectural edifice of civilization. The myth embodied what Robert Appelbaum terms the "food of wishes," a pervasive dream of transcendent abundance that became especially popular in times of deprivation, hunger, and starvation.[59] Neither labor of food preparation nor the economics of the marketplace have a place in this myth, because animals willingly sacrifice themselves for the human table. In Breughel's *Land of Cockaigne*, to take one example, sausages serve as fence posts, roofs are made of pies, pigs wander with knives in their sides, fowls fly in the air already roasted, and a goose voluntarily curls up on a silver platter. Rather than celebrating this myth, however, Breughel employed it to offer a scathing critique of sloth and gluttony. As such, his painting famously included unconscious humans, satiated in food comas, as casualties of a land of excess. Jonson's poem "To Penshurst" more uncritically draws elements from the Cockaigne myth, couched as it is within an encomium to the Sidney family. Jonson portrays the harmonious natural state of their estate in Kent, a place devoid of antagonistic social divisions. At Penshurst, fruit falls from the trees and fish leap from the water to provide an aristocratic supper. Jonson writes:

> The purpled pheasant, with the speckled side:
> The painted partrich lyes in every field,

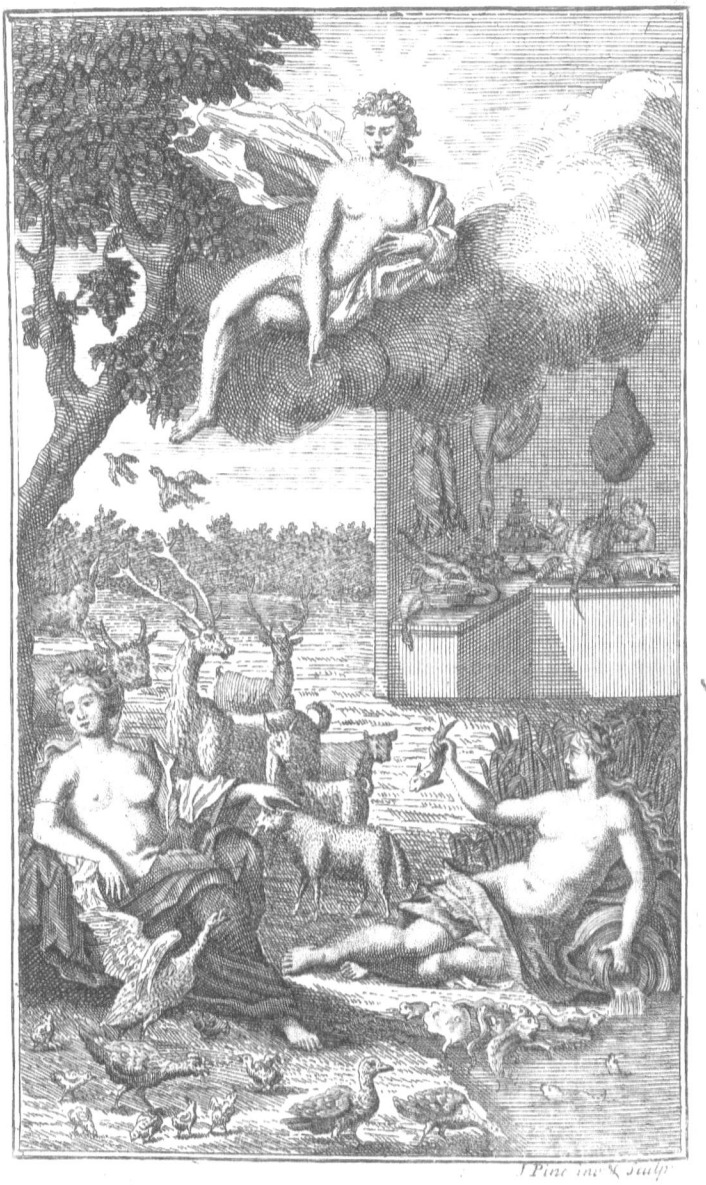

FIGURE 17. Frontispiece engraved by John Pine, in John Nott's *The Cook's and Confectioner's Dictionary; or, The Accomplish'd Housewife's Companion* (London, 1723). Beinecke Rare Book and Manuscript Library, Yale University.

> And, for thy messe, is willing to be kill'd.
> And if the high swolne *Medway* faile thy dish,
> Thou hast thy ponds, that pay thee tribute fish,
> Fat, aged carps, that runne into thy net.
> And pikes, now weary their owne kinde to eat,
> As loth, the second draught, or cast to stay,
> Officiously, at first, themselves betray.
> Bright eeles, that emulate them, and leape on land,
> Before the fisher, or into his hand.
> Then hath thy orchard fruit, thy garden flowers,
> Fresh as the ayre, and new as are the houres.
> The earely cherry, with the later plum,
> Fig, grape, and quince, each in his time doth come:
> The blushing apricot, and woolly peach
> Hang on thy walls, that every child may reach.[60]

In this utopian vision, the land and sea offer up their bounty for human use, and animals have complex personified intentions that allow them to make decisions and engage in social contracts. Partridges are "willing" to be caught, pikes "betray" their interests by swimming close to the surface of the water, and eels seek to imitate their peers. An animated natural environment similarly asserts agency within this world: "ponds" "pay tribute" to humans by offering up their fish, and an embarrassed apricot leans down to be picked. The erasure of human labor is key to this mythology; no one breaks a sweat to eat, because people can passively wait for fish to jump into nets and ripened fruit to fall into waiting hands. Yet, in Jonson's representation, this world is the product of human virtue and aristocratic hospitality, because it collectively emanates from the intrinsic worth and virtues of the Sidney family. Only the fantastical and somewhat absurd quality of the utopian world creates a strain that undermines the poem's praise of civil society. Unlike Jonson's poem, however, Pine's scene of culinary bounty is deliberately timeless and unmarked as private property. The figures are classically positioned and the scene is devoid of historical markers or names. And unlike Breughel's rendition, the recipe book engraving does not satirize the myth it exuberantly cites. Nevertheless the recipe book has imported the issues that have been so predominant in food discussions of the past.

It's hard to overstate how odd it is for a book producer to associate a recipe collection with a mythology that occludes and devalues the labor and technology of cooking. Indeed, Pine's engraving acknowledges this contradiction, for it jarringly interrupts the pastoral scene with an inlaid picture that intrudes abruptly into the right edge of the visual field. A floating spatial interior, laid like a palimpsest onto the natural panorama, portrays two male cooks at work in a kitchen, laboring beside a counter piled high with animal corpses waiting to be butchered. Hams and poultry carcasses, no longer willing players in a blissful natural ecosystem, hang from the kitchen walls, clearly registering the violence and whims of human consumption. One of the cooks hacks an animal into pieces while another appears to decorate a multitiered cake (though the image is very difficult to read). The juxtaposition of visual sites—indeed the spatial crowding and asymmetry of the bifurcated scene—introduces a discordant reminder of the reality of human labor within the central image's pastoralism. The two images also offer contrasting modes of representation, allegory in the central visual field as distinct from the naturalism of the inlaid interior.

There is much to say about how this image speaks to the recipe genre's ongoing negotiation of "nature" as a category accessible within a civilized domain that necessarily has altered it. And there is much that remains puzzling about how to explain the relationship between these divergent images. Does the juxtaposition of scenes create a nostalgic lament about the "fall" from natural harmony into cookery, with the central image reaching its sorrowful culmination in the inlaid view? Or do the two images showcase alternative perspectives on how nature can be positioned in relation to "culture," "art," and "cookery"? Do the chefs inhabit the same temporal domain as the pastoral scene? Or do they represent a different, perhaps historically remote, view of nature and culture? Is the embedded image at odds with the landscape representation or the realistic culmination that any good recipe buyer might expect?

These issues remain as elusively irresolvable as the mystery of Markham's heraldic carrot. They pose intellectual puzzles for the reader. And yet there is no doubt that Pine's engraving reassigns women's roles within the intellectual conundrums of domesticity. The housewife or lady is no longer central to the process of converting natural goods into foodstuffs and thus no longer an agent querying categories through practice. Placing timeless female figures in an idealized and conflict-free world divorces women from the reality inhabited by male chefs, who presumably undertake the tasks that the book is dedicated to teaching. Even as the image locates women within a world of natural bounty, it secures male-controlled expertise over the production of food and the culture it marks. Just as pointedly, *The Cook's and Confectioner's Dictionary* gestures away from the "thoughtful practice" of food by lodging the theorization of cooking in reading rather than in a reading-working experience. The pleasure of culinary intellect, in Pine's image, rests in contemplating a pastoral dream where no one has to wrestle with the complexities of labor, representation, or artifice. Indeed the chefs in the kitchen are not even aware of their intrusion into myth; they do not even look out the window to enjoy the view.

In the preface subsequent to this engraving in *The Cook's and Confectioner's Dictionary*, Nott positions food more conventionally as the object of human management endowed by God. He first self-referentially comments on the practice of writing recipe prefaces: "Were it not for the sake of Custom," he explained, "which has made it as unfashionable for a Book to come abroad without an Introduction, as for a Man to appear at Church without a Neckcloth, or a Lady without a Hoop-petticoat, I should not have troubled you with this."[61] Adhering to a fashion that he nevertheless holds up for ridicule, Nott departs from custom, he expounded, in refusing to praise his own performance or justify his subject matter. Instead he argues for the providential nature of English land, cuisine, and culinary artistry: "By the Disposition of God, and good Providence, our Lot has been cast in this happy Island of Great Britain, which, like another Canaan, may properly enough be call'd, A Land flowing with Milk and Honey." When Nott alludes to the natural abundance cited in Pine's engraving, he emphasizes the importance of proper stewardship of this bounty, an exercise that the recipes promise to teach. Nott presents methods for "ordering these things which nature has furnish'd us." The preface thus secures the meanings of "nature," which are ambivalently presented in the frontispiece; it is not only the substructure for human creation but also specifically the English iteration of the biblical Canaan: *a land flowing with milk and honey*. Cooking is not, as the initial image might have suggested, a sign of loss but its pious consummation, one devoutly to be wished. Nott's ideal reader might appreciate the wit of the self-reflexive preface while grasping the national utopian vision that rests on pragmatic (male) labor.[62]

Thirteen years later, Eliza Smith provided an alternative intellectual framework for placing food in relation to nature. In *The Compleat Housewife; or, Accomplish'd Gentlewoman's Companion* (1736), she countered Nott's account of cuisine. While applauding practical and plain culinary practice, Smith labors to identify English cookery as one of the arts of antiquity whose lineage she traces to the Bible. In her preface, she pointedly revises Nott's opening gambit:

> It being grown as unfashionable for a Book now to appear in publick without a Preface as for a Lady to appear at a Ball without a Hoop-petticoat, I shall conform to Custom for Fashion-sake, and not

through any Necessity. The Subject being both common and universal, needs no Arguments to introduce it, and being so necessary for the Gratification of the Appetite, stands in need of no Encomiums to allure Persons to the Practice of it; since there are but few now-a-days who love not good Eating and Drinking. Therefore I entirely quit those two Topicks; but having three or four Pages to be filled up, . . . I shall employ them on a subject I think new, and not yet handled by any of the Pretenders to the Art of Cookery; and that is, The Antiquity of it.[63]

Scorning rival recipe writers for relying on staid literary conventions such as prefaces, commendatory poems, and encomia, Smith places her text in dialogue with Nott's. In repeating his fashion analogy but eliminating the mention of men's neckcloths, she pointedly chooses to portray the world of custom as exclusively female. Mocking the pretension of a preface as an unnecessary petticoat, Smith hints that cookery is as basic as the (female) body beneath the fashion. Because people possess a natural "appetite," true food does not need supplementary rhetoric. She then rebuts the seeming trendiness of her subject by offering a manifesto on food's historical evolution. Dressing up, for Smith, means converting "fashion" into erudite knowledge. By opening with the image of female frivolity, Smith inhabits yet explodes expectations people might have had of a lady writer. The housekeeper with practical and historical knowledge emerges behind the figure of the petticoated lady, who is aligned with more superficial writers enamored with ornament.

Smith's preface concerns the longstanding history of cookery, which "did not arrive at a State of Maturity but by slow Degrees, various Experiments and a long Tract of Time" (A2v). In the Garden of Eden, she explains, people had no need to cook, because the inhabitants of the earth lived in close association with nature. As vegetarians surviving on healthy raw food, Adam and Eve needed neither artifice nor technology to prepare meals nor to heal bodies: "Apples, Nuts, and Herbs, were both Meat and Sauce, and Mankind stood in no need of any additional sauces. . . . Food and Physick were then one and the same thing," she explains (A2v; A3). As Smith imports an orthodox Christian account of food into the recipe world, she also locates household technical knowledge within the mythology.[64] It was only after humans were severed from a natural state and begin to dine on animals—as a by-product, we presume, of the fall from grace—that they needed to preserve and/or render foodstuffs artificially palatable; that is, cookery was designed to offset literal and spiritual corruption. Smith's biblical account shared common ground with the utopian image manifest in Pine's frontispiece and articulated in Ovid's account of the golden age: "And men themselves contented well with plaine and simple foode, / That on the earthe of natures gift without their travaile stood, / Did live by Raspis, heppes and hawes, by cornelles, plummes and cherries, / By sloes and apples, nuttes and peares, and lothsome bramble berries, / And by the acornes dropt on ground, from Joves brode tree in fielde."[65] Yet whereas Ovid and Pine emphasize the ease of a prelapsarian food life, Smith tweaks the story so that it celebrates a cookery based precisely on knowledge of the utility of natural substances. She does not lament the lost golden age as much as show the long-standing and legitimate craft of cookery as it evolved within a long span of time; that is, she offsets a traditional narrative of loss by emphasizing the Bible's interest in the *progression* of cuisine, which moves toward a state of near perfection.

Smith's interest in consolidating female control over food preparation within this mythology is clear: she cites the antiquity of cookery in order to authorize women to manage cuisine so that it balances nature and techne. Rudimentary seasonings and spices emerged, she suggests, to compensate for the physical deterioration of aging (in the individual) and the corruption of natural tastes (in the collective). Only later did "luxury" elevate cookery to a science (with seasonings) and then "to the height of an Art" (A3r). Smith traces this evolution through the story of Esau, who, though not the first cook, was the first person in Western history to care about dressing and preparing food. As did Rabisha, Smith alludes to Esau's exchange of his birthright for a pottage as a means of legitimating food's role in history, but she slyly interjects women into the account by observing that Jacob *may* have learned his culinary skills from his mother Rebecca: "it is a Question too knotty for me to determine," she mischievously observes. Even without the certainty of Rebecca as the original biblical chef, Smith provides a lineage for the "art" (traced through the Israelites) that she then defines as the purview of women, an art that functions as a corrective to overly artificial styles of cuisine. Identifying moderate food practices in antiquity allowed her to weigh in on current artistic, mythological, and culinary debates. Craving "whatsoever new, upstart, out of the way Messes some humorists have invented, such as stuffing a roasted Leg of Mutton with Pickled Herring, and the like," she argues, "are only the Sallies of a capricious Appetite; and debauching rather than improving the Art itself" (A4). In keeping with recipe writers of her era, Smith designates food conceits of the recent past as the product of ridiculous "humorists." Her story takes up the "knotty" problems of conceptualizing a "natural cookery," which was supposed to be everything: supplementary to the natural world, compensatory for past errors, and commonsensical. In the end, Smith turns away from the temporal and historical divide she narrates so that her "art of antiquity" serves as a means for distinguishing contemporary authentic foods from inauthentic modes of preparation.

Using the verbal and visual components of the book apparatus, recipe book writers and publishers of the eighteenth century took up the vexed questions that had previously been entertained through the preparation and consumption of foods and sweetmeats. These later texts invited readers to participate in long-standing philosophical discussions concerning the relationship of nature and culture while also contemplating the histories and myths underwriting these conceptions. Readers were cued to grapple with these issues through the intellectualized framework of reading rather than through domestic practice. As such cues, recipes promoted a mode of thought distinct from acts of making consistent with a newly emergent Cartesian dualism. Because recipes also represented cookery as labor rather than as leisurely work, they segregated the tasks of conceptualizing food from the kitchen work largely undertaken by servants. Ladies no longer aspired to experiment and showcase, as Jonson put it, "nature in a pot."

Despite the fact that the earliest published recipes in England required arduous labor, cookery conceits, as we have seen, were presented as a form of socially prestigious creative play, something akin to literary devices or rhetorical turns of phrase. In the previous chapter, we saw that the representation of confectionery and cookery as recreational was tied to the cultural capital that the printed recipe book offered to a widening reading public. In this chapter, we see that these modes of class aspiration also enabled intellectual inquiry. The recipe's ethos of culinary punning marked the domestic space a site of "play" akin to that offered by popular theatrical entertainments or sports; recipe culture thus participated in the ideological mystifications that critics have so richly investigated with regard to recreational forms in general. In marking domestic practice as cerebral amusement, recipe books evaded socioeconomic struggles taking place across households, commercial sites, and farms. They obscured from view the uneven wealth produced by global commerce systems and the colonial violence attending to trade ventures.[66] The recipe archive makes legible these ideological struggles only by what they did not say. Aside from listing ingredients, they offered few clues about the social stakes of the foodways, the costs of the work that they endorsed, or the brutal competitive struggles surrounding people's efforts to stay afloat as crops failed or family fortunes fell. Although recipes are not particularly helpful sources for mapping a socioeconomic landscape, they are tremendously important for our understanding of how the early modern domestic space provided women of means with a creative and intellectual license that has not been fully acknowledged in histories of reading and of labor. Indeed, as we see in the next chapter, they constituted distinctive yet unrecognized forms of literacy.

By the time Ann Peckham created her *Complete English Cook*, recipe readers no longer expected culinary delights and intellectual puzzles to feature within food practices. Instead they bought recipes in hopes of transforming themselves into English housekeepers or managerial ladies overseeing a proper home. Peckham presents herself as a dedicated worker rather than as a lover of art and ingenuity. Her forty years of experience, she explains, have left her wiser but in a near state of exhaustion. The only moment in which Peckham raises the specter of gratification is, ironically, in noting the "satisfaction" that talented audiences could take in *not* needing to heed the book's advice at all: "The most accomplish'd house-keepers, will have at least the satisfaction of seeing their own methods approv'd by one who is generally allow'd to be a competent judge," Peckham writes, "whilst they who have had less experience, will meet with suitable directions how to proceed in all cases with propriety and reputation."[67] A female reader might learn propriety, or she could take smug satisfaction in the fact that she already possessed approved domestic knowledge. Such were the delights for ladies in the new recipe landscape. Certainly Peckham and other recipe creators did not see the making of jellies and sweetmeats as "drudgery," as did Joseph Addison, but they did similarly divorce confectionery from what Addison saw as the "exalted Sphere of Knowledge and Virtue" to which, he allowed, women should be included.[68]

The evolution of recipe writing into a form that celebrated functionalism has made it hard for scholars to recognize an earlier historical moment when the technical and the fanciful shared a home together, because, from a modern perspective, practical writing and poetry handbooks have little in common. Early modern recipes, however, provide us with a way to savor their interconnection. "Hungrie I was, and had no meat," George Herbert writes in his poem "Faith":

> I did conceit a most delicious feast;
> I had it straight, and did as truly eat,
> As ever did a welcome guest.⁶⁹

In a poem about the instantaneous power of spiritual belief, Herbert trades on the capacious meanings of "conceit," which is imagined as a powerful operation crossing the poetic and the culinary. For the speaker, to think is to have and to eat: the material is implicated in the intangible. As we have seen, the recipe archive assumed the interconnections that Herbert experiences, the fused discourses that would later diverge so completely that modern readers find it hard to grasp their past shared terrain. Reestablishing the link between the *receipt* and *conceit*, we are able to appreciate the intellectual coordinates of an early modern recipe culture that placed high stakes on the joy of cooking. In the next chapter, we will reengage the materiality of domestic artistry and making, as we consider the multiple "literacies" involved in manuscript collections.

CHAPTER 3

Literacies: Handwriting and Handiwork

> Lord prosper thou the Works of our hands upon us: prosper thou our handy works.
> —Ann Fanshawe, *Memoir*

> But I wolde in no wyse that a woma[n] shulde be ignorant in those feates, that muste be done by hande: no nat though she be a princes or a quene.
> —Juan Vives, *The Instruction of a Christian Woman*

> The hand is an ideological formation.
> —Jonathan Goldberg

If you consult the online catalogue for the Wellcome Library in London, you discover bibliographer S. A. J. Moorat's description of an eighteenth-century text called *Her Book of Recepts* by Elizabeth Michel:

> 11411. 4to. 18 1/2 × 14 1/2 cm. Original calf binding worn. . . . Mid-eighteenth century. Purchased 1931. . . . Written on the rectos only, and by an illiterate hand. There are a few additions by later 18th century owners, one dated 1797 and the other 1801.[1]

This record seems conventional enough: it details the material features of the artifact, its provenance, and an early assessment of its value. You discover that multiple writers penned the text without writing on verso pages, that the book circulated to different owners, and that its originating hand was "illiterate." It is this curious term, "an illiterate hand"—as well as its implied converse, a "literate hand"—to which I turn my attention, in hopes that it might shed light on the relation of recipe work and textual production in early modern England.

Moorat's confident ascription of the work to Michel masks how challenging and ultimately inconclusive attribution of manuscript recipe collections can be—both generally and in this case. The challenge stems from the fact that most are collaborative and entirely or partially anonymous. Michel's text might seem to simplify the matter, for it offers two clear ownership marks. One, which reads "Dorothy Michel Daughter to the owner of this book," unusually asserts an affiliation with the book's owner. When writing in a recipe book to which she has access, Dorothy chose to name herself through a qualified proprietary claim: this book belongs collectively to my family, which gives me the right to set my mark on it. Inverting the book, the reader discovers the more typical inscription that has provided the authorship cited by the catalogue: "Elizabeth Michel her book of Recepts." The mystery is solved in part; Elizabeth Michel began a recipe book listing her favorite ways of making lemon cream, pickled oysters, dried apples, fricasseed veal, and boiled calves head. Her daughter Dorothy added to the book while still considering it her mother's property. The two hands register a familially united collective, a set of textually and biologically related hands.

We also notice that writers have covered the flyleaf to the Michel book with scribbles and words. Among the textual "graffiti," as Jason Scott-Warren calls such markings, we discover these words and phrases: "Eliz." (written six times), "Eliz. Fellon," "is my desire," "show me," "however honored," "To honored Madam," "M. Eliz.," "Hopes farewell a due to all pleasure," "All hopes farewell," and "Fellon," written as a name three ways.[2] Although we tend to see doodling as aimless scrawling and signs of unconscious fantasy outside the scope of recoverable meaning, we can identify the domain of significance for some inscriptions: they rehearsed bits of polite phrases, as if someone were thinking about decorum; they also tested fantasy signatures. Extrapolating from biographically supported evidence in other recipe collections, we can guess that "Fellon" is a maiden name and thus one of Elizabeth's self-identifications. The flyleaf indicates that the hands of the book and, perhaps, the identities of its writers were in process even as they intermixed and registered affiliation.

How might this hand, or these hands, be said to be "illiterate," as Moorat suggests? Certainly the book was not written by someone "ignorant of letters or literature; without book-learning or education," as are common understandings of the term.³ Michel not only could read and write, but also could fashion proportionate and regularized letters. Moorat's use of the term might reveal his personal assumption that recipe manuscripts were, by definition, "illiterate," because written by a person whose hand had not been trained formally (literacy thus signifying an orthodox learnedness). Rather than merely singling out Moorat's phrasing to exemplify a bias against domestic documents or women's writing, I see his term as also productively hinting at the nuanced range of subjective cultural meanings that filter into definitions of "literacy." If a "hand" (meaning handwriting) could be illiterate, then "literacy" cannot refer to a clearly defined expertise (reading or writing) that signifies proper learning; it instead designates variant and subjectively assigned knowledges and skills. Moorat's phrase ironically exposes the capacious, evaluative, and contested nature of literacy itself. With alphabetic competency shown to be less a clear-cut skill than a social construct, it becomes possible to investigate the diverse literacies generated within particular social institutions surrounding recipe writing, some of which do not fit neatly within commonsensical definitions of the term.

Scholars have hotly contested how best to assess literacy in the early modern period. Basing his influential work on the analysis of signatures, David Cressy estimated female literacy as extremely low—only 10 percent in 1640.[4] On the basis of this research primarily, there has until recently been a widespread belief that few English women of the period could read or write. Yet because standard measurements of literacy have been inferred largely from evidence of a person's ability to write (but have only inadequately assessed an ability to read), scholars have begun to question not only the methods used to ascertain literacy rates but also the terms we use to describe a fairly wide range of practices. What do we call someone who signed one kind of document but not another (a household account book but not an oath, for example)? What about someone who could read but not write? Someone who could read italic but not secretary hand? A woman who demurred from writing in public? Those who could write with charcoal on a wall but not with ink? Or a woman such as Mary Radcliffe who signed her name early in life but only used a mark later in her will?[5] Might even a narrow definition of "literacy" hopelessly entangle alphabetic facility with other cognate knowledges?

As Frances Dolan observes, the binary of literate/illiterate has stalled a full understanding of the diversity of competencies around written expression: "Refusing that simple distinction," she argues, "makes it possible to see that reconsidering definitional categories may be more important than proving that women belonged in one category rather than the other."[6] If handwriting can be illiterate (an assertion that I entertain heuristically) it opens up a central and fruitful question: what movements of the hand might constitute "literacy"? Pamela Smith grapples with this issue when she defines "artisanal literacy" as knowledge gained by experience and labor; for she edges the word away from its root etymology in "letters."[7] Scholars often maintain but elasticize the term by devising categories that invite reconsideration of the social conditions defining writing practices, including "partial," "private," "shared," "graphic," "gendered," "resistant," or "selective" literacy.[8]

Literacy, as Keith Thomas, Margaret Ferguson, Frances Dolan, Eve Sanders, and Heidi Brayman Hackel have argued, can be seen as a social relation and a site of contest over something insufficiently answerable by empirical research. In her analysis of the relationship between literacy and empire, Margaret Ferguson uses the work of John Guillory to counter the pragmatic definition of literacy as the ability to read and write in one vernacular language: "*Literacy*, in my usage," she writes, "almost always connotes 'literacies' and points to a social relation that has interpersonal, intercultural, international, and interlingual dimensions. Instead of asking, 'What is literacy?' we might ask, rather, 'What counts as literacy for whom, and under what particular circumstances?'"[9] Recipe books can thus allow us to do more than revise statistical assessments of who could read or write; they broaden the spectrum of meanings that fall under this term. In particular, they offer differently tactile ways that literacy might signify, and they dramatically expand the scene of literacy formation. Recipes enable us to define "taste literacies" within a broader sensorium, competencies that locate the formation and consumption of letters in proximity to tasting, eating, smelling, and swallowing. Along with expanding understanding of embodied learning, attention to recipes can alert us to previously unrecognized mechanisms by which social status and value were assigned in the early modern world.

My analysis of early modern kitchen literacy is built on—and expands—frameworks established by scholars who have rendered histories of reading as material acts. Peter Stallybrass, Roger Chartier, Carla Mazzio, Bradin Cormack, Heidi Brayman Hackel, and William Sherman have shown ways that early modern book use constituted physical as well as cognitive acts, and, by expansion, ways that acts of reading signified in the culture.[10] Margaret Ezell pioneered a mode of scholarship that showcased manuscript sources as ways of unthinking assumptions about women and authorship. Unearthing scribal communities rather than relying on printed sources, she argued, revises claims about literacy and letters in the period, particularly as they pertained to women.[11] Recent scholars have made similar critiques with regard to conventional studies of reading practices. Newly examining physical marks of all sorts left in a variety of books, Hackel and Rebecca Laroche have helped us to understand better who had access to which books and how reading itself took place in the early modern period.[12] Such inquiries go far in offering a heightened understanding of "reading" and "writing" as activities situated in lived experience. Adding the recipe archive to the mix provides a new perspective on how textual production was intertwined with specific labors that women undertook; it also brings to light literacy formation as bound up with the artistic and intellectual reflection seen in previous chapters.[13]

My subject matter might, at first glance, seem somewhat marginal to histories of reading or of textual production because cooking is a practice thoroughly immersed in oral culture and hands-on learning. Doesn't a person genuinely learn to cook by rolling dough, seeing mother make cheese, or experimenting with seasonings? As we have seen in earlier chapters, however, a dynamic world of textuality shaped the act and understanding of the hands that brewed and baked and fricasseed and boiled in the kitchen. As early as 1529, humanist trained tutor Juan Vives advised literate women to keep a "lytle boke" of receipts "diligently written."[14] Over the course of the sixteenth and seventeenth centuries, more and more women took up the practice of creating and maintaining personal or family recipe collections. Study of these "lytle" books provides a window into the ways that "writing" deeply informed household knowledge—not only as a co-extension of reading—but also as a feature of a craftswoman's physical skill extending in and out of other household work.

And this is where the idea of materiality comes into play. In *Graffiti and the Writing Arts of Early Modern England*, Juliet Fleming argues that Renaissance "writing" was seen as a physical praxis that could not be abstracted from its medium and material situation.[15] A culture that encouraged people to paint sayings on parlor walls and scrawl words into pots embraced the materiality of language as it was distributed across the physical world. Fleming's articulation of early modern writing as inextricable from its physical manifestation helps us to reconceive domestic space itself as a site of potential inscription. Lady Anne Clifford, known diarist, epistolary writer, patroness, and tireless negotiator for her affordances under the law, provides a somewhat spectacular instance in this regard, for she was reported to have projected "her rich Store-house" of remembered sayings and quotations all over her household. She created, in effect, an ephemeral library by pinning papers to beds, walls, curtains, and furniture.[16] Clifford expected her servants to do as she did: to "read" (or learn to read) their inhabited space as they navigated through their daily space or undertook household chores. More common forms of domestic artistry included stitching alphabetic samplers, embroidering decorations on furniture, etching sayings on trenchers (serving boards), and limning pictures on glass. These graphic traces not only offer evidence of "women's textualities" or the "wrought" entities so ably theorized by Susan Frye, but also document domestic incarnations of early modern writing as taking meaning from their inscription *on* particular substances. If the early modern world "lacked a systematic bifurcation between real and thought objects, and consequently apprehended matter not as that which is deprived of meaning but as a principle of structure that underpins all meaning," as Fleming argues, then manuscript recipes provide a perfect case for understanding the inscriptional tenor of all representation (21). Handwritten recipes, I argue, enhance our understanding of the particular instances in which specifically domestic matter structured meaning; they offer a gender-inclusive writing matter whose subject itself was artifaction.

In this chapter, I examine early modern recipe collections to understand how "writing," in its broadest and most material senses, intersected with domestic practice. While they recorded ways to prepare foods and medicines, recipe books, I contend, served as instructional manuals and draft pads for honing the mechanical skill of crafting letters and developing penmanship styles. Recipes were not only a distinctive tutorial for displaying a particular "hand," but also the manifestation of the physical, creative, and organizational handiwork of the home—a condition of domestic thought. While traditional tasks that we define as "housewifery" (including carving and confectionery) trained hands in the disciplined motions that underwrote writing, they also signified in their own right as unrecognized types of "writing." Recipe collections thus illuminate ways that women (as well as men) engaged in tactile handiwork in the home across different media, demonstrating a kitchen literacy that is too often invisible in the scholarly record. The story that these collections tell about early modern literacy's artifactual character, I argue, contradicts the claim that domesticity and handwriting instruction largely served regulatory ideologies stemming from what is termed the civilizing impulse. Instead this archive makes visible a broader spectrum of literacies through which domestic writing signified and opens up new possibilities for imagining writing as a sign of domestic expressivity.

Writing Lessons

> The true office of the Hand is to apprehend or to holde ... (for *Hand* and *Holde* are Conjugates as we term them in Schooles).
> —Helkiah Crooke, *Microcosmographia*, 1615[17]

Scholars have recently assembled evidence documenting that literacy training took place outside of formal institutions in early modern England. While most schools and centers of learning in late sixteenth-century England were limited to boys from affluent families, a wider range of the population had access to grammar schools and to unofficial sites of instruction. Governesses, tutors, and writing masters home-schooled elite girls; some local statutes allowed girls lower on the social spectrum to attend free grammar schools. Boarding schools and writing schools for both genders became popular and more affordable throughout the seventeenth century. Prior to this broadening of access, girls and boys (and male and female servants) had been educated on an ad hoc basis within and outside of households. In her mother's advice book, Dorothy Leigh revealed that she took this to be a standard procedure in civil households; she reminded her sons of the important duty of teaching all members of households to read. Writing masters, merchants, and household mistresses also informally taught maids and apprentices to wield a pen; and household guides instructed mothers to teach literacy skills as part of religious education.[18] As writing teacher Edmund Coote acknowledged, wives of day laborers and small craftsmen, seamstresses, and widows offered lessons in reading and writing.[19] Coote addressed *The English Schoole-Master* to "such men and women of trade, as Taylors, Weavers, Shop keepers, Seamsters, and such other as have undertaken the charge of teaching others."[20] Gentlewomen and merchant families sought instruction in writing and mathematics as a means of advancing professionally and socially. In the late sixteenth century, Jane Tutoft, for instance, implored a cousin to oversee her daughter's education in a program of housewifery that included accounting and literacy: "let hyr lern to wryt & to rede & to cast acount & to wash & to bru & to backe & to dres meat & drink & so I trust she shal prove a great good huswyf."[21]

In the second half of the seventeenth century, domestic manuals and printed recipe collections attributed to Hannah Woolley classified penmanship as an integral component of housework. *The Gentlewomans Companion* emphasized reading, writing, hygiene, polite conversation, deportment, letter writing, fashion choices, proper exercise, table manners, and piety as fundamental components of the "right Education of the Female Sex" (B1r).²² This guide included over 160 specific medical, culinary, confectionary, and dairying recipes. After a brief overview of the manual's subjects, the author turned to what governesses should teach girls. "Letters undoubtedly is the first step to the perfection of knowledg," the text explained, "by which means they come to improve their own understandings by the help of others" (7). After championing the importance of reading (even romances!), the writer concluded by admonishing women to undertake another "literate" act—the practice of the "pen" that underpinned home decoration: "Having qualified [girls] for reading, you should so practice them in their pen, as not to be ignorant in a *Point de Venice*, and all the Productions of the Needle, with all the curious devices of *Wax-work*, *Rock-work*, *Moss-work*, *Cabinet Work*, *Bengle-work*, &c. and in due time let them know how to Preserve, Conserve, Distill; with all those laudible Sciences which adorn a compleat Gentlewoman" (9). It's worth noting that this taxonomic system grouped reading and writing as handiwork. But even more telling is the notion that being practiced "in the pen" was a rubric that included manipulation of a certain class of instruments. Whether paintbrush, stylus, quill, or needle, the generic tool called the "pen" facilitated writing as well as other types of craftwork, including "rock-work" (a sewing stitch and a candied dessert), "moss-work" (garden adornment), and "wax-work" (the reproduction of fruits and designs in colored wax).²³ The mention of this latter activity reminds us that writing in many eras was seen as slicing marks *into* wax tablets that could then be erased. As Frye discusses, early modern pens were sewing as well as writing implements; they were used to design needlework patterns, prick designs onto cloth or other materials, and/or apply paint to create patterns. In early modern recipe books, the housewife, gentlewoman, and/or servant were enjoined to use a stylus to engrave onto matter. As *The Gentlewomans Companion* indicated, supposedly non-literate activities practiced girls "in the pen," all grouped as part of the "laudible Sciences" of housewifery (9). In *A Supplement to the Queen-Like Closet*, Woolley emphasized the importance of epistolary writing for women. Attaching Woolley's name to a text targeted a clientele of aspiring readers: she had become famous for rising in the world from lowly roots. Indeed Woolley modeled for readers the use value for domestic workers to be practiced in the pen, having transformed her career from household servant into professional writer.

When *The Gentlewomans Companion* offered advice on the proper way to request favors, offer congratulations, or chastise others in a letter, the author interrupted a discussion about composition to offer tips on the mechanics of letter writing: "Have especial care of blotting your paper, giving it a large Margent; and be curious in the cutting your Letters, that they may delight the sight, and not tire the Reader. Lastly, be curious in the neat folding up your Letter, pressing it so that it may take up but little room" (229). The reader needed to blot the paper with sand and to pay attention to typographical layout. She should "be curious" about shaping physical letters and folding paper, because these details ensured the reader's pleasure. I will return later in this chapter to the significance of seeing writing as a form of cutting, but here I emphasize the attention that the recipe book gives to writing as a component of housework.

The Compleat Servant-Maid, a popular text attributed to Woolley, further specified the handwriting styles that those in service should learn. It offered young maidens in search of employment "directions for Preserving, Conserving, and Candying, for Writing the most usual hands for Women, as Mixt Hand, Roman and Italian Hands" (the mixed hand combined roman and italic script to form the "round hand" that evolved into modern cursive).[24] When the formal secretary hand waned in popularity in the late sixteenth century, emergent scripts competed to become the most fashionable style of writing. As Nicolas Barker observes, "Calligraphic exercises, the ability to write the several current scripts, 'command of hand,' the dexterous construction of flourishes and even pictures with a single movement of the pen and the design of large fancy capitals for use in the headings of documents, were all part of the basic education of the literate."[25] Making a bid to perfect prestige styles of writing was thus not just an enterprise for courtiers; handwriting lessons were increasingly identified as a pragmatic and commercially advantageous talent that could profit people of many social stations.

The Compleat Servant-Maid complicated the relationship of lettering to labor by conveying its instructions on handwriting in the *form* of recipes. After fifteen recipes for conserving and candying, it presented seven *recipes* for handwriting, each following the format used for culinary instruction in terms of placement on the page, typeface of titles, and length of prose: "How to make a Pen," "How to hold Your Pen," "How to sit to Write," "Necessaries for Writing," "Directions for Writing of Mixt Hand," "Direction for the Roman Hand," and "Directions for the Italian Hand" (1683; 23–26). The book additionally provided two double foldout templates that displayed varying italic alphabets (the new prestige form of writing) accompanied by calligraphic designs of animals and hearts, ornate capitals, and rhyming epigrammatic moralisms penned in a sample hand. One of the adages to be copied hinted at the connection between the alphabet sampler and its recipe format; for it identified "soveraign Ingredients" for a good life, "sovereign" being a common adjective used to guarantee efficacy for medical recipes (e.g., a sovereign water for the gout). Given that "soveraign" and "ingredients" were part of a recipe idiom, the saying signaled the conceptual overlap between manual making and the abstract fashioning of a good life. In heeding recipes—for writing, cooking, or virtuous being—the reader was to see practical skills as character-building exercises, in both senses of the term "character." Simultaneously affirming definitions of virtue and the correct imitation of physical letters, the writing *subject* seemed a product that could be made by actualizing a formula.

The Compleat Servant-Maid included a second copy-text that was similarly self-conscious about its inscriptive lessons. This maxim compared nature to a divinely written text imperfectly copied by mortal hands: "The Worlds a booke writt by th'Eternall art / Of The great maker Printed in mans heart / Tis falsely printed tho divinely penned / And all th'Errata will appear at th'end" (Figure 18).[26]

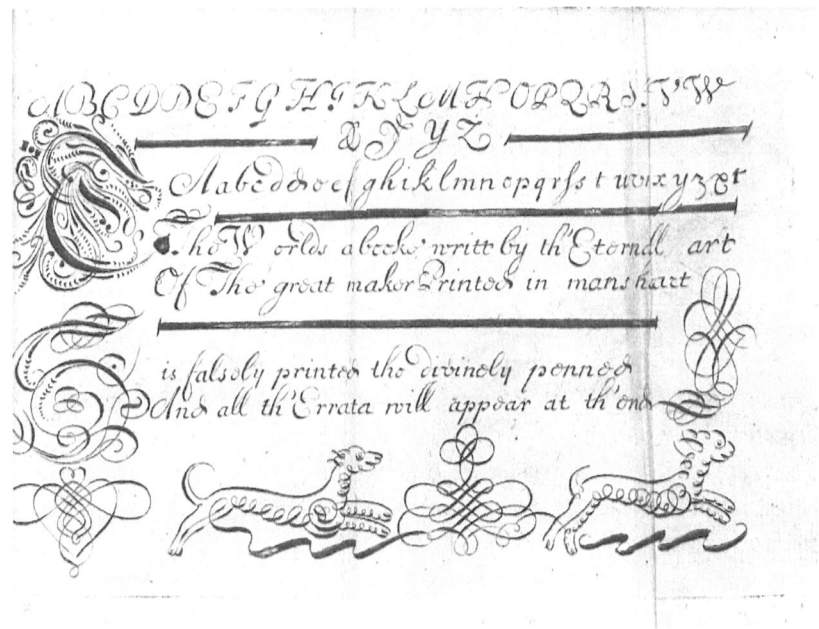

FIGURE 18. Copy text for learning writing, in *The Compleat Servant-Maid*, attributed to Hannah Woolley (London, 1685), A3v, insert between 24 and 25. Beinecke Rare Book and Manuscript Library, Yale University.

This commonplace, which a few years later appeared in a book of witticisms published by Francis Quarles, portrays the world as authored perfectly by God before becoming "falsely printed" through human sin; the original text-creation devolved in its incision in a frail and imperfect form. As the repetition of the word "printed" made clear, "printing" did not oppose writing or penning but instead referenced inscriptions in various states of mediation: it constituted the natural world and then secondarily was etched into the human interior. (I'll come back below to printing as a term specifically for stamping confections.) In this analogy, the error, or textual errata of the mortal realm, is hidden from human perception until the revelation of the apocalypse's final publication. Because Woolley's readers were to copy painstakingly the lettering of this saying as they contemplated the spiritual limitations of their endeavor, they were to gain a mechanical mastery tethered to a humble sense of their own insufficiency. Though virtuous, handwriting, the text implied, could only offer an imperfect measure of control over waywardness.

This maxim and copy-text steer us to see codified household writing instructions in terms of the story charted by Norbert Elias and told specifically with regard to penmanship by Jonathan Goldberg. The "civilizing process," according to Elias, was a program that bolstered emerging nation-states by fashioning a "cultured" class with particular structures of psychological management. Spurred by Erasmus's 1530 book on civility in boys, which was reprinted throughout Europe for two hundred years, the book market generated numerous works devoted to defining bodily propriety and civil behaviors for the upper and rising middling classes. Materializing as hierarchies of medieval feudal society were loosened and an emergent modern state formation was consolidated, these treatises cultivated self-consciousness about manners, including body carriage, gestures, dress, and facial expression.[27] While codified manners were certainly not invented in the Renaissance, they were newly emphasized and instrumental, as Elias notes, in the acceleration of the "social circulation of ascending and descending groups" (1:68). The result was a new elite, composed of bourgeois and aristocratic elements, predicated on self-restraint and disciplined behavior. Woolley's copy-text, complete with its moral coding of bodily control through writing and its proximity to advice on table manners, might, at first glance, seem a domestic incarnation of the civilizing process, a household manifestation, as Goldberg terms it, of submission to the regime of writing. Domestic writing lessons might seem part of the production of a seemingly sovereign subject who internalized ideological constraints in fashioning a regimented "female hand."

But did practice match prescription in recipe writing lessons? We do not actually find evidence that recipe readers copied sayings in recipe books verbatim, which makes sense given that informal writing exercises were relatively unmonitored. In the copy of the 1683 *Compleat Servant-Maid* housed at the British library, for instance, one reader changed the content of the copy-text by inscribing a different adage altogether, although the writer did choose a saying popular in early modern girl's samplers: "Delight in Larning Soon doth bring A Child to Lerne the hardest Thing."[28] While exhibiting wisdom and handwriting proficiency, the inscriber proclaimed pleasure to know the secret of good pedagogy. But tellingly this reader did not imitate the sample text's italic style, choosing pointedly to create darker, more upright versions of letters with secretary features. On the flyleaf to this same copy, another reader ignored the copy-text verse and practiced her handwriting by repeating an italic signature and proprietary claim, "Arabella best her book."[29] What makes this ownership mark interesting is the fourth "signature" in a different but related hand, which interposes "best of harabella." Arabella (or a later reader—the evidence is not clear) free-associated and reshaped the signature to unearth its buried, boasting superlative (the "best of" even as it played with an alternate spelling). Rather than generating a submissive posturing of a hand, the writing lesson generated a playful idiosyncratic practice of the pen.

The large leather-bound folio that is known as the *Maddison Family Recipe Book* tells a similar story. Family members over the course of two hundred years used the collection as an occasion for honing writing proficiency (with the bulk of the writing stemming from the seventeenth century).[30] As Janet Theophano has pointed out, a young girl named Mary Maddison inscribed the flyleaf with cascades made up of the letter "M"—tested over thirty times in different styles of writing. Mary then playfully signed the book, "Mary Madcap," a nickname that she repeated elsewhere in the text with the date, 1679 (Figure 19).[31] Rather than offering an orthodox ownership inscription, Mary stylized a mischievous self-identification. Holding, reading, writing, and/or using the family cookery book, she editorialized herself as a "madcap," someone reckless, impulsive, extravagant, or zany.[32] While being tutored on making preserves and medicines, Mary Maddison—like Arabella Best—lightheartedly experimented with mechanical and intellectual turns of the letter. From these case studies, we see that when collections sharpened writing proficiency, they also enabled familiarly estranging literacies that hardly accorded with handwriting pedagogy's regulatory functions.

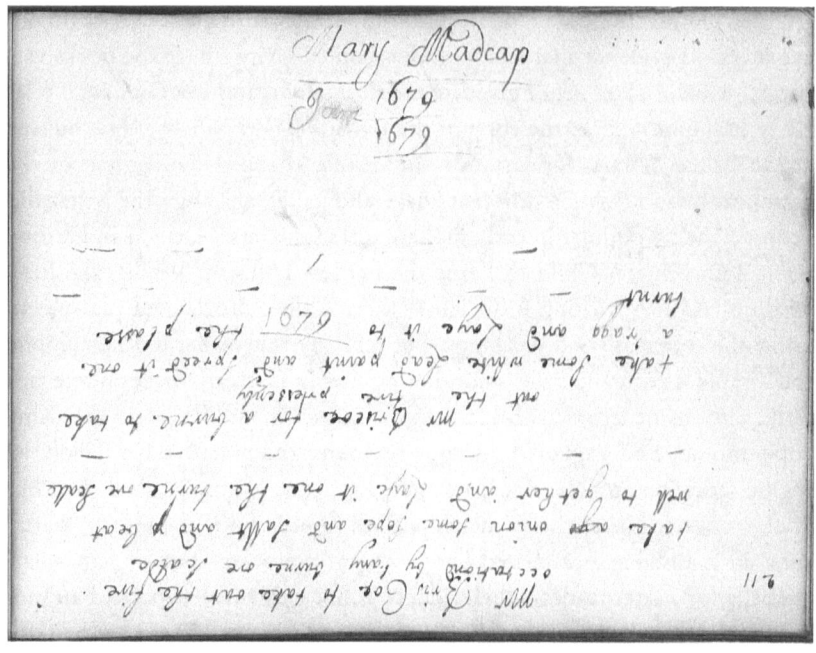

FIGURE 19. "Mary Madcap." Inscription in the *Maddison Family Recipe Book*, ca. 1600–1710. Esther Aresty Collection, MS codex 252, 211. Kislak Center for Special Collections, Rare Books and Manuscripts. University of Pennsylvania Libraries.

When Woolley's guides began to classify handwriting as housewifery in the later part of the seventeenth century, they merely articulated the previously unspoken ways that domesticity intersected with a culture of writing. (This was the case, to some degree, as I discuss later, even when a family employed a scribe to record recipes.) While we cannot establish with any certainty the provenance and precise routes of circulation for the astonishing number of handwritten recipe books that have survived from early modern England, we do have evidence that people from a wide swatch of the social spectrum had a hand in their composition: noblewomen, gentry wives, schoolmasters' and merchants' wives (and in one case an actor's wife), clergy, and yeomen wrote, read, annotated, cited, and exchanged recipes as part of daily life. Indeed the very existence and sheer number of these extant collections might seem unexpected, if we believe the statistics cited for early modern women's literacy.

Lettice Pudsey used the occasion of her seventeenth-century recipe book to boast of her ability to form letters, a feat perhaps as important to her as knowledge of puddings, pies, and wafers. Her 170 medical and culinary recipes, begun in the unjoined italic hand commonly used by women in the first half of the seventeenth century, introduced readers to rabbit fricassees, eye ointments, oysters, puddings, laxatives, mutton disguised to look like venison, carp gutted alive, kidney stone cures, herbal horse dung drinks for internal bruises, fritters, perfumes, face washes, an antidepressant,[33] a vegetarian Lenten stew, cakes, creams, preserves, and the period's equivalent of aspirin, "Dr. Steven's Water." Pudsey, about whom we know nothing, signed the book by bragging: "Lettice Pudsey, her Booke of recipts, these following are written with my owne hand" (F7v) (Figure 20).[34] The possessive and possessed hand emerges here as at work in the kitchen *and* exhibited through writing, marked by the use of what is called the "his-genitive" possessive (altered to "her-genitive" form by female possessors). Pudsey later re-asserted her claim to have written

FIGURE 20. Lettice Pudsey, commenting on her handwriting in *Lettice Pudsey Her Booke of Receipts*, ca. 1675, the Folger Shakespeare Library, MS V.a.450, F7v. Reproduced by permission of the Folger Shakespeare Library.

the core of her recipe book by scribbling this annotation beside an added recipe for biscuits in a different hand: "W. Oldfeld His Writing" (F43v). It was highly unusual to differentiate and attribute handwriting in recipe collections; marking the prescription as "his" writing, not hers, Pudsey revealed her investment in possessive claims to both writing and content.

Other writers loosely associated proprietary claims with an ability to sign. On one flyleaf a writer poetically scribbled: "Jane Buckhurst her book and yf this booke chances to bee lost and any one do find the same I [praye] restore this booke again to her that heare hath sette her name."[35] Variations on this type of inscription were common among university students, who inscribed their books with rhymes beseeching, threatening, or cursing people who might discover their lost texts.[36] Domestic records of how to make candies or ointments thus created a site in which writers staked a claim to self-possession and possessive ownership (e.g., "my owne hand," "her book") not necessarily concerning the originality of the content (which was often freely borrowed from family sources or recycled from guides) as much as its technical making. Signing the recipe book could mark a moment when one had and held what one's hand created; it claimed a self-possessed hand, complete with its capabilities and dispositions.

Recipe compilations sometimes served as draft pads where rudimentary writing skills could be tested, perfected, and/or exhibited. If we return to the Maddison family codex, we find that its compilers did not all have the same exuberant relationship to writing that Mary Madcap displayed. One writer, identified by Theophano on the basis of internal evidence as Mary's mother, struggled to record a cure for the dropsy (an edema or swelling); she broke off in midsentence with a note in a simpler italic hand, "I cannot write it right" (40). It is not clear whether her frustration stemmed from lack of medical knowledge, or, as the material evidence of shifting writing styles indicates, difficulty with lettering. But the two tasks fused in the written document. Her apt phrase, "writing it right," signaled a mechanical and expressive goal at issue for recipe producers and consumers, who often became the texts' next-generation compilers.

As those who have jotted their names on notebook pages in adolescence might remember, the crafting of a name can be an identity experiment carried out by variant handwriting styles. A woman named Rhoda Fairfax indulged in this experiment. We do know something about Fairfax: daughter of Thomas Chapman of London, Rhoda married a Lincolnshire gentleman, Thomas Hussey, and suffered a loss of money and standing when he was killed in the civil war. She then regained position in the world in her second marriage to a parliamentarian army officer and peer, Baron Ferdinando Fairfax of Cameron II, who lived only two years after their marriage. The initials R. H., luxuriously stamped on the book's cover, marked a prized possession, one that she inscribed with her first married name "Rhoda Hussey." She then re-signed the book with her new married name ("Rhoda Fairfax") and fantasized herself as the object of address by another, "Madam Rhoda Fairfax."[37] Mary Miller also presented herself alternately as "Mrs. Mary Miller" and "Lady Mary Miller" in her recipe collection. Well aware that recipes would circulate to future readers, compilers toyed with the form in which their identity would be received, as they undertook the conjoined projects of displaying letters, crafting signatures, and asserting rank. In "making a mark," they expressed, at the very minimum, what Fleming sees as "the graffito's most simple and paradigmatic instance, 'I was here'" (72). "Sarah Justice" thus comes to life momentarily amid pages of the Eyton family collection as the confident producer of a thick upright script combining italic letter-forms with secretary features (Figure 21).[38] Jane Staveley, on the other hand, was more cavalier, as she scrawled her name casually in a 1693 receipt book using a sloping italic hand without decoration or flourish (Figure 22). Miller, who tested out different addresses, is introduced by a decorative naming,

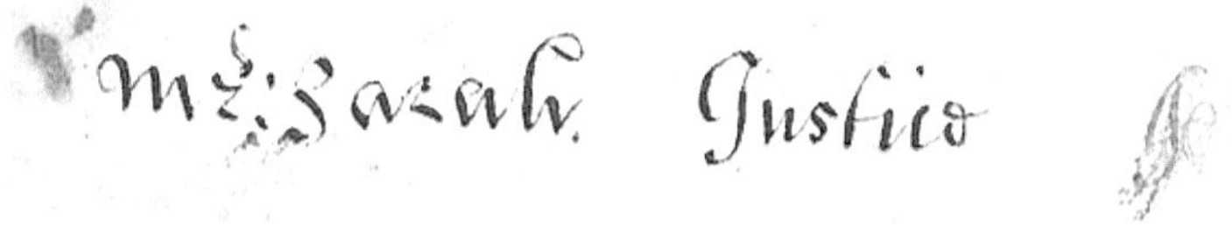

FIGURE 21. Sarah Justice's signature on the endleaf to Amy Eyton's *Collection of Cookery Receipts*, 1691–1738. Wellcome Library, MS 2323.

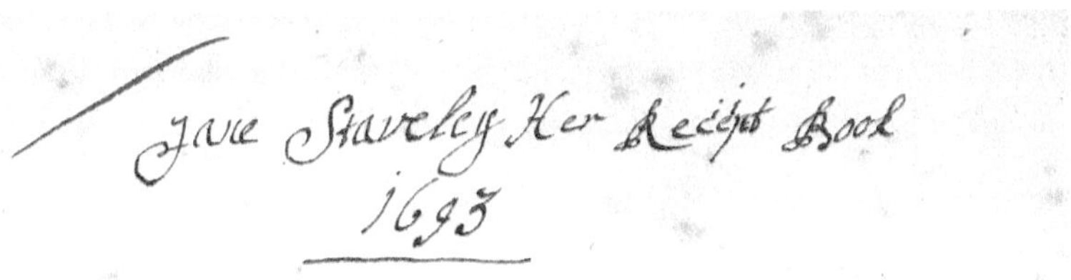

FIGURE 22. Title page to the *Receipt Book of Jane Staveley*, 1693–94, Folger Shakespeare Library, MS V.a.401. Reproduced by permission of the Folger Shakespeare Library.

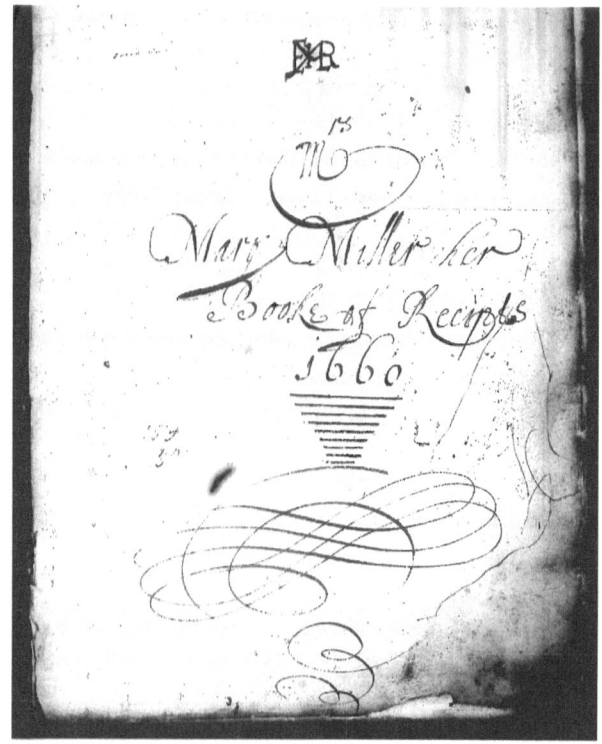

FIGURE 23. Title page to Mary Miller's *Booke of Receipts*, 1660, Wellcome Library, MS 3547.

complete with centered text, lined design elements, swirling accents, and curling descenders (lines traveling downward in letters) (Figure 23).

A large, well-used, and anonymous culinary and medical manuscript housed at the Folger Shakespeare Library opens with a recipe oddly exhibiting three different handwriting styles. Various men and at least one woman signed the collection between 1634 and 1683, inscribing in it remedies for scurvy, colic and constipation; directions for making preserves, jumbles, dried fruits, muttons, and puddings; a page of Latin medical terms; an inventory of household items; a record of someone in service; cross-referencing of recipes; and records of debts. The opening recipe for an herbal panacea called the "water of life" calls for the reader to distill sack with rosemary, rue, thyme, sage, rosa solis, liverwort, bugloss, lavender hyssop, elecampane root, horehound, mouse ear, savory and wormwood, licorice mace, nutmeg, dates, sugar, seed pearl, and gold paper. Extravagant but not unusual, the recipe is noteworthy centrally because its composing hands change twice *within* a single recipe, a fact made stranger by its location as the initial recipe in a collection (Figure 24).[39] The recipe for "water of life" begins in italic, shifts to a mixed secretary and italic hand in mid-sentence, and then alters once again to a *different* italic script.

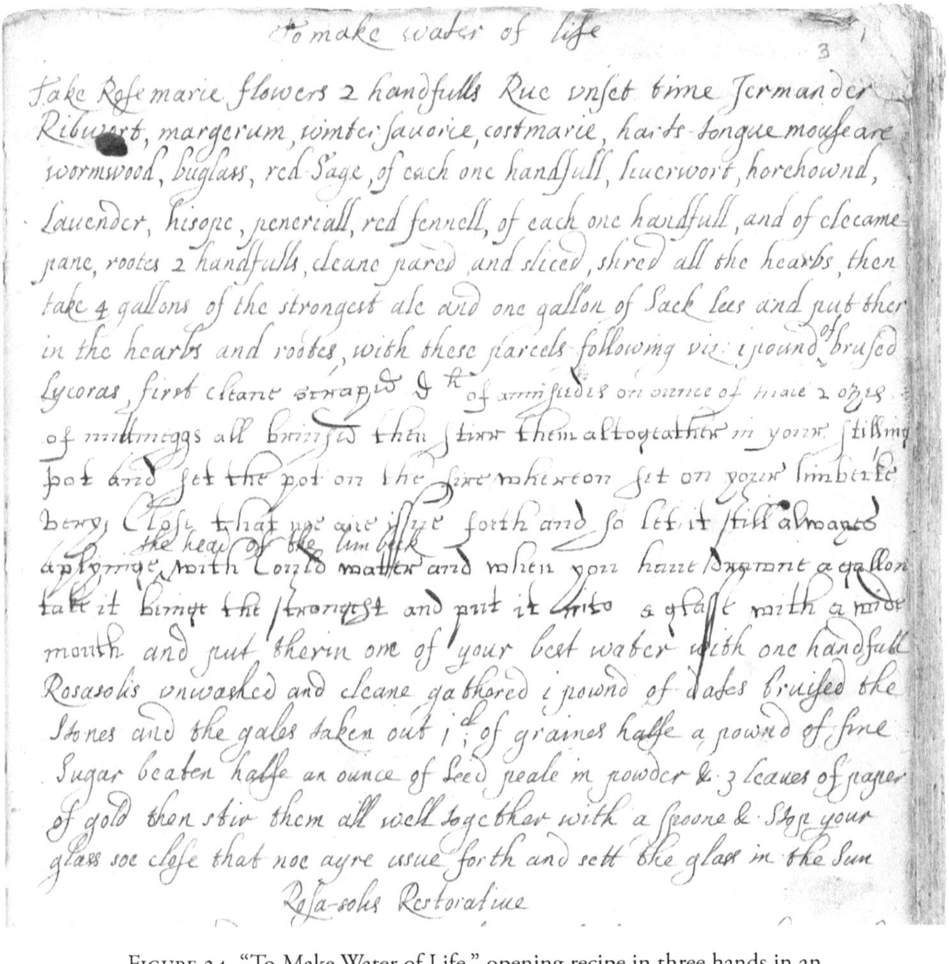
To make water of life 3
Take Rosemarie flowers 2 handfulls Rue unset time Jermander
Ribwort, margerum, winter sauorie, costmarie, harts tongue mouseare
wormwood, buglass, red Sage, of each one handfull, liuerwort, horehownd,
lauender, hisope, peneriall, red fennell, of each one handfull, and of elecame
pane, rootes 2 handfulls, cleane pared and sliced, shred all the hearbs, then
take 4 gallons of the strongest ale and one gallon of Sack lees and put ther
in the hearbs and rootes, with these parcels following viz: 1 pound of brused
Lycoras, first cleane scraped & of annisedes one ounce of mace 2 ounces
of nutmeggs all brused then stirr them altogeather in your stilling
pot and set the pot on the fire whereon set on your limbecke
being close that noe aire issue forth and so let it still alwayes
the head of the limbeck
applying with cold water and when you have drawne a gallon
take it being the strongest and put it into a glasse with a wide
mouth and put therin one of your best water with one handfull
Rosasolis unwashed and cleane gathered 1 pownd of dates bruised the
Stones and the gales taken out 1 d of graines halfe a pownd of fine
Sugar beaten halfe an ounce of seed peale in powder & 3 leaues of paper
of gold then stir them all well together with a spoone & Stop your
glass soe close that noe ayre issue forth and sett the glass in the Sun
Rosa-solis Restoratiue

FIGURE 24. "To Make Water of Life," opening recipe in three hands in an anonymous collection, 1678–ca. 1689, Folger Shakespeare Library, MS V.b.13, fol. 3. Reproduced by permission of the Folger Shakespeare Library.

What situation could have eventuated this oddity? Did three different writers collaboratively take turns writing the recipe, deliberately handing the book around with interruptions in midsentence? Or did a single writer consciously alter his or her script as part of a personal amusement or challenge? This odd phenomenon recurs in the third recipe, which offers directions for an herbal restorative, where the hand abruptly modulates from italic, in the eighth line, into a secretary that persists for the next few recipes. Although we cannot account for these handwriting changes, we can appreciate that the manuscript served as a copy-text sampler for future readers. Readers who opened the first pages became aware that lettering was important to the collection.

As was typical of manuscript writing in this era, recipe collections accreted inscriptions, took on new functions, and expanded as they traveled to family and friends. Evidence of their textual circulation is plentiful, with some collections marking the specific routes of their voyage through a clutter of recorded names. Abraham Sommers enlarged Mary Baumfylde's 1626 collection, a text that Katherine Thatcher then coauthored one hundred years after its inception. Ann Clayton readily supplemented Mary Bent's recipe book. Years after it was written, Catherine Sparks joined Fanny Richardson as "authors" of "Miss Caldwells Book"; Thomas Pyborne and Katherine Annal each owned a recipe book that had been in the possession of Katherine Brown; and Cisilia Haynes directly wrote, "Lady Anne Lovelace Gave me this Book.'"[40] Compilers often anticipated future readers beyond a close circle of acquaintances, people who might need lexical aids to make sense of their recipes. In addition to marking status through their knowledge of fashionable dishes and methods, writers must have imagined that their *handwriting* would signify socially as their books traveled. The physical lettering of recipes "marked" a person to those temporally and geographically afar, while exhibiting and promoting specific styles of writing. The social, epistemological, and intellectual features of recipe circulation that I discuss in other chapters thus bear on the texts' function as exercise tablets and primers. As readers mined their inherited collections for tips on making cordial waters, ointments, and sweetmeats, they were invited to notice whether previous compilers had chosen to use the angular features of secretary script, integrated roman upright non-connecting letters, toyed with long looped descenders as flourishes, or demonstrated minimal pen lifts.[41]

We might presume that the labor of writing became disconnected from domestic work when scriveners were hired to create recipe collections. It was, after all, common for people of means to hire amanuenses to handle correspondence or transcribe texts.[42] Three recipe collections that I encountered in my research explicitly identified mediating scribes: Lady Ann Fanshawe's collection is signed "by Me, Joseph Averie"; Lady Borlase's compilation is written by "her servant" Robert Godfrey; and Ann Smith's collection is "Written by Tho: Barnaby Gent Of Reading."[43] Other recipe texts are so ornate and carefully lettered that they are assumed to be the work of professionals. The collection attributed to Hester Denbigh, wife of Basil A. Earl of Denbigh, for instance, is one such case. A masterpiece of calligraphy and visual design and bound in expensive red morocco, the title page presents intricate graphic designs nested within three rectangular boxes. Ornate letters formed with equivalent pressure emanate from peacock feather-like swirls spelling out "Hester Denbigh: / Anno Domini / 1700"[44] (Figure 2). Among the recipes, the reader discovers a hand-drawn lady holding a flower and an eagle comprised of pointillist dots. The capital "A" in the recipe for "Whole Apricocks" becomes a calligraphic event, with descenders that spiral into a human face. The deliberate physical construction of this display copy rivaled if not subsumed its functionality.

The governing assumption has long been that seventeenth-century manuscripts, including those few recipe collections noticed by scholars, were the product of scribes. In the last decade, this assumption has been challenged by the discovery of materials in which women mention writing, by reconsideration of the methods for establishing literacy rates (which I have discussed above), by the discovery of female ownership marks in printed materials, and by increasing skepticism that so many published books would be targeted to illiterate women. In the course of writing this book, I have encountered numerous scholars who assume recipe collections are the product of professional scriveners unless there is extrinsic or intrinsic evidence to the contrary. My working assumption, by contrast, is that the question is up for grabs and has to be settled on a case-by-case basis or left undetermined.

As a test case, we might consider Elizabeth Fowler's 1684 collection, which includes recipes for potted venison, fricassees, "the best sausages that ever was eat," egg pie, calves head hash, wines, and candied lemons. On a spectrum, the book falls at the far end in terms of care of presentation: the page layout is neatly ruled, the first hundred pages are heavily flourished, and the title page uses decorative interlaced capitals like those appearing in calligraphic manuals (Figure 25). Given the similarity of the majuscules in Fowler's name to those in popular writing masters' guides, the text has been assumed to be the product of a scrivener. But what then are we presupposing as the definition of a "trained" scribe? Might it include men and women informally trained at home

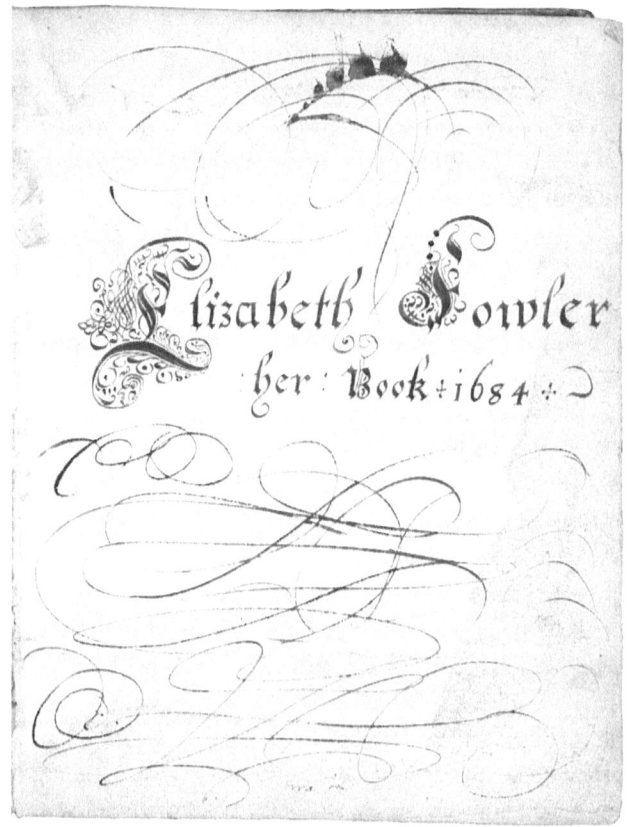

FIGURE 25. Title page to *Elizabeth Fowler Her Book*, 1684, Folger Shakespeare Library, MS V.a.468. Reproduced by permission of the Folger Shakespeare Library.

who sought to cultivate an elegant hand to obtain patronage, courtly reward, or commercial gain? Might it reference those amateurs to whom writing manuals were addressed?

While we cannot definitively determine who wrote Fowler's name and her recipes, we discover clues in the collection, for here *traces* of writing blur the line between personal and professional penmanship. In the doodles on the end flyleaf, where someone has scribbled, "The Fear of the Lord," "amen," "made," and "commandment," we see lacework designs similar to those forming the majuscules in Fowler's name (Figure 26).[45] If the title was the work of a scribe, then a later reader has sought to reproduce this calligraphy and thus has used the text to learn the professional art of making "fair copy." But it is just as possible that

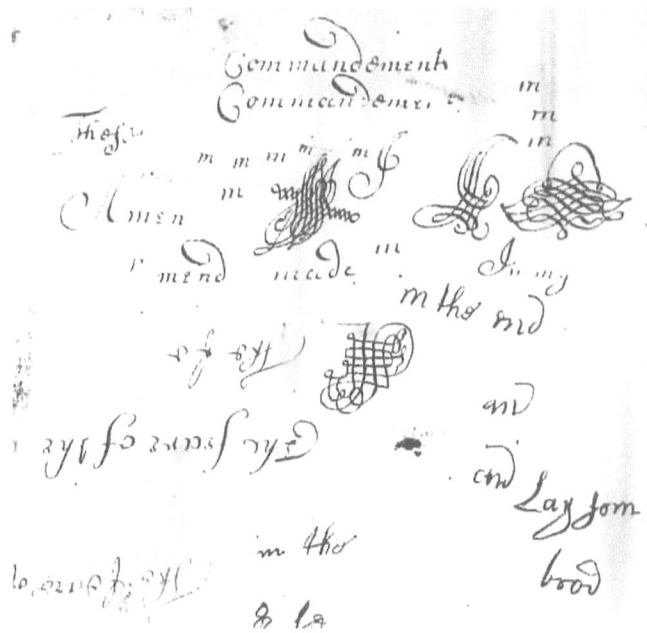

FIGURE 26. Doodles on the end flyleaf of *Elizabeth Fowler Her Book*, 1684, Folger Shakespeare Library, MS V.a.468. Photograph by Wendy Wall, from the collection of the Folger Shakespeare Library.

the "professional scribe" was instead an amateur, perhaps Fowler herself, who practiced the lacework lettering on the flyleaf before creating the signature title. It is clear that the decorative design work on the recipe pages is not perfected. The cursive spirals used to separate recipes are of an uneven quality, with some carefully proportioned and others hastily scrawled (Figure 27). Some titles are punctuated by isolated and asymmetrical lacework designs; some titles, though elegantly written, are so poorly spaced that additional words had to be crowded above the letters. Perhaps Fowler, we might guess from this evidence, was just a faster learner than other amateur calligraphers. My hypothesis finds support in other collections, where we see readers overtly attempting to perfect letter writing. A reader of Elizabeth Hirst's recipes, for instance, become intrigued by the letter "B" in "Balme Water" (Figure 28) and attempted two versions of the letter in the margin.[46] When later owners added a cucumber or pudding recipe to Jane Newton's recipe collection, whose index is tellingly called "The Alphabet," they were tasked with choosing whether or not to imitate the flourished lettering of

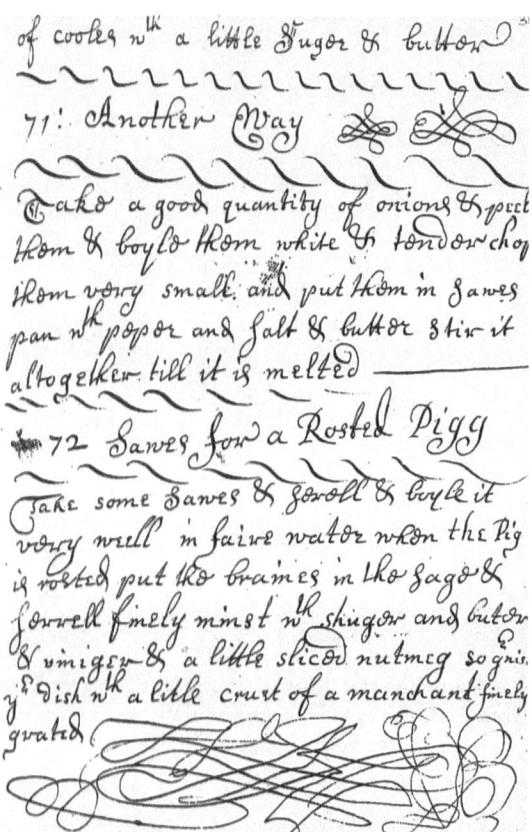

FIGURE 27. *Elizabeth Fowler Her Book*, 1684, Folger Shakespeare Library, MS V.a.468. Photograph by Wendy Wall, from the collection of the Folger Shakespeare Library.

the titling. While we can only speculate about who wrote Fowler's collection, we see that it incarnated refined handwriting that was shown to be in a state of progress elsewhere in the book.

Lady Anne Percy's collection gives us a glimpse of how recipe work nurtured other bibliographic skills. Percy, daughter to the Earl of Northumberland and wife to Philip Lord Stanhope, incorporated her recipes with those of her family and friends. Her husband inscribed her collection by calling attention to her holograph: "These receits are writ in my dear wifes the Lady Anne Pircies own hand," he stated, "and have long been kept as secrets in the Northumberland family."[47] Next to a recipe for apricot paste, in her "own hand," Percy drew a pointing hand, a highlighting symbol that bibliographers term a "manicule,"

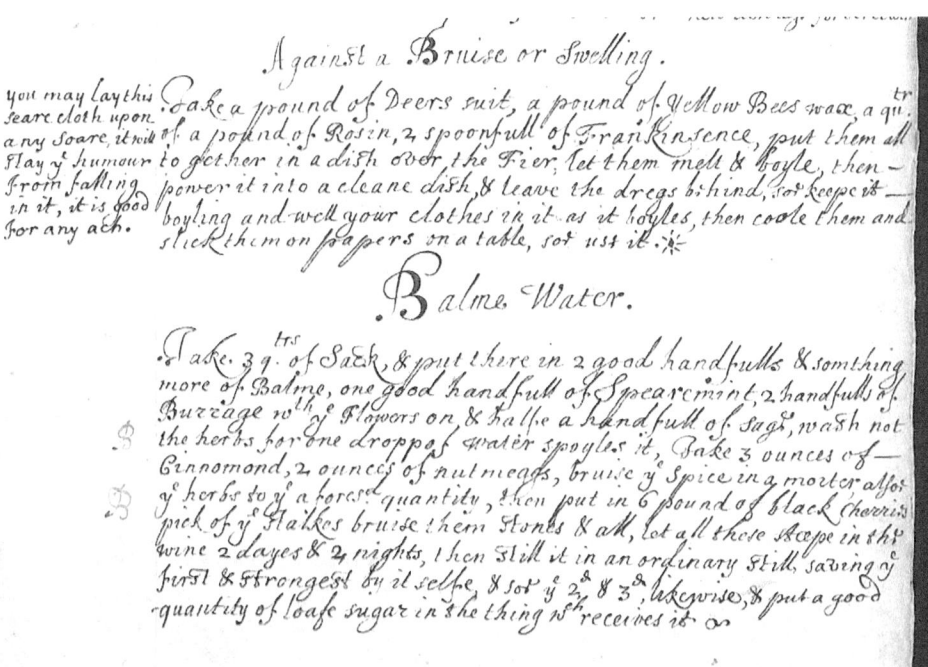

FIGURE 28. Practice letter work in Elizabeth Hirst's *Medical and Cookery Receipts*, 1684–1725, Wellcome Library, MS 2840, p. 7, fol. 5.

an "index," or simply a "hand" (Figure 29). As William Sherman has so richly explained, medieval and Renaissance readers frequently created highly individualized manicules to highlight noteworthy sections of texts.[48] Recipe collections are no exception: the Granville family collection presents a deliberate drawn hand, with slim proportioned fingers emerging from a shirt sleeve, pointing directly to an ink recipe written in Spanish; the writer of Grace Blome's collection deploys a quickly drawn angular hand to mark a potted venison recipe (Figure 30); and Jane Jackson's collection is littered with so many manicules that they lose their purpose as highlighters and become all-purpose design features (Figure 31). While Percy's recipe for apricots is fairly unremarkable, her manicule, drawn imperfectly almost to resemble a bird or feather, uses crudely shaped fingers to point *away* from the text (100). Percy's attempt at personalizing her marginal notation has gone askew, or rather, it represents an unskillful hand in several senses of the word, pointing not to a particular recipe but to its own still unfinished or "illiterate" form.

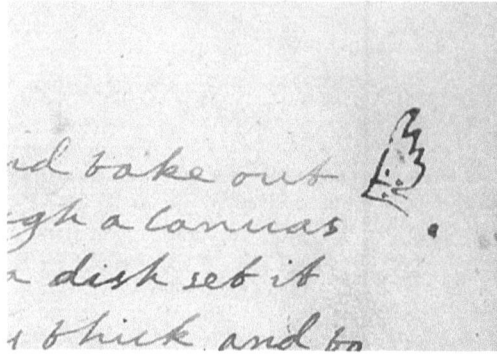

FIGURE 29. Manicule (pointing hand) in Lady Anne Percy's *Manuscript Cookery Book*, 1650, Whitney Cookery Collection, MssCol 3318, vol. 2. Manuscripts and Archives Division, the New York Public Library, Astor, Lenox and Tilden Foundations.

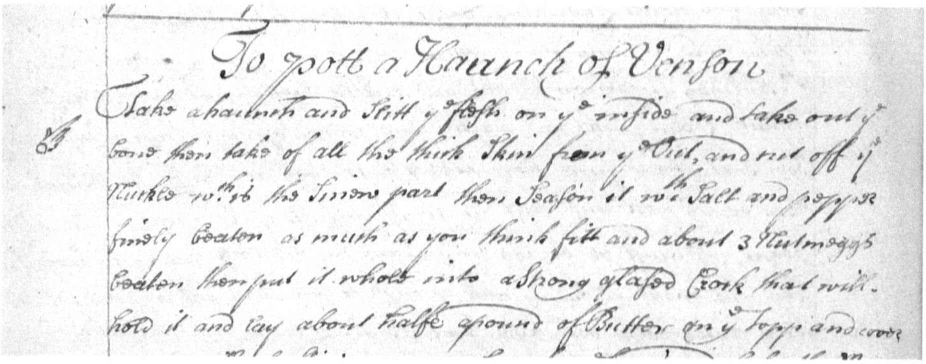

FIGURE 30. Manicule in Grace Randolph Blome's *Cookbook*, 1697, Folger Shakespeare Library, MS V.b.301, 80. Reproduced by permission of the Folger Shakespeare Library.

In their interests in hands and handiwork, recipe collections function like embroidered samplers that taught the art of calligraphy and alphabet styles. Recipe collections could thus be multiply pedagogic—teaching a reader how to make a posset, while enabling the writer (and later writer-readers) to develop a uniform or particular hand, the sign of learned, elite, and literate status. Knowing how to "smear" a rabbit the French way (which involves making the rabbit stand upright in a puddle of butter, nutmeg, mace, and broth) might have exhibited cultural capital, but so did the self-possessed hand inscribing that knowledge. Recipe books thus offer more than a window onto

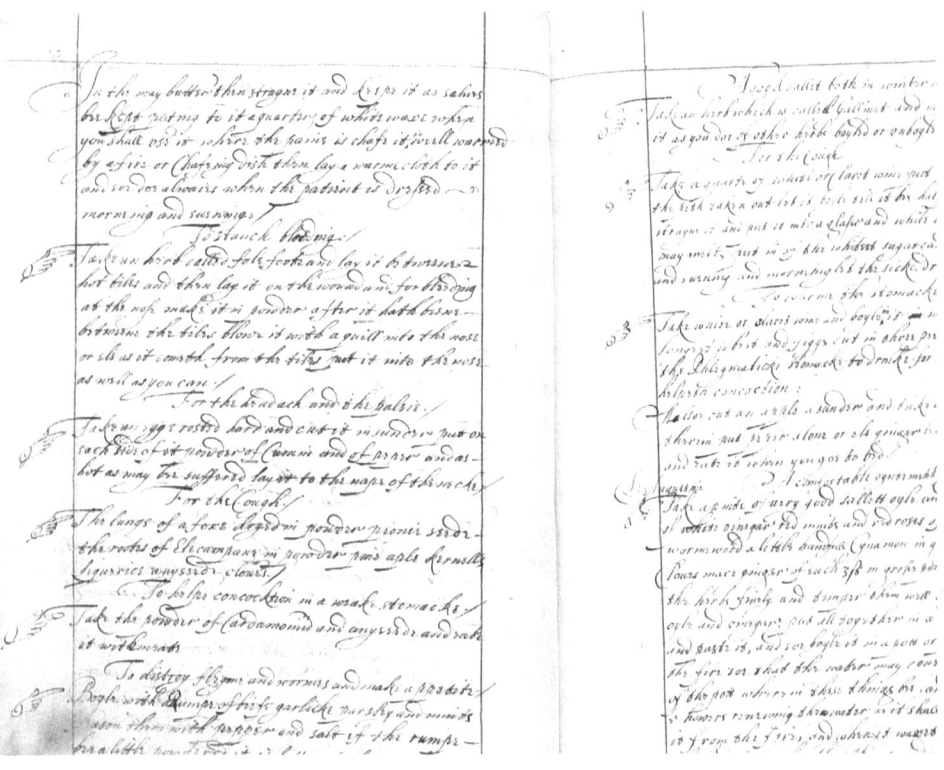

FIGURE 31. Manicules in Jane Jackson's *A Very Shorte and Compendious Methode of Phisicke and Chirurgery*, 1642, pp. 35–36. Wellcome Library, MS 373.

the lives of early modern women or a peek into their dining practices. They constituted, displayed, and circulated literacies in and around the kitchen.[49]

Handiwork: Cutting, Knotting, and Lettering Confectionery

> Fashion & finish [sugar plate dough] only with your hand and pincers, but if you want handiness ... then you must hae mouldes of tynne.
> —John Murrell, *Delightful Daily Exercise*, 1617[50]

It's not saying anything particularly new to observe that manuscripts in the early modern period served as guides, catalysts, and exercise sheets for the production of writing. Recipes were distinctive, however, in being available to women and in being nestled within domestic space and work. How might the content of recipe collections be relevant to the literacies they fostered? One way to address this question is to think about how "handiwork" within the domestic environment involved different but related movements and dispositions of the hand. Housework shared a skill set with early modern penmanship, especially when we remember that writing began with the cutting of the quill and ended with what was commonly called the "cutting of letters." *The Compleat Servant-Maid*, the domestic guide that we discussed previously, began its writing lessons by offering technical details about how to make a pen: "Having a Penknife with a smooth, thin, sharp edge, take the first . . . quill of a Goose wing and scrape it, then hold it in your left hand with the feather end from you, beginning . . . in the back, cut a small piece off sloping, then to make a slit enter the knife in the midst of the first cut, put in a quill and force it up . . . fashion the nib by cutting off both the sides equally down, then place the nib on the nail of your left hand thumb, and to end it draw the edge into it slanting" (1683: 23). Learning to write, early modern style, might involve defeathering a goose and isolating one of the first four flights of feathers (a task executed, perhaps, in the kitchen where the goose was to be prepared for dinner). As this guide explains, the would-be writer had to sharpen the wing (or *penna*) through a sequence of cuts to form the correct sized nib (different for secretary and italic scripts). Schoolboys learning to write used a penknife to scrape marks into and off parchment. Later in the guide, the maid is to pick up her knife again, this time to tackle the innards of the goose: "cut off the Belly-piece round, close to the lower end of the Breast," the guide instructs, "lace her down with your Knife clean thorow the brest, one each side two Thumbs bredth from the Brest-bone" (36). Slicing and slashing were key components for tasks that were not just related metonymically.

Jonathan Goldberg argues for the violence of early modern subject formation by reading crossovers between the figurative and visual representation of tools in penmanship manuals.[51] The transference of agency and objecthood—from the penknife carving the quill, to the quill that seems to slice ink into paper, to the seemingly amputated hand trying to control these instruments—formed a semiotic pattern, according to Goldberg, whose menacing alienation was part and parcel of the newly emerging civilized subject. Goldberg points to the fact that the quill was metonymically linked visually and verbally to sharply bladed tools in writing manuals, where human hands, seemingly detached from bodies, appear to be engraved by characters on the page. While I will argue that the practices described in recipe collections cannot be accounted for by the story of the civilizing process, I recognize that they do bespeak the sinister violence haunting handwriting lessons, as carving quill and letters interchanged with carving animals.

When placed next to the tasks of dismembering carcasses that women were to perform in the kitchen, the tactility of cutting-in-writing becomes especially pronounced. In *The Accomplished Ladies Rich Cabinet of Rarities*, John Shirley advised, "In Writing, beware that you blot not your Paper, but imitate your Copy in cutting your Letters fair and even."[52] Writing master John Davies drew out the potentially injurious nature of "cutting," which involved applying manual pressure to the quill. "Never saw I yet a woman that could write our English secretary hand lively," he warned, "though the *Romane* or *Italian* handsomly: because they naturally lack strength in their hand to perform those full strokes, and (as it were) to bruise a letter as men can do."[53] Davies's devaluation of female strength aside, his description of writing as the act of bruising a letter posed a salient reminder of writing's physicality. In recipes, writing's proximate link to bodies that required injurious healing and animals that required precision slaughtering was underscored. Make your hand literate, domestic manuals seemed to say, by learning to cut with strength, curiosity, and care.

Recipes show everywhere that housework required manual dexterity, exact surgical incising, and physical force. Women were coached to wield knives with exactness so as to chop root vegetables, etch designs onto pastries, and carve at the table. In "unlac[ing] or carving a Coney" (rabbit), the housewife, according to *The Compleat Servant-Maid*, should brandish a knife like a surgeon: "pull the leg open softly with your hand: but pluck it not off, then thrust in your Knife betwixt the Ribs and the Kidney, slit it out, then lay the legs close together" (1677: 34). Constance Hall's recipe for making "scotch collops" (thinly sliced meat in a stew) pointed to the differentiated degrees of manual control that we expect in modern cooking (27v). The cook was to "take a Legg of vele and cut the Fleshey parte into Thin Slices as a Shilling and as broad and as Long as your fore finger."[54] Measured cutting then gave way to brute force: "then hack and beat them with the Back of the Knife then fry them Browne" (28). Knives had to be positioned accurately to control the depth, width, and shape of various cuts. Lady Borlase sees the penknife, the very utensil used to cut quills for writing, as a kitchen utensil. "Turn them forth with a pen-knife uppon glass sheetes," she advises in her recipe for fruitcakes, "& cut them into what fashion you please" (158). In fact, "cut" and "print" were commonly used as interchangeable verbs for designing pies and pastries. Confections were to be "cut" or "printed" as the reader pleased.[55] "Handiness," according to Murrell (cited in my epigraph), involved the production of form through acts of incision (F3).

Carving, the most socially visible form of household cutting, was primarily performed by servants and noblemen in the medieval period but was newly opened to household mistresses in late sixteenth-century England.[56] Guides directed to male readers are our best source of information for appreciating the intricate knowledge of anatomy and social decorum required in carving. According to *The Genteel House-Keepers Pastime*, carving "teaches its Practitioners to know the Dissection of Parts, the scituation of Joynts and Ligaments, and the true position of the . . . emininent Muscles. Nor does it shut out the most excellent Sciences of Arithmetick and Geometry: for the skillful Carver knows how to proportion his several dividends of Services according to the number of Guests at the Table, and . . . [to] dispose the best of Delicacies to the most eminent Persons."[57] Acknowledging that women had joined male servants and householders in the spectator sport of carving, recipe books for women explained its procedures and protocols. In *A New Booke of Cookerie*, Murrell republished verbatim parts of a 1508 carving book that had been formerly directed to male butlers. Seventy years later, Giles Rose put forth a guide, perhaps too literally translated from the French as *A Perfect School of Instructions for the Officers of the Mouth Shewing the Whole Art of Carving*, which he described as of "singular use for Ladies and Gentlewomen."[58] By the time Woolley took over as the leading writer of domestic guides in the later seventeenth century, she saw it as standard to tutor women and male servants about the art of dressing and serving meat.

Carving, for the mistress as well as the male servant, encompassed skill and shrewd social knowledge. *The Gentlewomans Companion* for instance, advised the young gentlewoman or housekeeper: "Thrust your knife into a Leg of Mutton a considerable depth, above the handle . . . in the joint on the other side, is a little bone to be presented, and in great estimation among the Curious" (67). Exhibiting knife skills for an admiring audience at the table, the carver was to isolate prized bones and joints, show a careful discrimination of taste (an ability to identify with "the Curious"), and display exacting mechanical aptitude. Failing to identify the treasured small bone hidden in the mutton, numerous witnesses warned, created an embarrassing social gaffe. As such, carving functioned as an expressive mode of social communication, categorized as what John Donne called a "mechanic" skill of the hand, which included the capacity "to write, to carve, to play."[59] Given the insistently material nature of early modern inscription, it is not surprising that the Old English word "carve" was, in fact, held to be cognate with the Greek *grafein*, to write.

Domestic handiwork overlapped conceptually with writing, but the metonymic argument has to be made as well, because, as we've seen, the quill and penknife doubled as materials for writing and cooking. Other items in the kitchen would have been at home in a library: pages of books were on hand to line pie pans or to wrap spices, fish, preserves, or tobacco; "pensells" (brushes) were used to moisten foodstuffs and to make inscriptions; and bread crumbs could be used not only in making pies but also in erasing mistakes written in black lead. To create a popular chicken dish called "Spread Eagle," the cook used a quill to slit the chicken's throat, remove its craw, and blow the flesh from the bone.[60] To cure sight problems (using Mrs. Rebekah Ash's remedy), the reader was to use a quill to blow an aluminum, sugar, and fish mixture into the eye.[61] Almost every respectable collection, as I discuss in Chapter 5, had to include a good ink recipe. The knife, stylus, quill, pencil: these incised form out of chaotic matter, whether parchment, animal flesh, or sugar dough.

From the domain of shared tools, we return to shared skills. The art of making sets of interlacing and interconnected lines, called "knots," was fundamental to both the literate hand and to domestic craft. In household confectionery, oblong braids or intricate pretzel-like ringed designs served as the basis for fashioning sweetmeats such as cracknels, gimbals, or jumbals. The names of these edibles corresponded to their formal features, the cracknel having a curved hollowed shape; the "gimbal" formed by connecting links or rings; and the "jumbal" constructed of interwoven shapes (not a disorderly mixture, as the word signifies today). In *The Queens Delight* (supposedly the sweets lovingly prepared by Queen Henrietta Maria), W.M. offered a recipe for fruit jumbals that emphasized their visual presentation: "Take the Apricocks or Quinces, and coddle them tender; then take their pulp and dry it in a dish over a Chafing-dish of coals, and set it in a stove for a day or two; then beat it in a stone Mortar, putting in as much Sugar as will make a stiffe paste; then colour it with Saunders, Cochinele or blew Starch, and make it up in what colour you please, rowl them with battle-dores [wooden paddles] into long peeces, and tye them up in knots, and so dry them."[62] Attending to the texture of the glutinous paste as well as the color palette of natural dyes, W.M. assumed that readers already knew requisite patterns—from simple braids, to lover's knots, to the elaborate intertwinings featured on coats of arms.[63] Recipes to make "Knotts with Almonds," or jumbals "exceeding well moulded and then

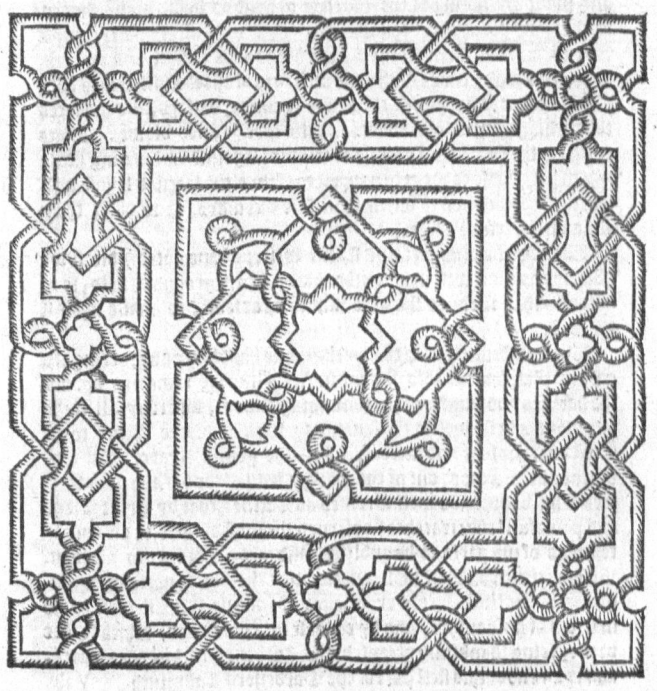

FIGURE 32. Knot garden design in Thomas Hill's *The Gardeners Labyrinth* (London, 1594), 80. Beinecke Rare Book and Manuscript Library, Yale University.

rowled out, tied in knots and put on flowered plate," for instance, hinted that dough was to be coiled, looped, tied, ringed, plaited, or wreathed into patterns.[64] "Tye them up in knots" recipes commanded. Knots, of course, were ubiquitous as designs in landscape gardening, as fasteners in seamanship, and, as I will discuss later, in sewing patterns. Thomas Hill's *The Gardeners Labyrinth* not only promised to model for housewives ways to "set forth divers Herbes, Knots and Mazes, cunningly handled for the beautifying of Gardens," but also provided illustrations for knot garden designs (Figure 32).[65] William

Lawson's *The Countrie Housewifes Garden* (1618) offered ten "formes, mazes and knots" for patterning functional, small-scaled kitchen gardens.[66] Ladies of means were expected to blueprint plans for Italianate formal gardens, complete with symmetrical walkways and shaped topiary.[67]

Historians of women's labor have not fully appreciated the fact that "knotting" was a basic component of an expansive array of domestic work including confection-making as well as refined handwriting.[68] One hundred and fifteen different writing manuals appearing between 1570 and 1700 highlighted knot-making as a critical stepping stone for learning cursive writing.[69] In William Comley's *A New Alphabet of the Capitall Romane Knotted Letters, Fit and Ready to Set Any Manner of Hand To; with Knots vnto the same; for the vnskilfull to practise by*, knots "set," or founded, handwriting styles. "Knots," in this context, referred both to specific styles of lettering and to the steady circular motions that underpinned joined or cursive writing (Figure 33).[70] Recipe compilers employed these design elements in marginal borders and title decorations. A compilation attributed to "Rose Kendall & Anne Cater," for instance, presents an initial thirty-page group of "core" recipes adorned with patterned swirls—from simple connecting links, to double-linked embedded circles in contrast-

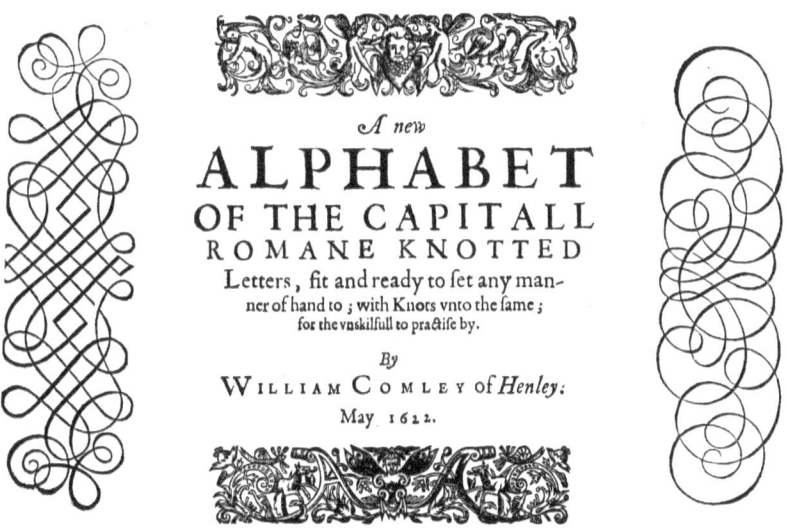

FIGURE 33. Title page to William Comley's *A New Alphabet of the Capitall Romane Knotted Letters* (London, 1622). Plimpton Collection, Rare Book and Manuscript Library, Columbia University.

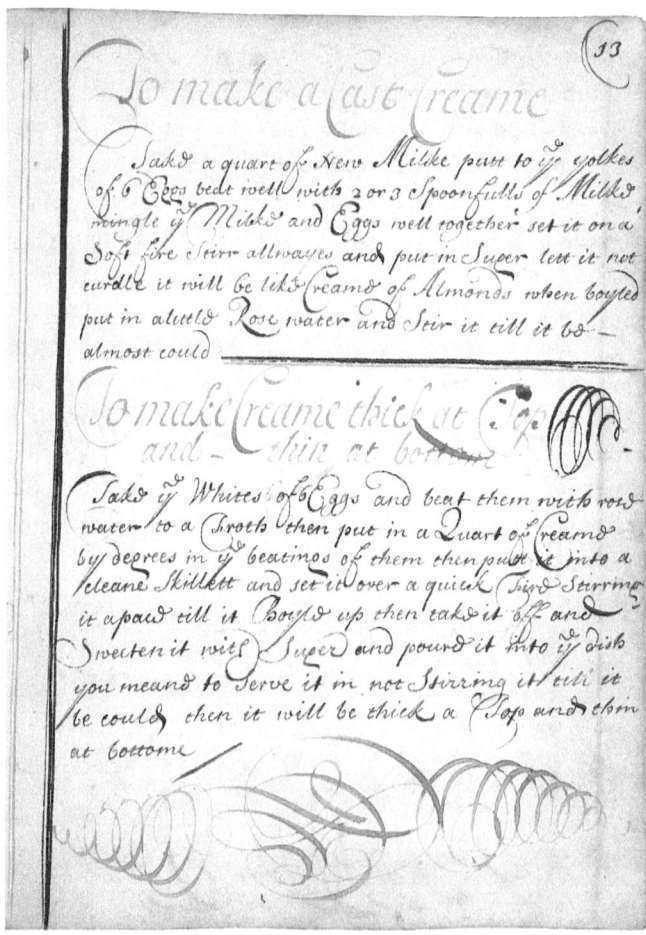

FIGURE 34. Ornamentation in Rose Kendall and Anne Cater's *Cookery and Medicinal Recipes*. 1675–ca. 1750, Folger Shakespeare Library MS V.a.429, fol. 13. Reproduced by permission of the Folger Shakespeare Library.

ing inks, to elegant laceworked majuscules (Figure 34). The spiral punctuating Lady Sillyard's recipe for whitening cloth mutates gracefully into the figure of a woman's face, a design that calligraphers such as William Comley recommended precisely for practicing minimal pen-lift figures (Figure 35, Figure 36).[71] Compilers who later continued the Kendall/Cater collection became acquainted with the Countess of Warwick's way to make almond butter but also her refined style of writing. In other recipe books, writers converted descend-

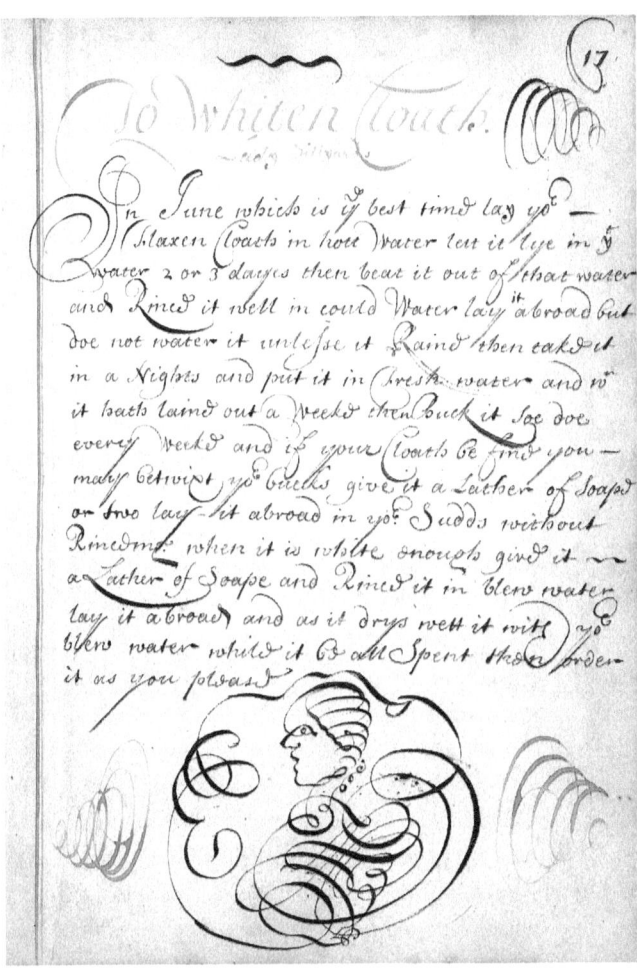

FIGURE 35. Calligraphic "face" design in Rose Kendall and Anne Cater's *Cookery and Medicinal Recipes*, 1675–ca. 1750, Folger Shakespeare Library, MS V.a.429, fol. 17.

ers into human faces and experimented with amateurish laceworked capitals that morphed into images of the sun (Figure 37).[72]

Confectionery, knife-work, and carving might have trained a hand for writing, but it is precisely the assumed sequencing of the developmental model that the recipe archive forces us to reconsider. Why not consider foodwork as constituting writing in and of itself? In *Delightes for Ladies*, Plat identified "letters" as one of the curious "fancies" that the reader might stylize

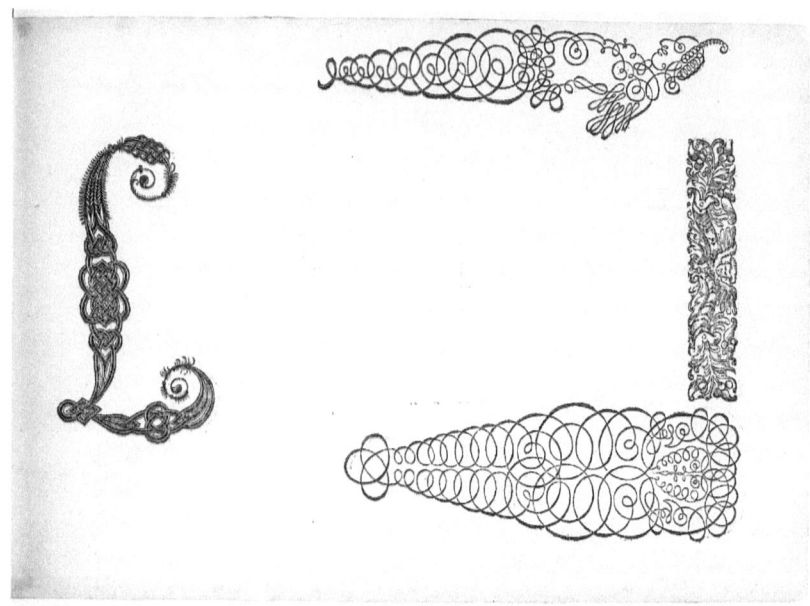

FIGURE 36. Practice pen lift "face" in William Comley's *A New Alphabet of the Capitall Romane Knotted Letters* (London, 1622). Plimpton Collection, Rare Book and Manuscript Library, Columbia University.

in the kitchen. Marzipan could be adorned with comfits (sugar-coated spices) but the reader who had time and skill might shape them into "letters, knots, Arms, Escocheons, beasts, birds, & other fancies."[73] Letters were thus one of the conceits that home confectioners were encouraged to include within their repertoire, forms that, as we have seen in previous chapters, carried intellectual and social dimensions. Shakespeare's *Cymbeline* reflects on this practice when Fidele, the cross-dressed Innogen, plays the "housewife" to Arviragus, Belarius and Guiderius in their exile from civilization (4.2.44). Exclaiming over the "gentle" quality of their houseguest, the men praise Fidele's singing voice, nourishing medicinal broths, and "neat cookery": "He cut our roots in characters," Belarius marvels (39; 50; 51). The brothers are astonished to find that a wandering starving youth can fashion alphabetic letters even in homely roots.

In *A Delightfull Daily Exercise for Ladies and Gentlewomen*, John Murrell offered a detailed and elaborated view of culinary lettering. He offered de-

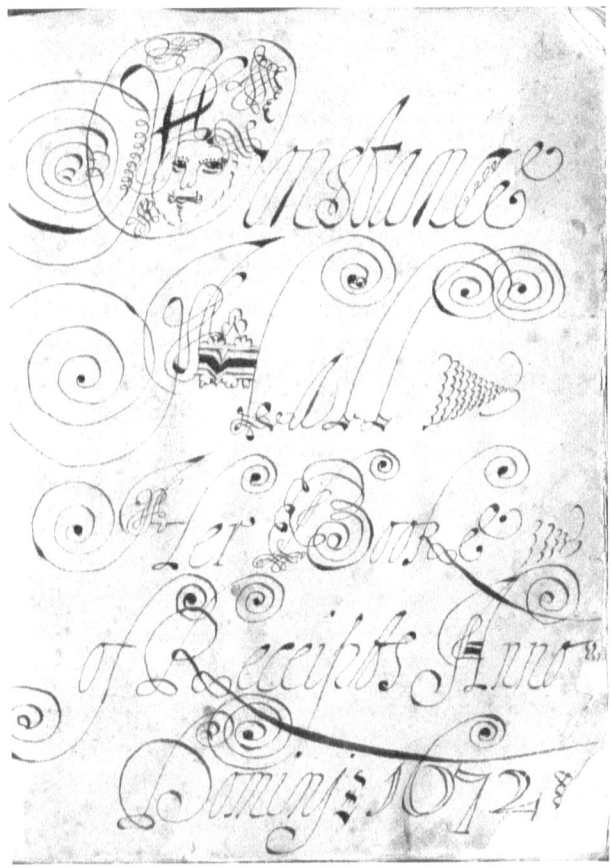

FIGURE 37. Title page to Constance Hall's *Receipt Book*, 1672, Folger Shakespeare Library, MS V.a.20. Reproduced by permission of the Folger Shakespeare Library.

tailed instructions for making "letters and knots in almonds," as if the two forms occupied the same conceptual category.[74] After forming and slicing pastry dough, Murrell explained, the reader should roll the mixture of crushed almonds, sugar, musk, and rosewater into a paste, "turn" the dough "into letters and knots," and then bake the pastries on buttered paper. Murrell's similarly named *Daily Exercise for Ladies and Gentlewomen* included a recipe entitled "To make Letters, Knots, or any other Jumbell," in which the reader is offered two methods for concocting sugar alphabets: she can harden boiled rosewater and sugar in premade molds or cut a mixture of crushed almonds, sugar, gum dragon (a resin), and rosewater into "double knots" or "capital letters" (1617; F4).[75] While early modern handwriting manuals conceptualized knot-making as a developmental stage in the mastery of lettering, Murrell's recipe books portray them as alternative and contiguous designs that a kitchen worker might use. His recipe for "Cinamon Letters" shows that recipe workers had to have a detailed understanding of letter genres, for desserts should take the form of "faire capitall Romane letters according to some exact pattern" (#89). The reader, that is, must distinguish capital letters (majuscules) from lowercase minuscule, roman from Gothic and italic fonts. Would the "exact pattern" that Murrell directs the reader to consult be found, we might wonder, in

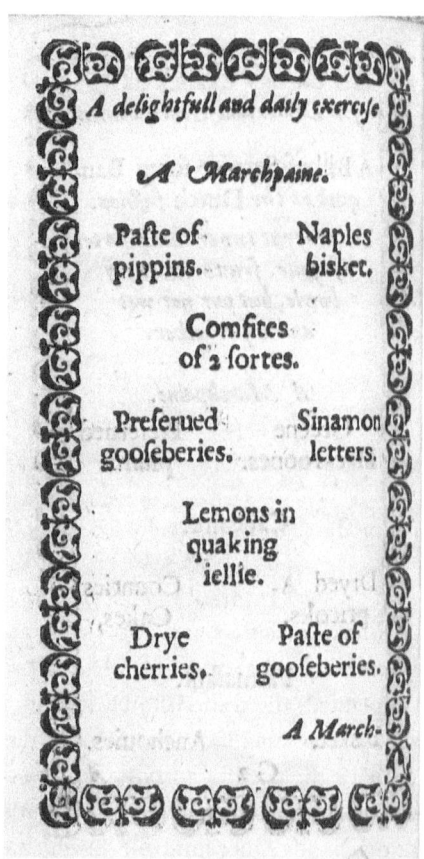

FIGURE 38. Cinnamon letters in a table arrangement in John Murrell's *A Delightfull Daily Exercise for Ladies and Gentlewomen* (London, 1621), G2v. Reproduced by permission of the Huntington Library.

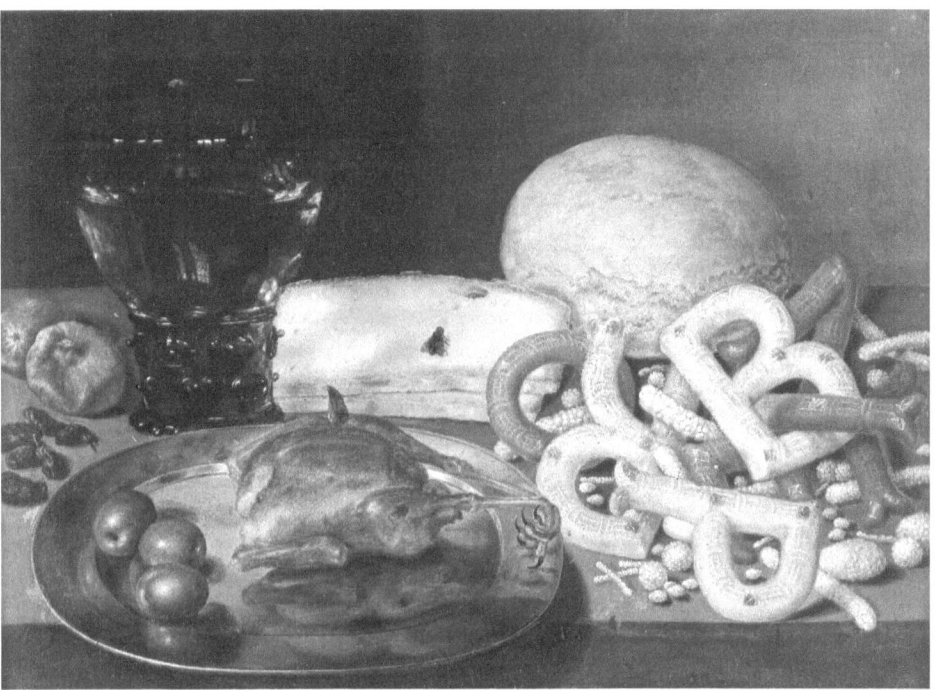

FIGURE 39. Peter Binoit's *Still Life with Letter Pastries* (Stilleven met lettergebak) ca. 1615. Collection Groninger Museum, photograph by John Stoel.

any printed book or specifically in a writing manual? Would the recipe worker need to have lettered material at hand as she tackled her sugar paste?

Recipe books offer frustratingly little evidence about how culinary letters looked when served to diners. Two diagrams in Murrell's *Delightfull Daily Exercise* place edible letters alongside other extravagant sweets in banqueting courses (Figure 38). His "cinnamon letters made by art" were to be served beside dried fruits, jellies, spiced comfits, biscuits, cakes, pastes, jumbles, candied roses, and marzipan. By referring to the dish as "letters," Murrell suggests that his cinnamon alphabets were not ordered into words. Peter Binoit's contemporaneous Dutch painting, *Still Life with Letter Pastries*, confirms this serving style in its portrayal of food-letters heaped in a pile on a table next to a loaf of bread, decanter of wine, capon, olives, and comfits (Figure 39). The tactile and sensual elements of the letters, as we see, trump any semantic meaning.

Although Binoit's letters are not ordered into a meaningful sequence, they do hint at the artist's name ("P," "B," "T," and "R" are clearly legible). In this way, the painting suggests that diners might have been presented with culinary versions of the name and word games prevalent in early modern texts and entertainments. Anagrams and acrostics, games that foregrounded the materiality of the signifier, were ubiquitous in early modern English culture, appearing in one domain in epistles to printed books that used tantalizing initials to tease readers into guessing the identity of authors. In Shakespeare's *Twelfth Night*, Malvolio satirizes such games by struggling to "discover" his name in an epistle, while making salacious puns about the shape of Lady Olivia's letters. *Five Hundred Points of Good Husbandry* plays a more informative word-game; the book "speaks" in the opening poem whose initials that spell out "Thomas Tusser Made Me."[76] A female reader inscribed her copy of the 1599 quarto of *Romeo and Juliet*, as Jason Scott-Warren reports, with a signature anagram that doubled as a complaint: "Elisabeth Rotton: Her lot is to b neat."[77]

Recipes encouraged readers to translate signatures, monograms, and word clues into edible form. We thus return to the heightened materiality of the letter that Fleming and other scholars have theorized: the gross substantiation of page, letter, and word in the early modern world.[78] Recipes give us a glimpse of new sensory qualities for the tactile signifier; for letters could have been experienced as crisp, doughy, aromatic, gooey, sweet, and/or spiced, even as they provided flavorful acrostics, monograms, or anagrams. In addition to the pleasure and intrigue of being ingestible, that is, food-writing could be tasted and experienced by the tongue. The modern world has retained traces of the pleasures of consumable letters, chiefly in the form of alphabet soups and cereals (ostensibly directed to children) and cake writing (a special holiday release from dining norms). In the early seventeenth century, edible letters were, by contrast, the hallmark of elegant dining and a source of intellectual contemplation. Pudsey, the woman who proudly marked her recipes as written in her "owne hand," saw alphabetic shapes as a possible form for her gooseberry cakes. After instructing readers to mix scalded and strained gooseberries with candied sugar, she advised: "Turne them out with your knife [on] a pie plate . . . doe somwhat on them: ether letters or what you please & lett them stand till thay be dry: then box them" (fol. 20v). *Do somewhat on them*: the inscription will register the reader's pleasure. Pudsey's offhand comment indicates that letters were among the classic shapes that readers might have selected when they followed recipes urging them to "print" and mold confections as they pleased.

Murrell's cinnamon letters also afford a clue about how edible alphabets might have been made to signify in their early modern setting. When directing his reader to insert "a cross in the beginning" of her "capital roman letters," Murrell steers her to create a simulacrum of a hornbook, the alphabetic primer used in grammar schools. The hornbook was comprised of parchment or paper affixed to a wooden paddle; the small cross preceding the displayed letters—the Christ-cross or crisscross —generated the English nickname for the alphabet. This visual icon had come to signal a directive: "let it be printed" on the memory of students.[79] In his advice on how to teach reading, Erasmus had offered a pedagogical rationale for the lip-smacking literacy that Murrell recommended; for Erasmus advised baking letter-shaped treats to familiarize pupils with the alphabet. The master could reward a student by giving him permission to eat his lesson.[80] Early modern recipes suggest that banqueting dishes might imitate educational instruction, with the housewife moving between the role of pupil (who must learn how to stylize capitals) and instructor (who puts diners through the paces of a marzipan hornbook, complete with catechism). The woman who purchased Murrell's recipe book was invited to manufacture a fairly complicated domestic representational role as she fashioned letters.

Murrell's clever dessert hornbook returns us to the domestic handwriting instructions seen in guides attributed to Woolley; his fanciful iteration of education points to the unstable line between subscription and parody that pervades the recipe world. Would an edible hornbook render its instruction as "substanceless" as a world of sugar? Did recipes echo vernacular drama, which routinely caricatured the regimented structures and obscure knowledge cultures of formal education? In plays on the London stage, flogging teachers and incomprehensible academics were often the subject of farce. Shakespeare's *The Merry Wives of Windsor*, to take one example, comically has a linguistically errant housekeeper, Mistress Quickly, interrupt a seemingly superfluous Latin language lesson with her eroticized vernacular mistranslations. Murrell's sugar-plated primer created dining theatrics that might have similarly lampooned educational instruction, even as it offered an alternative (and ideologically distinct) site of literacy acquisition.

Recipe consumers were taught traditional modes of food literacy as well as parodies of scenes of instruction. *A Closet for Ladies* published instructions for how to fashion a sugar paste trompe l'oeil walnut that seemed to be real. When the diner took a bite of this already witty dessert and discerned its sweet substance, s/he also discovered a second surprise: a "pretty Posey" that the confectioner had "written" and secreted within (1608; 33–34). Creating an early modern version of the fortune cookie, women created "poesies" as they baked, a term that referred to visual emblems with mottos, epigrammatic sayings, or short verses. Posies appeared in a variety of environments and media; early modern people memorized and circulated versified adages in and on commonplace books, plate ware, glass, rings, bracelets, and household walls. Poesies inscribed on objects included short mottos such as "I love and like my choise" (as one seventeenth-century wedding ring announced);[81] or "as a ring Go Round and hath no end / So Is my Love unto my friend," a verse Abigail Rand attached to a headache remedy in her recipe collection. Trenchers and knives were so frequently engraved with sayings that they gave rise to the terms "cutler's poetry" and "trencher-poets" to signify less prestigious domains of writing.

In his key rhetorical manual, *The Arte of English Poesie*, George Puttenham indicates that writing was as much at home in dinner party culture as rhetorical theory. He explains that it was customary for compressed versified sayings to be "printed or put upon their banketting dishes of suger plate, or of march paines, & such other dainty meates as by the curtesie & custome every gest might carry from a common feast home with him to his owne house, & were made for the nonce [for the occasion], they . . . never contained above one verse, or two at the most, but the shorter the better, we call them Posies, and do paint them now a dayes upon the backe sides of our fruite trenchers of wood, or use them as devises in rings and armes."[82] Poesies printed onto food constitute the "void verse" that moralists denounced. Whether carried home as a party favor or eaten at the banquet, confectionery was, in Puttenham's thinking, constituent of and framed by a type of writing that was experientially different from that consumed in book culture. The production and consumption of sweetmeats were delicious acts of social display and performance. Yet food texts were—as Plat's recipe for engraving "armes, posies, or other devises" on eggshells demonstrates—valued precisely because of their ephemerality and fragility. Plat's assurance that his miraculously versified eggshell would amaze beholders chimes with Puttenham's story of the occasional nature of food-writing.[83] We can speculate about how the media of food might have inflected poesy writing. For example, if someone transcribed the motto "My beginning and my end" (found on a gold gimmel wedding ring)[84] onto transient sugar paste, how might those enduring bonds signify in this evanescent form? Would the posies' anticipated disappearance nullify the declaration? Stage its "end" comically? Eroticize the bond by delivering it in a form that could be taken orally into a body? Or would the dessert simply rearticulate the poem's meaning in another, albeit tasty, realm? Desserts provided new and challenging arenas in which housewives and gentlewomen might inflect the meaning of verses when framing them within a new material "reading" experience. These edible texts, the equivalent of early modern fortune cookies, are not the bathetic exception but virtually a staple of food culture.

In order to contextualize the meanings of early modern lettered food, we might turn to Ben Jonson's poem "Inviting a Friend to Supper," which embeds the consumption of poetry within the consumption of food in two distinct ways. Echoing classical invitation poems, the poet beckons a friend to a sumptuous dinner that offers unfettered fare as well as unfettered speech. The fantasy of unlimited food and conversation strains against the modest offerings that the host reasonably can provide. Food and words serve as commensurate gestures of hospitality and are thus metonymically associated. The speaker pledges to have a servant read pieces of classical literature to inspire free commentary: "Of which, we'll speak our minds, amidst our meat."[85] Yet the literal inscription of verses onto food creeps into the poem, in a passage that requires some glossing: "I'll profess no verses to repeat: / To this, if aught appear, which I know not of / That will the pastry, not my paper, show of" (ll. 24–26). In enumerating the enticing liberties of his meal, the speaker promises not to bore guests by reading verses (presumably his own). The now conventional reading of these lines, first offered by Roger Cognard and now appearing in glosses to most editions, is that the pastry is unwittingly imprinted by the recycled book pages used as food wrappers by merchants. Writers in many eras—Horace, Martial, Pope, Swift, Dryden, Fielding, Byron—lamented the indignity they suffered in knowing that their books could easily descend to become casings for greasy pies or waste paper to plug holes in barrels.[86] Jonson's poem, straddling the line between fantasized extravagance and deliberate moderation, imagines the humbling fate of his unsold pages appearing without his permission, in degraded form, at his banquet.

Joseph Loewenstein reads Jonson's mention of imprintation as a sign of authorial anxiety about the commercial iteration of print. For Loewenstein, Jonson saw in food the prospect of any potentially "fugitive" printed words that could unwittingly escape authorial control.[87] An equally plausible reading views these lines from the perspective of the poem's final celebration of liberty, which appreciates the unfixed nature of printed language. The pastry wrapper will be discarded after its greasy baptism and thus, like potentially seditious table talk, evade the punitive measures of spies ("Pooly" or "Parrot," two spies are mentioned in l. 36) or censors: "Nor shall our cups make any guilty men: / But, at our parting, we will be, as when / We innocently met" (ll. 37–39). The poem's insistence that there will be no conversational leftovers supports an interpretation of the speaker as celebrating the disintegration of language and larks. Whether as a form of liberating evanescence or a degrading rejection of value, the wrapped pastry points to a food-writing that guests enjoy at a remove from the more restrictive environment of book reading. While numerous writers lament that their pages might serve as functional commercial and domestic products, few mention the possibility that food might be inadvertently marked by words. Jonson's poem interestingly raises the prospect of early modern tarts as ephemeral commonplace books bearing letters, ink stains, phrases, and sentences. In this culinary recycling, words disassociate from their written or printed context and are recast as fragments re-experienced in the particular moment of biting into a lamb pie or quince tart.

But there is another way to interpret these lines, which I hope will be obvious by now: the speaker might refer not to iterations of printed words on pastry created by a wrapper but to food marked with writing by the cook. The fact that the speaker imagines verses "which [he] know[s] not of" suggests that the poems might not be his at all but instead the "devises" that recipe books urged readers to "print" onto sugar paste and marzipan. The fact that the pastry is made the agent of presentation ("that will the pastry. . . show of") supports this interpretation. The difference is significant. Instead of language reused by people who no longer care to read the pages, this supper proudly exhibits food-authored letters and designs. In this interpretation, Jonson's speaker does not reference the threat of the commercial print marketplace or bemoan the loss of authorial control with pretended humility. He instead registers a hitherto unrecognized liberty of the meal: poesies made by a cook (at home or purchased from a confectioner's shop) might enter the space of freely exchanged discourse. And Jonson's poem allows for both readings: it might refer to the fleeting phrases and pages circulating around London foodstuffs *and* to inscribed dishes common at the table.

When John Donne added a commendatory poem to the many mocking poems prefacing Thomas Coryat's travel book, he mentions the practice of recycling book pages. Connecting the author's travels to the personified book's recirculation in print, Donne commands Coryat:

> Go bashful man, lest here thou blush to look
> Upon the progress of thy glorious book,
> To which both Indies sacrifices send;
> The West sent gold, which thou didst freely spend,
> (Meaning to see 't no more) upon the press.

> The East sends hither her deliciousness;
> And thy leaves must embrace what comes from thence,
> The myrrh, the pepper, and the frankincense.
> This magnifies thy leaves.[88]

The material resources spent in producing the book (both the cost of travel and the cost of having the book printed) are contrasted with the exotic spices that the reused pages will "embrace" after the book is discarded, a set of interactions that Donne teasingly portrays as moments of global cultural contact. Inverting the usual complaint that great words descend into household garbage, Donne celebrates this evolution as a component of the rich cycle of textual production. Coryat's leaves will be "magnified," enlarged, and enriched by their intimacy with sacred medicinal spices. The speaker then moves down the food chain to imagine Coryat's text enfolding medicines, cheap shop goods and, finally, home-made wares:

> If they stoop lower yet, and vent our wares,
> Home-manufactures, to thick popular fairs;
> If omni-pregnant there, upon warm stalls,
> They hatch all wares for which the buyer calls;
> Then thus thy leaves we justly may commend,
> That they all kind of matter comprehend. (ll. 43–48)

The tone here is hard to interpret, because the poem so thoroughly ridicules Coryat's excesses at points. But the proliferation and ennobling of *matter* that Donne imagines in pages that "comprehend" (behold, understand, embrace) other substantial forms does not seem ironic (and here we might be guided by Donne's other evocative poetic meditations on substantiality and meaning). The housewives who sell pastries and confections at fairs keep in circulation a significant mode of production as the book amplifies in its reuse.

The practice of having printed pages wrap foods is significant for understanding food writing, even if Jonson's poem means to evoke the conscious food-imprint by the cook. For Donne's poem, certainly part of an authorial roast that mocks Coryat's buffoonery and pretension, reflects a serious early modern understanding of the substantiality of text, letter, and language, a topic most recently excavated by Jeffrey Masten. Asking why so many eroticized naked boys populated historiated capitals, Masten speculates about the possible psychic and social relations structured around capitalized letters: "A printed early modern letter might be seen as something that combines features for which we have no single term: a rebus, a body, a character (with a character's desires, habits, social relations), a pictogram, an ideogram." Masten suggests that early modern printers and publishers had "identifications and fantasies through the practices of the letter that we would think of as psychically structured."[89] The cinnamon capitals that women fashioned are no longer here for our inspection (indeed this was precisely part of their thrilling consumable meaning); but clearly they functioned as sites for psychic and social identification, embedded as they were in freighted moments of hospitality, making, and consumption. As crunchy ideograms, they enabled the pleasurable display of conspicuously consumable commodities as well as the forging of patronage, erotic, and/or other social relations.

Even as it contrasted with the durability of other artistic forms, confectionery can be put on a continuum with early modern textile art, which, as Frye, Jones, Stallybrass, Bianca Calabresi, and Jennifer Munroe have argued, formed a central component of aristocratic women's "writing."[90] Early modern women embroidered stories, scenes, shapes, designs, knots, verses, and—most notably— varying scripts and "hands" onto fabrics as they created expressive crafts.[91] Two enormous "commonplace books" or "copybooks" (for lack of better classifying terms) created by Thomas Trevelyon at the beginning of the seventeenth century offer spectacular examples of sewing designs.[92] The Trevelyon text displays exquisitely drawn, multicolored, and detailed patterns of gods and goddesses, English kings, plants, trees, animals, weaponry, and geometric shapes. It includes six different alphabets, some with complex latticework and others where weapons, gargoyles, and animals flow from letters. As in modern fonts offered by computer software, these samples presented creative options for those eager to manipulate the alphabet in thread and fabric.

Given that needlework, writing, and confectionery were rendered through a shared lexicon and were proximate household tasks, it's reasonable to think of these pattern books as offering templates for those who wanted to inscribe food. The Trevelyon manuscript, that is, might well register the sensual literacy of the banquet table. "Cutwork," the term seen on the title page to the 1634 guide *Schoolhouse of the Needle*, referred to openwork embroidery designs or appliqué patterning.[93] *A Book of Curious and Strange Inventions*, a sixteenth-century English reprint of a Venetian text, similarly described needlework patterns as "singuler and fine sortes of Cut-workes."[94] Given this vocabulary, it's telling that Lady Borlase collected a recipe for how "to make paste for a lace tart or to make Little Cakes cut in works," for she implies that the same "cut" patterns might be applied across media—fabric, strings, walls, embroidered jewelry cases, bed hangings, table linens, or sweetmeats (65). The expressive, social, political, and artistic acts that scholars have recovered from textile objects lend insight to the way edible "devices" functioned.

In *The Anatomy of Melancholy,* Robert Burton recommended women's domestic practice as an early modern antidepressant; he saw labor and sociality as staving off melancholy. Burton approvingly described how women use "curious needleworks, cutworks, spinning, bone-lace, and many pretty devices of their own making, to adorn their houses, Cushions, Carpets, Chairs, Stools . . . confections, conserves, distillations, &c. which they shew to strangers."[95] Burton's ambiguous phrasing allows for the possibility that the same "devises" used to adorn furniture and wall hangings were printed onto kitchen confections. After all, Woolley described food work (such as pie-shaping) as part of home décor, along with embroidery, picture-framing, and table arrangement. In *A Supplement to the Queen-Like Closet,* Woolley offered tips for how "to adorn a Room with Prints," which involves stenciling figures, landscapes, mythological gods, and stories onto glass plates, flowerpots and walls (1674; 70–71). She gave advice on how to make waxworks, including realistically rendered fruits, imprints of body parts, or even death masks (home-made wax molds of a corpse's face).[96] Scholars have appreciated that sewing and embroidery were principal female arts, though they have only recently understood the intellectual and social negotiations of these labors. Recipes allow us to see an early modern world of female food "writing," one that might have included experimentation with letter forms and flourishes as well as acrostics, anagrams, signatures, monograms, and poesies. Yet these displayed luxury items principally took value from their perishability. As such, recipes expand our grasp of the media used in domestic making, where "writing" was imagined to have dimensionality. Recipes also provide a crucial impetus for rethinking the developmental models often assumed in studies of literacy. Rather than seeing carving and confectionery as preparatory or initial stages in a progression that culminated with etching words on paper, we should reconceive these "literate" activities as overlapping and intertwined spheres of competency. In writing recipes into collections, women transferred expertise in confectionery onto paper, but they also might have used the design work and letter types of their printed and written materials as blueprints for imprinting pastries, cakes, and desserts. The elaborate design work in Elizabeth Fuller's recipe book might well have provided a

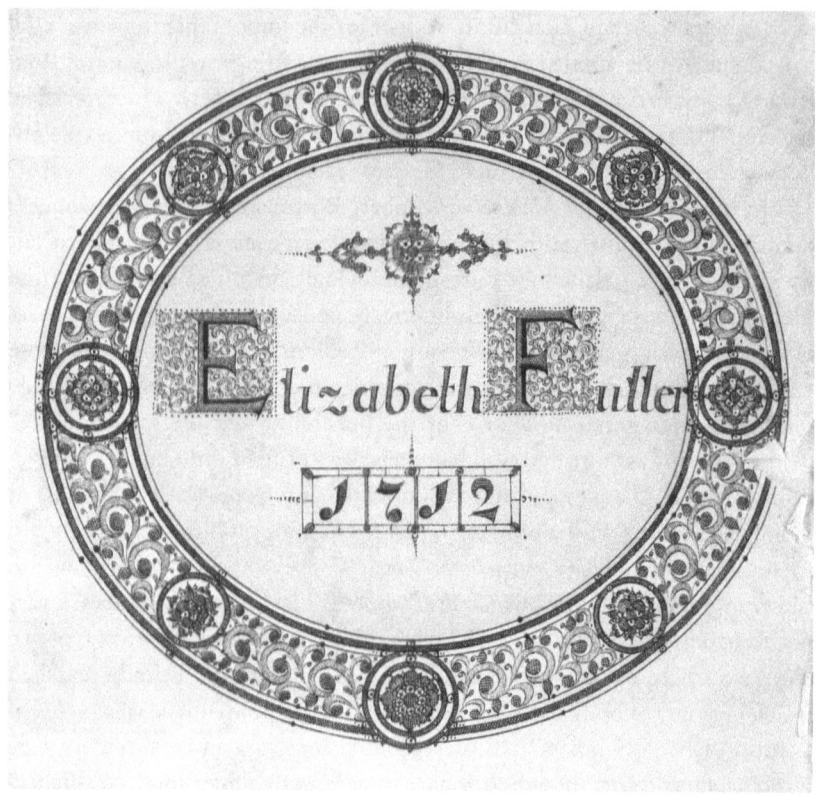

FIGURE 40. Title page to Elizabeth Fuller's *Collection of Cookery and Medical Receipts*, 1712–1822, Wellcome Library, MS 2450.

template for other domestic designs, on food or other materials (Figure 40). Food work, that is, was a desired "literate" endpoint. From the burst of initial recipe books in the late sixteenth century until the mid-seventeenth century (when recipe users no longer created posy-inscribed pastries), the domestic world was filled with inscribed, engraved, and printed objects that included edible visual signifiers. In a culture in which language was offered repeatedly (however skeptically) as a bulwark against mutability, culinary writing ironized that general cultural project by producing signifiers that would not and could not outlive their local moment. Culinary literacy not only provided a different sensory experience of letters, but also new meanings emanating from their particular substance.

People of "Letters"

While I have thus far emphasized ways that recipes contribute to the revisionary project of broadening and redefining literacy itself, they also might conventionally signal a "person of letters," the cultural accomplishment of being learned, knowledgeable about letters, or well-read. Recipe writing was in dialogue with other forms of writing recognized as literate. Bridget Parker's recipe book, for instance, included a twenty-eight-line set of rhymed couplets, the ending of which adapted lines from one of John Donne's poems.[97] A collection attributed to Mary Baumfylde (but composed by many hands) interspersed metrically challenging poems among advice on medicines and foods. Grace Blome Randolph's recipe collection, as we will see in Chapter 4, included a Pindaric ode heralding the death of Lady Oxendon, a tribute that circulated in prestigious female poetic circles. According to Jayne Elisabeth Archer, poetry had an affinity with recipe writing that made these textual collisions more than coincident. "The recipe and the poem were, to use terminology employed by Susan Fry in a related context, "'wrought' texts," as Archer writes, ones "operating at the interface between mind and matter, the recipe expressed the human desire to remodel the material world."[98]

In addition to edging into conventionally recognized "literary" writing, some recipe collections displayed other recognizable intellectual skills. Sarah Hughes offered a dual language translation of a Spanish recipe collection, complete with running commentary on the difficulty of linguistic translation. For Hughes, the subject of cookery and medical care provided a means for comparing grammatical forms used in Spanish and English recipe writing as well as an index of culturally distinct methods and practices. Other recipe compilers included religious and political satire. "How to make a right Presbyterian in two days," a recipe found in a collection of foods and medicines, purported to metamorphose an ordinary person into someone who could run down the church, delude the people, and foment rebellion. The writer commands:

> Take the herbs of hypocrisie and ambition of each two handfuls of the flowers of formality two scruples of the spirit of pride and malice two drams each of the seeds of contention & stubbornness of each four ounces of the cordial of reflection and lyes of each fifty ounces, of the root of moderation as small a quantity as you please. Drink the cordiall, chop the herbs, powder the seeds, slice the roots, bruse

them all together in a morter of vainglory with pestles of contradiction & deceit, put them in a pan of canting water to be infused over a brimstone fire of fained zeal . . . when lukewarm take the person that is to be made a Presbyterian take two spoonfulls night and morning, and when [he] is full of this hellish compound let him make wry mouths and squeese out some tears of dissimulation.[99]

Like the similarly minded mock recipe "How to make a Jacobine," which was inscribed on the flyleaf to an eighteenth-century manuscript collection, this recipe loosely followed the satirical tradition exemplified in the publication of *The Court & Kitchin of Elizabeth, Commonly Called Joan Cromwel[l], the Wife of the Late Usurper* (1664), recipes designed to show Elizabeth Cromwell's failed, vulgar, and overly frugal domestic practices.[100] And recipe texts could range from religio-political satire to the verbal witticism that we saw, in the previous chapter, exemplified in playful food dishes. Witness the family teasing memorialized in a recipe explaining "how to collar a pig," which is glossed, "Grace Forster Junior is the Hogg in question."[101] Like the punning "best of harabella" spun out of a name, Forster offered a playful jab at a family member's pig-like behavior while contemplating collaring pigs and making puddings.

It is precisely the tension between the drive to create socially decorous food and the playful, literate, intellectual, and expressive productions of the recipe world that makes this archive so ideologically evasive and interesting. The most prominent scholarly avenues for thinking about writing in a domestic context have emphasized its regulatory functions. Until recently feminist scholars have assumed that early modern domestic productions, textual or otherwise, were inherently politically disempowering. To be "domesticated" has often been assumed to be synonymous with loss of political agency or conformity to socially normative strictures; the simple fact of being located within a household has been read as marking exclusion from a supposedly "public" or "economic" sphere. Elias's account of the "civilizing process" has also shaped interpretations of handwriting and of domestic practice as part of disciplinary regimes designed to police internal self-regulation and bolster an emerging modern state formation. Whether one accepts Elias's larger conclusions or not, his master narrative does help us to see that handwriting and housewifery were *prescriptively* codified as part of a drive to harness unruly passions as part of the experience of early modern selfhood. Manuals teaching manners and penmanship tried to shape the mind (the "character") as something made "manifest" in deportment, bodily movement, and the "hand" (another term for "character"). "Minde, hand, and eye, must all together goe," wrote schoolmaster Peter Bales.[102] The hand that learned to write, Goldberg argues within an Eliasian framework, was simultaneously written; it was materially formed within institutions that constrained and subjected personhood. Goldberg's emphasis on prescriptive manuals rather than practice, much like feminist work relying on widely circulated domestic ideals rather than evidence of uncanny household experiences, leads to an overemphasis on the regulatory nature of handwriting.[103] What, I ask, of the relatively less supervised food writer and recipe user in the household? We might refine scholarly understanding of the ideological effects of literacy instruction and domestic labor by conscripting a new archive as the basis for evidence. Signs of practice reveal the provisional nature of the hand's regulation, moments when writers failed to attend properly to linguistic and social disciplinary codes and instead produced unorthodox motions of the hand.

I am arguing that recipes unearth a domestic set of experiences and competencies that were potentially at odds with the prescriptive idealizations of the "good housewife." As I have discussed elsewhere, the idea that housework inevitably bridled women's intellectual ambitions or curbed their unruly wills was only one fantasy among many in the early modern world. While numerous conduct writers urged women to undertake domestic labor so as to avoid idleness, suppress imaginative waywardness, and shape their submission, others recognized the liberatory potential of household labors and productions. Introducing Margaret Roper's 1526 translation of Erasmus, for example Richard Hyrde contrasted the disciplinary modality of education to the domestic realm, where a woman's mind was free to "compasse many pevysshe fantasyes."[104] To get a sense of the tension between the mannered dispositions of the hand and the license such dispositions could be imagined to afford in the domestic realm, we might return to the art of carving. Although still undertaken by male servants in the upper echelon of noble households, carving was a task increasingly assigned to housekeepers and ladies in the seventeenth century. As a theatrical social display, carving offered women and aspiring serving men the opportunity to exhibit markers of social grace through manual skill. When cutting meat, fish, and fowl, the housewife was warned to mask her appetite and restrain her bodily movements; she was also to make precise cuts to allow the best portions of flesh to be allocated to people of highest rank at the table. Serving meat tested bodily control, composure, and manners. *The Gentlewomans Companion* describes a grotesque dinner scene in which a gentlewoman fails the test by intermixing her sweat and saliva with the juicy meat she carved: "I have been invited to Dinner, where I have seen the good Gentlewoman of the House sweat more in cutting up of a Fowl, than the Cookmaid in roasting it; and when she had soundly beliquor'd her joints, hath suckt her knuckles, and to work with them again in the Dish; at the sight whereof my belly hath been three quarters full, before I had swallowed one bit" (65). As sweat lubricates the dish and the gentlewoman's "joints" blend with the "joints" of meat, the line between human and animal/food blur. Instead of refinement, the carver reveals her connection with the sweaty kitchen maid and gooey meat.

In its prescriptive incarnation in guides, carving thus seems to fit the "civilizing process" narrative. It reveals "domestication" as part of the history of manners, including the regulation of appetite, the propriety of body deportment, and the internalization of social stratification. But the lexical range of the early modern term "carve" brings to the fore the unruly potential of the practice, for the term was used figuratively to indicate a person's expressive agency. When Laertes warns Ophelia about the limited choice that a prince has in his erotic life, he says of Hamlet: "He may not, as unvalued persons do, / Carve for himself" (1.3.19–20). Carving for oneself, as Laertes implies, was an assertion of will. When pertaining to women's labor, this power was predictably expressed as sexual agency. In Shakespeare's *Merry Wives of Windsor* the debauched knight Falstaff declares his attraction to Alice Ford by interpreting her "carving" as flirtatiousness. In a vulgar rendition of "can she carve or can she carve?" Falstaff states, "She discourses, she carves, she gives the leer of invitation" (1.3.38–39). To Falstaff's mind, carving advertises an expressive power associated with desire. Alice Ford's display of apportioning food and discriminating among her guests in Windsor bespeaks an erotically charged domestic authority. Could carving for diners as a part of social display imply carving for oneself? Did carving letters on paper and sweets reveal the ideological tensions evident in carving at the table? Did "handwriting" and "handiwork" constitute similarly regulated functions whose potential for going pointedly awry was recognized?

When recipe collections trained the hand in unsupervised settings far from centers of learning, they generated estranging literacies: hands that lent moral sayings unexpected meaning because cut into extravagant and ephemeral substances; hands that toyed with signatures and claims of self-possession; hands that tested writing styles and designs across food, paper, and walls. Even in the drive to acquire recognizably prestige penmanship, recipe writers deployed inventiveness in determining the *content* of their writing; they registered what Hyrde might have identified as the "pevysshe fantasyes" stretching across domestic literacies.

We detect evidence of domestic license in early modern textual doodles, which Sandra Sherman theorizes as having an intimate, though not exclusive, connection to the recipe form: "As a type of off-the-cuff, not fully deliberated performance, the doodle acknowledges the text's power to induce spontaneity. . . . Though doodling is a parody of the text's utility, an act of conspicuous idleness, it is also an objective correlative of how one can visit the [recipe] text, using the text to suit one's impulse."[105] Whether or not one agrees that the recipe's invitation to action necessarily creates "spontaneity," Sherman's provocative analogy points us to think about the "impulse" evident in recipe textual graffiti. The doodler of spiral designs and words in cursive italic on the opening pages of Penelope Patrick Jephson's recipe collection, for instance, unwittingly called attention to recipe work as an artifactual production. Near Jephson's signature, the words "to make" float in a space isolated from any sentence (Figure 41).[106] Because this unassuming infinitive serves as the opening command in most recipes (for example, "to make collops of veal"), it makes

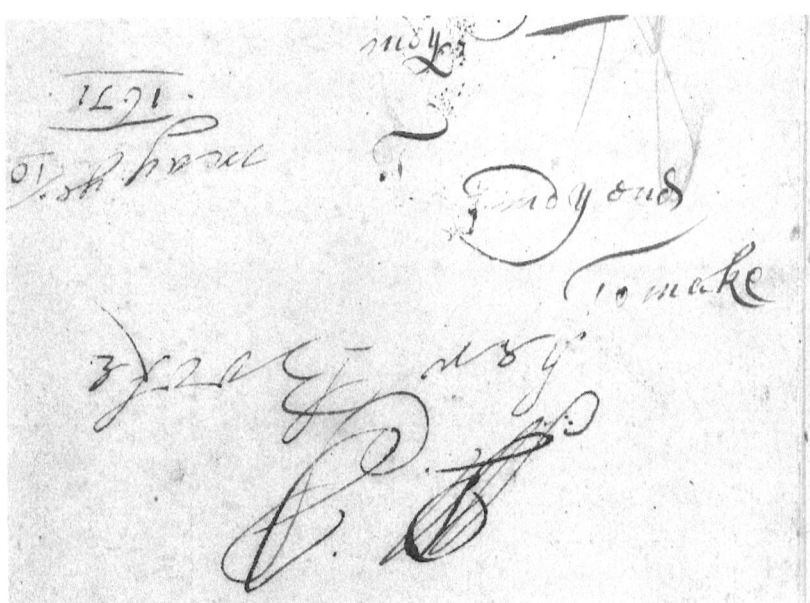

FIGURE 41. "To Make," practice writing in Penelope Patrick Jephson's *Receipt Book*, 1671, 1674–75, Folger Shakespeare Library, MS V.a.396, part 2, fol. 2. Reproduced by permission of the Folger Shakespeare Library.

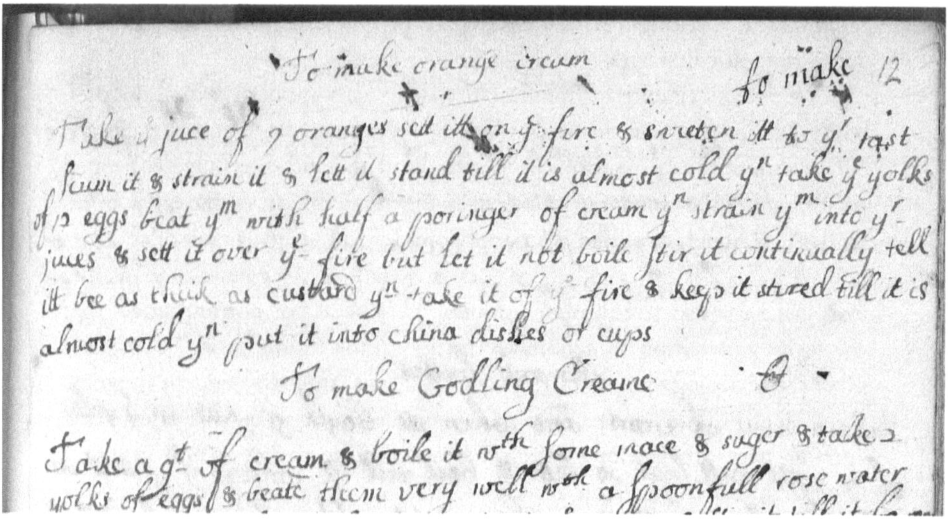

To make orange cream   to make

Take y juce of 9 oranges sett it on y fire & sweeten it to y tast
scum it & strain it & lett it stand till it is almost cold yn take y yolks
of 12 eggs beat ym with half a poringer of cream yn strain ym into y
juces & sett it over y fire but let it not boile stir it continually tell
it bee as thick as custard yn take it of y fire & keep it stired till it is
almost cold yn pout it into china dishes or cups

To make Codling Creame

Take a qt of cream & boile it with some mace & suger & take 2
yolks of eggs & beate them very well with a spoonfull rose water

FIGURE 42. Elizabeth Brockman, *Receipts and Exercises*, ca. 1674–87, British Library, MS 45199. Reproduced by permission of the British Library.

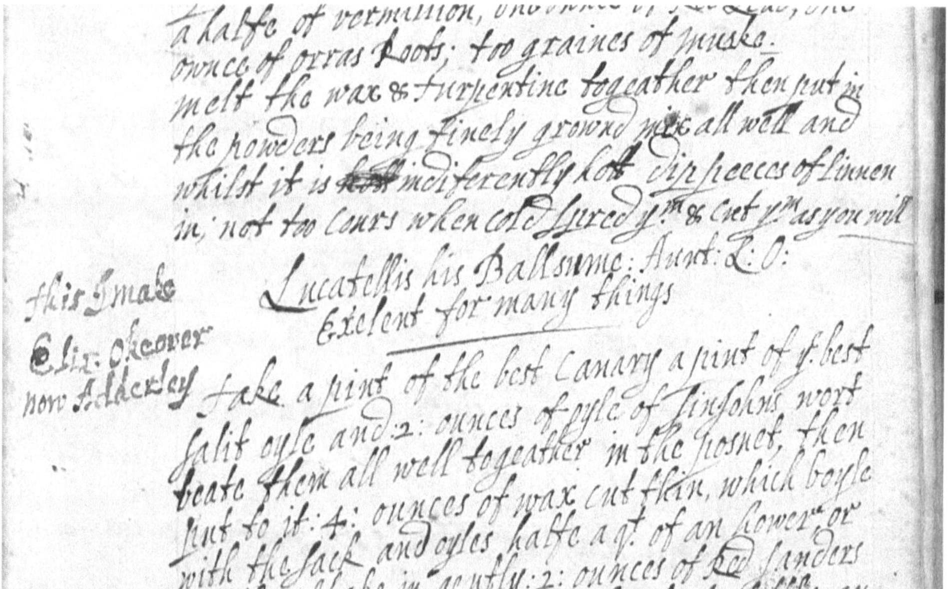

a halfe of vermilion, one ounce of [...], one
ounce of orras roots; too graines of muske.
melt the wax & turpentine togeather then put in
the powders being finely ground mix all well and
whilst it is indifferently hott dip peeces of linnen
in, not too coars when cold sized ym & cut ym as you will

This I make   Lucatellis his Ballsume : Aunt: E: O:
Eliz: Okeover   Exelent for many things
now Adderley   take a pint of the best Canary a pint of y best
            salit oyle and 2: ounces of oyle of St Johns wort
            beate them all well togeather in the posnet, then
            put to it: 4: ounces of wax cut thin, which boyle
            with the sack and oyles halfe a qt of an hower or
            more shake in gently: 2: ounces of red sanders

FIGURE 43. Elizabeth Okeover, *Collection of Medical Receipts*, ca. 1675–ca. 1725, Wellcome Library, MS 3712.

sense that a recipe compiler would want to form these particular words with care. After all, in several recipe books, including those attributed to Amy Eyton and to Elizabeth Brockman (Figure 42), compilers and/or readers have etched the word "make" on the flyleaf. Yet this phrase, drifting free of any semantic framework, could attach to grand aspirations. In his *Defense of Poesy*, Philip Sidney asserted the classical definition of the poet as a maker, elaborating the fact that the Renaissance word for poet derived from the Greek word for "maker" (*poiesis*). "Making" was often the verb used in Renaissance poetry to describe artistic feats. When a character in Spenser's *The Shepheardes Calendar* wonders about his friend's "skill to make so excellent," the reader knows that he is talking about poetic talent.[107] Jephson did not mean, of course, to present herself as a laureate artist when she recorded recipes for orange marmalade and face washes. Neither did Elizabeth Okeover when she boasted, "This I Make. E.O." in the margin of her collection (she probably only wanted to signal a favorite recipe (Figure 43).[108] Yet the choice of the word "make" carried meanings. While compilers did not imagine themselves as makers in the sense embraced by humanist poets and thinkers of the day, they participated in a world where representation was itself artifactual and material. Devices and poems were "made" rather than thought. As such, the lexical crossing between *poiesis* and kitchen posies cannot be dismissed. The governing assumption of writing-as-making in this period created the imaginative conditions for understanding textualized domestic interiors and objects.

By 1750, published recipe books, as we have seen in previous chapters, assigned cooking to servants, leaving the woman of refined taste to remove her hand from the kitchen. Ladies of the house were no longer applauded for knowing the details of manual labor. I want to return to Glasse's 1775 *Art of Cookery*, which, I argued in Chapter 1, staged this division of labor in its engraved frontispiece. This image presents a recipe-reading lady of high fashion positioned outside of the kitchen, coiffed and attired in a manner that signals her leisure (Figure 44). We are now in a position to notice that the fowl being butchered in the kitchen is tellingly separated spatially and conceptually from the quill that rests on the mistress's writing table, as she copies a recipe and hands it to her servant. Through the doorway on the left, another servant works with the carcass of a dead goose or duck; in fact, the folds of the dress extending out of the recipe-receiving servant's arm blur into the animal corpse in the kitchen. This image beautifully contrasts the role of hands, which have drifted apart conceptually and practically: the hand writing the

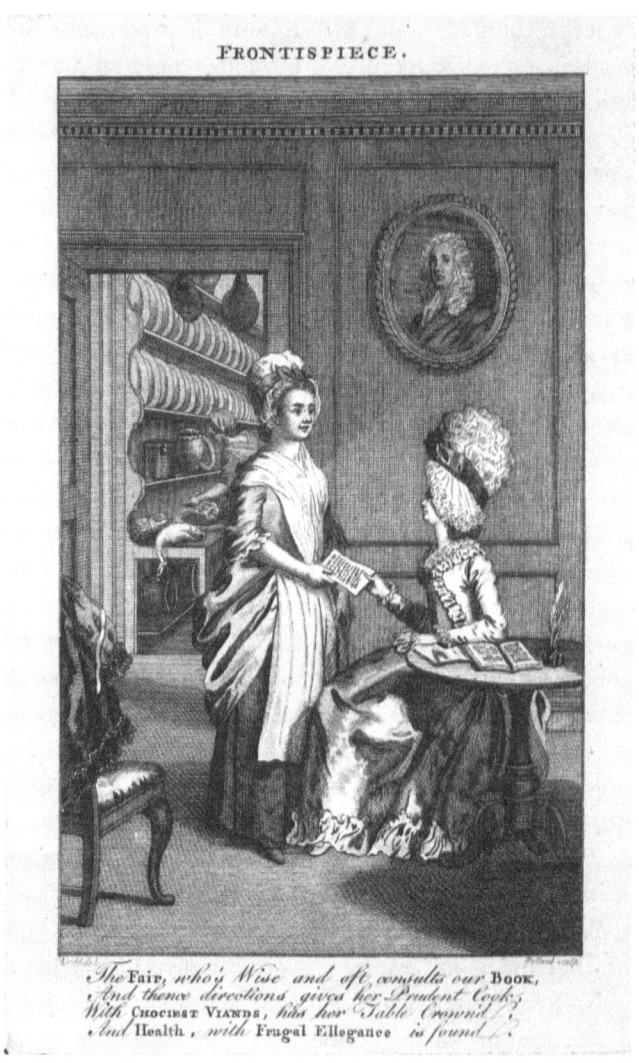

FIGURE 44. Frontispiece to Hannah Glasse, *The Art of Cookery* (London, 1775). By permission of the British Library.

recipes no longer carves flesh or incises meaning into edible substances. This later disjoining, with its implications for redefining handiwork and literacies, makes it all the more important to recover earlier manuscript sources, where joined hands disclosed household material inscriptions that crossed paper and food.

CHAPTER 4

Temporalities: Preservation, Seasoning, and Memorialization

> The Cook in *Plautus* . . . did not account it sawcinesse to call himselfe . . . The preserver of mankind. The Great Authour [of this book] . . . shewes you the Excellency of Kitchin-physick, beyond all Gally pots, and their Adherents. He doth in this Book teach you . . . To improve a Porters dinner into a Dish fit for a Princes Table, To make badde meat good, and good meat better. This Book is a Save-all; It suffers nothing to be lost. It will teach you to keep good houses, by keeping good things in them.
> —Theodore Mayerne, introducing a book of recipes, 1658

> The true economy of housekeeping is simply the art of gathering up all the fragments, so that nothing be lost. I mean fragments of *time*, as well as *materials*.
> —Lydia Maria Child, *The American Frugal Housewife*

What does a recipe allow a person to "keep"? Early modern recipe compilers and readers were invited to meditate on this question as they produced, circulated, and, occasionally, critiqued generic and broad fantasies of preservation. "Housekeeping" involved learning the nitty-gritty practices designed to conserve household resources as well as reflecting on the recipe's status as a written document created to endure over time. As people went about the practical tasks of making and managing material goods, they indulged in dreams of a world where humans might prevent or retard loss in a capacious sense. When the recipes of court physician Theodore Mayerne were printed in 1658, for instance, the publisher grandly identified them as techniques for rescuing and improving the sensible world. He did not feel that he needed to explain why a physician would offer advice about sweet cakes and jams rather than traditional remedies. Instead he assumed that his audience would understand the inclusivity of acts that "preserve[d] mankind." In this chapter, I explore what preservation meant as it emerged at the intersection of early modern domesticity and temporality. In this discursive register, recipes functioned as a site where material and abstract notions of preservation converged. They not only invited readers to manage the physical world through the artful reconfiguration of natural bodies and substances but also constituted textual forms that reiterated and duplicated those processes. As a textualization of domestic acts of salvage, the recipe archive was implicated in a process that "suffer[ed] nothing to be lost."

The key to understanding the management of time in recipe writing lies in investigating the early modern discourse coalescing around the lexical terms "seasoning" and "preserving" (and, to a lesser degree, "distilling"). These terms, I argue, not only named specific technical practices but also underwrote the philosophical categories through which people theorized their work. In order to tease out the intellectual puzzles of recipe writing, I examine figurative uses of recipe terminology in Shakespeare's *All's Well That Ends Well* (a work that showcases a recipe in its plot), in two Shakespearean sonnets, and in recipe writing. Reading forms that placed a premium on figurative denseness and associated meanings alongside "technical" writing demonstrates the crossover of semantic and intellectual inquiry carried out in each of these genres. From this broader perspective we are able to pinpoint the philosophical concerns about temporality enacted in domestic labor and recipe writing. This examination lays the groundwork for an analysis, in the final section, of the recipe as a written storage file of personal and collective events, one that compilers and readers placed in relation to time.

'Tis the Season

Shakespeare's early seventeenth-century play *All's Well That Ends Well*, begins with two powerful men dead and a king gravely ill. In the opening scene, the Countess of Rossillion introduces her ward Helena by praising Helena's tears as externalizing virtue and preserving a dead father's memory: "'Tis the best brine a maiden can season her praise in. The remembrance of her father never approaches her heart but the tyranny of her sorrows takes all livelihood from her cheek," states the countess (1.1.42–45).[1] The Riverside edition's representative gloss on "season," as to "preserve, a culinary image," suggests that Shakespeare introduces Helena through the quaint image of her pickling—or preserving—abstractions, both her father's memory and her immaterial qualities, which are manifest in and made durable by her briny tears.[2] Readers familiar with Shakespeare's works might think of Shakespeare's *Twelfth Night*, which opens with a similar image. Valentine describes the Countess Olivia in mourning:

> Like a cloistress, she will veilèd walk
> And water once a day her chamber round
> With eye-offending brine—all this to season
> A brother's dead love, which she would keep fresh
> And lasting in her sad remembrance. (1.1.27–31)

While Olivia is imagined to use her conserving tears as a conscious and ritualistic means of reanimating her passionate memory of her brother, Helena is seen as inadvertently brining her *own* virtues by spontaneously weeping over the loss of her father. Both texts might appear to be making a gently devaluing analogy between mourning and cookery through the use of the term "seasoning." Yet these texts are instead alluding, I argue, to a complex process that involves managing time by tempering substances.

What does this culinary trope imply? In *All's Well*, Helena's seasoning figures an act of preservation as well as an enhancement of value. This meaning of the term registers prominently in recipe writing, which disproportionately featured preserved foods made from a variety of fruits (cherries, apples, gooseberries, raspberries, grapes, apricots, and quinces), nuts, meats (potted, salted, and dried), flowers, and vegetables. Preserves were by far the most popular subject of recipe collections. In a world without mass-produced canning or refrigeration, it was especially imperative to devise homemade methods for delaying the expiration date of produce from the garden or market. Often a reader of printed or manuscript recipes would turn the pages of thirty consecutive recipes that repeated the reassuring mantra: "this will keep." Elizabeth Fowler concluded more than a dozen recipes with variations of the phrase, "keep them for your use." Mary Baumfylde boldly said of her roses, "keep them for long as you please" (fol. 21). Susannah Packe claimed that her China oranges (as opposed to bitter Seville oranges) might serve as an "excellent Sweetmeate" although "they will not keep long." "Yet I," she could not resist boasting, "have keep them halfe a yeare very good" (7). And, as we have seen previously, Ann Goodenough effused about the pleasure of freezing in time— or rather in sugar—blooming flowers when she advised on "how to Candy Violetts or any other [f]lowers and Keepe them that they will looke as Fresh as when they are first gathared."³ Clearly the attraction of these foods was not merely their tastiness and visual complexity but the simple fact that they allowed for seasonal variety. As a functional luxury good, preserves attenuated, even as they marked, the problem of existing as beings in time.

For Plat, whose *Delightes for Ladies* was important in shaping recipe discourse, the mimetic features of confectionery were intricately linked to the kitchen's power to supplement and surrogate nature. As we have seen, Plat waxed eloquent about the representational power of sugar works and the ideologies of taste that these enabled. We can now appreciate the fact that his love of culinary illusions was bound up with his belief that conserves signaled a triumphant human mastery of nature. Plat zeroed in on how domestic work could interrupt the destructive temporal cycles that he imagined within the ubiquitous language of "consumption." In the lofty poem prefacing *Delightes for Ladies*, Plat theorized housework as providing a limited exemption from the natural world, as he grandly proclaimed, in mock heroic couplets, that housework could translate winter into summer:

> When chrystall frosts hath nipt the tender grape,
> And cleane consum'd the fruits of every vine,
> Yet heere behold the clusters fresh and faire,
> Fed from the branch, or hanging on the line.
> The walnut, small nut, and the Chesnut sweete,
> Whose sugred kernels loose their pleasing taste,
> Are here from yeere to yeere preserved,
> And made by Arte with strongest fruites to last.
> Th' artichoke, the apple of such strength,
> The Quince, the Pomgranate, with the Barberie,
> No sugar us'd, yet colour, taste, and smell,
> Are here maintain'd and kept most naturally. (A3)

In semiparodic and semiearnest tenors, Plat claimed that his recipes could undo time and reverse the "chrystall frost" that so blithely seemed to have devoured the tender grape. As a personified force, winter competed with humans who paradoxically used "arte" to "maintain" the organic world "naturally." Plat then tellingly chose to open his guide with "The Art of Preserving," a section whose seventy-three recipes far exceeded those offered in the other units: "Secrets in Distillation" (twenty-five recipes), "Cookery and Housewifery" (forty-one recipes), and "Sweet Powders and Ointments" (thirty-seven recipes). I will return to Plat's particular language in these lines, but here I want to stress Plat's theorization of practice as combating temporality precisely by means of "keeping."

Seasoning did not solely, however, serve a preservative function. "Seasonal knowledge" was a broad, complicated, and inclusive category in domestic guides and recipe books. As home herbalists, gardeners, and pharmacists, early modern women were instructed to *submit* to time by fully understanding and inhabiting the rhythms of change over the year. It was vital to learn the rules governing the organic world so as to understand the precise months and times of day when plants and herbs had potency and when particular foodstuffs were beneficial. Recipe readers were thus continually invited to endorse the seasonal elements of their knowledge. For the most prominent writers of technical guides, the harvesting of herbs constituted *the* foundational knowledge of housewifery.[4] Partridge's *Treasurie of Commodious Conceits* devotes an entire section to the "special time" of herbs (D7v). Markham opened the cookery section to the popular *English Housewife* with an excursus about the proper year, day, moon, and weather for cultivating plants (1623; 57–59). What the housewife had to grasp in her medical-culinary practice were flows of time, or, as a text held by Lady Marquess Dorset suggested in a mnemonic device, "the vertue of hearbs att all seasons."[5] Recipe writing issued an urgent injunction: one had to vigorously labor to *do* in the right instant so as to manage being in an organic world. In order to be effective as a restorative, the herb rosa solis had to be gathered only in June or July, observed Mary Doggett.[6] Elizabeth Okeover specified that fresh oranges for preserving could be harvested in February (fol. 178, p. 12). It is this meaning of seasoning—that of actively dwelling within the world of natural temporality—that underwrites Portia's assertion about virtue and aesthetics in *The Merchant of Venice*: "How many things by season seasoned are," she declares, "to their right praise and true perfection!" (5.1.106–7). Rather than using art to outmaneuver time, household workers, in this register of the term, sought to create value precisely by parsing time's elements with care. Imagined discursively within the work of the kitchen, humans were compelled to identify substances within their appropriate temporal location as the basis for a transformative knowledge. It is against this paradoxical concept of nature that we can better read the dramatic fantasy of preservation that saturates recipe writing, seen so clearly in the litany of assurances that the world, if apprehended correctly, will not slip by.

Recipe discourse had an equally pressing concern for *temporizing* as well as temporality. And here we need to think about the multiple meanings of *seasoning* and its cognates, which often collapse. As a verb, "to season," is derived from the Old French *saisonner*, "to ripen, to render (fruit) palatable by the influence of the seasons." This developmental meaning was then elaborated to describe the act of making a dish "palatable by the influence of a savoury ingredient" (1a), and it ultimately surfaced in the definition of seasoning as tempering a substance or person in order to make them "fit" (4) or fortified (4c). When Hamlet demurs from killing the praying Claudius because he seems "fit and seasoned for his passage" (3.3.86), he understands Claudius as tempered or readied spiritually for mortal harvest. We see that when tempering meant adding flavor to a dish (1a and 1b), the cook appropriated from Time the job of rendering materials palatable. While modern usage tends to separate these meanings grammatically, with *season* and *seasoning* as verbs pertaining centrally to flavoring, and *season*, as a noun, indicating a period of time, early modern usage blurred their meanings. The noun "season" occasionally took its verbal partner's meaning as flavoring; and to be "seasoned" could mean being flavored, fit for use or matured, or existing in proper time.[7] In recipe writing, the "season of meats" could strikingly modulate to refer to the time of year when animals were best slaughtered, the correct spices to be used to enhance meat's flavor, or the ingredients necessary for tempering meat to make it durable.[8]

In its meaning as flavoring, early modern seasoning was conceptualized within the physiological model of humoralism. In Galenic physiology, organic entities were constituted by properties corresponding to four fluid humors of the body. Because diet was one chief way in which the body's humors were balanced, maintained, and healed, cooking and medical care were structurally conjoined, more so even than in the modern world, where diet is imagined as the motor of good health. Early modern food preparation thus involved a temporizing process; one had to counter the attributes of particular ingredients with opposing features from others. As dietaries of the day articulated and recipe books assumed, the cook worked within the structural dynamic of humoralism to balance the properties of bodies with the foodstuffs they consumed. Assimilating ingredients in the kitchen, as Ken Albala has explained, meant reflecting on how to combine edibles with dissimilar properties, with an eye to negating and correcting the tendencies of an individual diner. Pepper, as a "hot" food for instance, could offset the coldness of ducks or of fish and stabilize people with phlegmatic constitutions.[9] When Markham recommended that a fresh water fish called a tench be seasoned with pepper, salt, nutmeg, oranges, and vinegar, he did not explain the theory driving his recommendation (1623; 93–94), but he understood that a "cold" fish needed hot and dry condiments. Seasoning was thus a *relational* process in which the characteristics of plants, foodstuffs, and persons had to be transacted with care. Rather than merely supplementing the organic world to make a dish tasty, the cook had to settle its potentially agonistic elements. In the sense of manipulating flavor and function, seasoning thus bore precisely opposite meanings: the act of intensifying flavor was simultaneously a moderation of an ingredient's effects.

Given that recipe writers did not distinguish medical from food recipes, domestic workers classified humans as one of the organic entities in need of "keeping." Humoral theory put humans squarely within an ecosystem, where the properties of animals, plants, herbs, and metals had to be brought into equilibrium as they were transferred into human bodies (which then added other variables to the project). Astonishingly, the word *preserve* is used in recipe collections as much in reference to humans suffering from ailments as it was to fruits and vegetables. In medical recipes, "preserving" could indicate three different aims: maintaining life by warding off disease, keeping people energetic, and eradicating the effects of aging.[10] While these tasks differed from preserving fruit (which sought to maintain cherries or the like over the course of a winter), they shared a structure and a vocabulary in recipes. In an herbal describing plants' benefits, the writer stated, "The conserve made of the floures of Rosmari is good for them that swoun & are week harted."[11] The conserve, a product tempered through the addition of sugar, could *conserve* the spirits (or energy) of those prone to fainting. Lettice Pudsey blended these meanings when she claimed that Dr. Stephen's water (the early modern Geritol) "preserveth helth: causeth long life: & is good against many desseases: . . . it is good against the shaking of the palsey: . . . it helpeth the conception of wemmen that bee barron: it killeth wormes in the belley: it cureth *the* cold & cough; it helpeth the tooth ach: helpeth the dropsy: it helpeth the stone & rines of the back: it cureth the stinking breath: & macketh one loock younge" (fol. 14–14v). Mary Doggett read preservation more narrowly as increasing longevity, while Mary Granville's prized recipe for distilled honey, as we have seen, promised to alleviate numerous ailments.[12] After heating and cooling white honey in a still until its color changed from "bloud" to "Rubie," it would undergo an almost alchemical transformation, as Granville described; it would

> be like to the coulor of gold, which then is most pleasant of savor, and soe sweet that nothing may bee compared like to it in fragrantnes of smell, [it] doth dissolue gold, and prepareth it to drinke. [It] is alsoe very comfortable to all those that are apt to have swounding fitts, and are used to faintings in the stomacke. . . . [L]ikewise if you wash any wound or stripe with this water, it doth in small time heale the same; this pretious water doth marvelously helpe the cough, the Rheume the desease of the Spleene, and many other deseases scarce to be believed; This water was administred, to a person sicke of the palsie for the space of 46 daies, and hee was by the mightie helpe of god, and this miraculous water, throughly healed of his desease, also this helpeth the falling sicknes, and preserveth the body from putrifying, soe that by all these wee may learne that this is as it were a divine water from heaven, and sent from God to serve unto all ages.[13]

Granville's distillation could be applied externally to wounds, used to freshen air or decompose gold, drunk to hearten weakness, and, most notably, taken to prevent the blood's putrefaction. In her ability to create a "miraculous" and "pretious" cure for coughs, fainting, palsy, and epilepsy, the housewife might assume the role of divine intermediary, possessing the alchemical and timeless power of the remedy itself (which was "sent from God to serve unto all ages").

In recipes, humans and edibles shared a structural place, as things in need of survival and duration. This substitutability was evident as well on the London stage, where characters joked that the housewife's passion to preserve the produce of the garden was saturated with eroticized fantasies about "keeping" humans for their pleasure. In *Il pastor fido* (a play known as *The Faithful Shepherd*), one character sarcastically urges women to use domestic know-how to manufacture secret paramours: "Learn women all from me this housewifery, / Make you conserve of Lovers to keep by."[14] "Keeping," in this register, points not only to a valued chemical transformation but also to a furtive possession (legible as well in the phrase "keeping" a mistress or lover). In John Crowne's *The Married Beau*, a character spins a cannibalistic vision of housewives' powerful transformations: "Conserve o' Man is more luscious," he notes, than conserve of roses.[15] By sexualizing and collapsing medical and preservative work, these comic allusions parody the preservation (with its attendant threat of destructive transformation) that housewifery entailed; they also eroticize the recipe's self-presentation of work-as-pleasure, discussed in Chapter 2, particularly the meanings available in the recipe phrase, "keep them as long as you please."

The idea that physical care was a modality of bodily preservation was a widespread sentiment that reverberated throughout early modern discourses. When Isabella Whitney, the first published female writer in England, declared the value of the popular versified adages she drew from (of all people) Hugh Plat, she employed, in a key moment, the metaphor of domestic preserving. In "A Sovereign Receipt," the poem used to finalize her presentation of 110 verses, she compares her "flowers," to moral ingredients that a reader should use to safeguard moral and healthy living:

> The Juce of all these Flowers take,
> and make thee a conserve:
> And use it first and laste: and it
> wyll safely thee preserve.[16]

In seeking to explain the use value of public writing, Whitney offers a poetic recipe in which reading preserves spiritual and physical being. She trades dually on the metaphor: the flowers should be taken out of natural time and made into a durable "conserve" which, when digested by the reader, could serve as a moral prophylactic against corruption. The reader is to be seasoned (tempered and rendered durable over time) through proper apprehension of the text; reading is a process of seasoning.

Because the decision of what and how to cook in the early modern period meant thinking about the physical complexions of household residents, recipe for carrots, cakes, and chickens could readily bring forth discussions of blood, retention, and organ inflammation. Cooking conjured up a world of "flesh" that united humans and animals within an economy of putrefaction. The realities of household butchery in an age before industrialization also meant that the live status of food and the mortal peril of food workers were often fully in view in the kitchen. As I argued in *Staging Domesticity*, domestic work's multi-purposing made mortality visible in everyday work.[17] Housewives were taught to slaughter animals so as to utilize their vital spirits and to convert "meate to puer blood."[18] In making medicine out of moles, Lady Borlase recommended that readers "Cutt *the* throats of them whilst alive & Let them bleed on a puter Dish or Plate as much as you can make them, then rip up *the* Bellies & take out the Lungs Gutts Young anes & all *the* Inards and Blood" and grind to a powder.[19] *The Compleat Servant-Maid* offers a similarly gruesome recipe for a restorative cockwater that began: "Take two Running Cocks, pull [pluck] them alive, then kill them, Cut them Cross on the Back, when they are almost cold take their Guts, and . . . break them all to pieces. "[20] The gory work of butchering, beating, and bleeding animals was not only part of life as usual but also a constituent element in the preservation of human health, part of the successive stages of destructive transformations that made up the ecosystem of health care. Is it any wonder that writer and philosopher Margaret Cavendish personified Death as a Cook who slowly roasts, boils, pickles, broils, sauces, jellies, stuffs, fricassees, stews, and dries people? "Death is the *Cook* of *Nature*," she wrote, "and we find / *Meat* drest severall waies to please her *Mind*. / Some *Meates shee* rosts with *Feavers, burning hot*, / And some *shee* boiles with *Dropsies* in a *Pot*."[21] Cavendish's horrific portrayal of diseased cooking has a counterpart in Shakespeare's *Titus Andronicus*, where the title character kills and "inters" his daughter's rapists into a pastry (commonly called a "coffin") to be consumed by their mother. The horrors of mortality that these fictions pathologize were glaringly visible in the kitchen.

Until the end of the seventeenth century, when humoralism was largely discredited, kitchen work made people aware of their location within a natural and cosmic food chain—a world in which a person, to paraphrase Hamlet, pointedly ate and was eaten. Determined acts of domestic preservation responded to what Julian Yates describes as the recognition of a nonanthropic general ecology in which human bodies are sites of (frightening) transformation by external agents; there is no human exceptionalism when the world is one great dinner in which everything, including humans, are "eaten" by organisms as they decay in the biosphere.[22] The food chain was literalized in epilepsy remedies that called for human skulls or *mummia* (liquid from corpses, made of decomposing human and embalming fluid).[23] Recipe labors sometimes exposed these issues as they attempted to suppress them. They participated in what Joyce Carol Oates has claimed that civilizing strategies always seek: to "obscure from human beings the sound of, the terrible meaning of, their jaws grinding."[24] Recipes partook of these "civilizing" strategies in attempting to hold at bay the consuming force of time even as they exposed the ultimate futility of their own measures. The lexicon of "seasoning" encapsulated this fraught process.[25]

In *Troilus and Cressida*, Shakespeare draws on the rich metaphorical potential of seasoning, laden with sexual innuendo and the taint of mortality. When Pandarus recommends Troilus to Cressida, he asks: "Do you know what a man is? Is not birth, beauty, good shape, discourse, manhood, learning, gentleness, virtue, youth, liberality, and so forth, the spice and salt that season a man?" (1.2.232–35). With looks, education, status, and morals going for him, Troilus is held up as a man perfectly developed and seasoned. Yet Cressida playfully refigures her uncle's terms: "Ay, a minced man—and then to be baked with no date in the pie, for then the man's date is out" (1.2.236–37). Punning on the word "date," a preserved fruit known for flavor and durability, Cressida renders her would-be lover "minced," chopped, and diminished. She imaginatively "unseasons" Troilus first by seeing him as a bland pie (with no tasty date), then as past his prime (his date is out). Tasting and time had to be intertwined in the culture for this joke to work; it plays on an association with clearly grimmer elements. "What sugar and spice really cured, in a word," writes Patricia Fumerton, speaking of aristocratic banqueting in the Renaissance "was mortality."[26]

The specter of death in the kitchen made temporality a pressing issue. Through repetition and juxtaposition of the related meanings of "seasoning," early modern recipes invited self-reflection about its contradictions and paradoxes. We find evidence of this self-reflection in Shakespeare's *All's Well*, a play that makes explicit the implicit puzzles revolving around temporality and seasoning in recipe writing. The play opens, as have seen, with the countess drawing a seemingly casual analogy between the main character's devoted weeping and the brining of memory and virtue. In the larger framework of the play, the French king is gravely ill, declared past hope by his retinue of formally trained doctors. Everyone is naturally skeptical when a young, untrained, nonaristocratic maiden marches into court and boldly offers a cure. In a riveting scene, the play's heroine, Helena, brokers a deal in which she risks her very life to gain the right to choose a husband and rise socially in the world. In a moment that departs from almost all other scenes of health care on the Renaissance stage, this "Doctor She," as she is called, succeeds; and a fairy tale–like story of riddles, sexual duplicity, false deaths, and covert pregnancies ensues (2.1.77).

Although critics have been interested in how Helena's unusual feat tests the limits of female agency as expressed in comedic form and in medical practice, they have largely ignored the fact that the secret of Helena's success is her expert wielding of a *written recipe*. It is this treasured text that allows Helena to reorient social/sexual relations, rehabilitate the polity, and make all end well.[27] Her dramatic moment of recipe healing is embedded, I argue, in the discourse of seasoning, a tissue of verbal associations that constellates the intellectual problems carried within manual labors. In probing the relationship between different meanings of *seasoning*, *All's Well* glosses ways that practitioners were invited to contemplate materiality in relation to temporality.

Influenced by Galenic and Paracelsian medical theories, the latter of which targeted symptoms rather than overall balance of humors, recipe collections commonly addressed the disease haunting the king in *All's Well*, the fistula.[28] Treatments for this tube-shaped ulcer or abscess (often located in the anus) took three primary forms: ingested herbal drinks,[29] externally applied ointments or bandages, and injected serums.[30] In a recipe attributed to his cousin Susanna Dutton, Archdale Palmer chose a pulverized onion-and-yeast fistula bandage that was effective precisely because it balanced opposing characteristics: "it will cure it, for one of these is of an hea[t]ing & the other is of a coolinge nature," he stated.[31] Palmer described his remedy as pairing, or seasoning, ingredients in relation to the properties of the abscess. Lady Barrett had her patient drink a purgative while she injected a wine mixture "as hot as possibly it can be endured" into the sore.[32] Mrs. Corlyon recommended that the reader "tent" the wound by inserting in it a resin-soaked bandage supercharged with "corrosive" mercury distilled in aqua vita.[33] "Tenting," as other recipes implied, involved using fingers and cloth to probe, search, and clean a wound.[34] Overall, these treatments necessitated not only technical knowledge of physiology, botany, and anatomy, but also intimate oversight of bodies and habits. "In the time of taking it," a fistula recipe in *The Queens Closet Opened* declared, "all Fish, white meats, fruit, wine, anger and passion must be avoided."[35] Probing, penetrating, and injuring the sovereign's body in what the play specifies as her "appliance" of the recipe, Helena might have been expected to regulate the king's behavior, diet, and emotions. She is to "temper" the king's temperament as she orchestrates the elements of his body.[36]

When the king declares Helena to have "preserved" him, he chooses a loaded term, one that trailed the capacious meanings that we have seen (*preservare*—to keep alive, prevent from harm, render durable, keep intact).[37] Preserving emerges as a form of *seasoning*, an operation that associates quickening, temporizing, and conserving. Given seasoning's meaning in recipe writing—as signalling a manipulation of time and a tempering of bodies—we can appreciate that its early appearance in the play inaugurates a verbal tissue whose complexity flickers into view in various scenes. The countess's trope of Helena as a self-seasoner, for instance, takes place in a scene where characters debate whether humans can effectively stay time or are subject to repetitions that only confirm loss. Will her son's act of leaving home *repeat* her husband's death? the countess wonders. This doubled and surrogated loss, articulated in a play known for its elaborate substitutions, is then connected to the afflicted king who has "persecuted time with hope" (1.1.13). The torture of time and the recursive repetition of the past spark the countess to think of her recently deceased physician, Gerard de Narbon, whom people see as having *almost* overcome mortality: "He was skilful enough to have lived still, if knowledge could be set up against mortality," Lafeu states (1.1.26–28). It is only after the scene has established a chain of associated losses and raised the possibility of human knowledge as a bulwark against temporality that the countess introduces de Narbon's daughter, Helena, whose tears brine virtue and preserve memory. Within this context, the countess's conventional trope of praise endows Helena with the ability to thwart ubiquitous deficits that haunt the fictional world of the play.

The fact that Helena only *seems* to mourn and remember her past tearfully (when she's really just desperately lovesick) is less important for my purposes than the language used by others to understand her character. For the countess tellingly repeats the word "seasoned" twenty lines later when warning that her son Bertram is, alas, "an unseasoned courtier" whose value must be produced over and through time (1.1.63). The countess means that Bertram has not been tempered or fortified yet, but the metaphor also introduces Helena's love interest as raw, unflavored material. With Helena identified as the agent who seasons and Bertram the material awaiting temporizing, the text establishes poles of activism and passivity important to the play, but these are immediately linked to two opposed modalities of time: Helena's way of "flavoring" is to grace the past in the present. The countess says of her: "I have those hopes of her good that her education promises; her dispositions she inherits, which makes fair gifts fairer. . . . She derives her honesty and achieves her goodness" (1.1.35–40). Helena seems to have paradoxically *achieved* her inherited virtue. Lafeu similarly tells Helena, "You must hold the credit of your father," which, the play later indicates, she does (1.1.72–73). Helena is discursively positioned as a force preserving the past in the present in ways that compensate for proliferating losses saturating the world.

Bertram's lack of seasoning is not just described as emotional inexperience but is pointedly the deferred paternal inheritance he has not yet assumed. His mother tells him that she hopes he will "succeed thy father / In manners as in shape" (1.1.54–55). As a person whose "birthright" is marked formally on him morphologically but not yet charactered within him, Bertram is positioned as having not yet properly imported the past into the present. "Thou bear'st they father's face," the king tells Bertram, "Thy father's moral parts / Mayst thou inherit, too" (1.2.19, 21–22). The moral and psychological lack that everyone recognizes in Bertram is that the inheritance etched in his natural body is not yet manifest in his character. Unlike Helena, Bertram is outer form awaiting a content expected to be unfolded in time; he is incomplete natural matter awaiting artful inner shaping, the thing but not yet its substance. The play's inscription of the younger generation thus distributes different modalities of time precisely by capitalizing on the expansiveness and paradoxes of a culinary trope.

In case we have failed to grasp the active philosophical categories underpinning the culinary discourse pressuring the initial scene, Paroles promptly offers a spirited argument against virginity using the same puns on dating that we saw in *Troilus*. "It is not politic in the commonwealth of nature to preserve virginity. . . . Your date is better in your pie and your porridge than in your cheek," he tells Helena saucily, "and your virginity, your old virginity, is like one of our French withered pears: its looks ill, it eats drily" (1.1.119–49). Having the date do double duty—as flavor and a sign of the clock ticking—Paroles makes people the agents and objects of a food-saturated temporality. Better to eat the flavorful date than to embody it, he suggests, lest one become the withered pears that English recipes found unappealing. Departing from the reputedly French practice of drying plums in boxes, English recipe books catered to upwardly mobile readers who preferred fruit steeped in sticky and sweet syrups to form marmalades, jellies, or crystallized candies. English methods for preserving de-accelerate deterioration through a simultaneous conversion to sweetness. Although Paroles draws on numerous tropes and metaphors when mocking the nonsustainability of virginity, his references to self-consuming cheese, dried pears, and date-flavored pies particularly echo with the countess's trope of preservation. In *All's Well*, the commonplace problem of time's erosion and losses—a manifestation of the play's noted nostalgia—is expressed in part as the quandaries of seasoning: he is "dieted to his hour," the First Lord later declares of Bertram (4.3.28).

When Helena tells the audience about her wondrous recipe, then, *All's Well* has already utilized the discourse of seasoning to establish categories and concerns that now materialize as a plot feature. The connection between the king's healing and food work might not be legible to modern readers who typically segregate culinary from medical care and who fail to grasp the deep-structural relationship of early modern disease to food. In her soliloquy at the end of the first scene, a speech that critics cite as key to understanding her agency, Helena rhetorically mixes eating and healing: "Our remedies oft in ourselves do lie. / Which we ascribe to heaven. The fated sky / Gives us free scope," she states, immediately turning to complain about a desire that she "cannot feed" (1.1.199–201, 204). The "remedy" for love, she decides, the way to *feed* appetite, lies in a restorative recipe. This is self-medicating at its finest: her cure for her lovesickness blurs into a venture to temporize, or temper, an amorous relationship, but only *indirectly* by "quickening" an intermediary body. Her balancing of the king's body becomes additionally complicated by the fact that "quickening" meant enlivening, conserving, and, strikingly, rendering sexually potent. Helena's healing of the fistula, which, as we have seen, could involve intimate physical contact, is explicitly eroticized. Lafeu describes their meeting as a sexual tryst. "I am Cressid's uncle," he declares, "that dare leave two together" (2.1.96–97). In her soliloquy, Helena, having lamented that she cannot *embody* her ardent wishes, turns to her sovereign's diseased body as a way to feed, cure, probe, penetrate, and body forth unfulfilled desire. What she envisions as the tempering "kiss" of opposites, the king imagines as a "ransom" of "nature" (1.1.206, 2.1.116). At the end of the play, Helena's pregnant body, resurrected from the dead, is produced as the solution to a riddle: "one that's dead is quick" (5.3.300).[38] This complex of linguistic associations routes temporally reprocessed bodies back to the opening trope of conserving tears.

In calling the recipe the "dearest issue" of her father's practice, Helena explicitly links the recipe's powers of preservation with a temporal materialization of the past (2.1.104). She sees herself, that is, as reproducing her dead father by materializing his recipe-progeny. Named as the king's "preserver," the play then literalizes the countess's trope of Helena as offering pickling tears, drawing out the dual function "preservation" played in fortifying foodstuffs and humans. Helena's seasoning seems to makes good on her father's failed promise to "set up" "knowledge" against "mortality" (1.1.27–28), as she triumphs in the war against time to which her father had succumbed. Cast as the animating performance of a recipe script that is itself a text from the past, Helena doubly thwarts linear temporality: she brings to life a past knowledge whose content involves the reversal of putrefaction. *All's Well* rhetorically meditates on a curative/culinary project that culminates in the "artful" ransoming of time and nature, a miraculous feat that plays out the logic of Helena's opening tears.

The play's plot and figurative glossing of events helps us to understand what was at stake in recipe work. Sanctioned to manipulate temporal cycles and natural matter, Helena seems remarkably free of the ideological binaries that defined womanhood. As both submissive good wife *and* tenacious aggressor, she confirms Kathryn Schwarz's reading of the early modern paradox of the female will.[39] Indeed, these two seemingly opposite positions are mutually implicated—the tenacious, aggressive, even predatory seasoning of Helena is part and parcel of her ferocious desire to be a subservient good wife. My analysis of seasoning, then, complements Schwarz's interpretation by showing the ideological capaciousness of the "housewife/huswife," a figure whose orthodox activities licensed the violation of orthodox gender roles articulated in discourses in the period.[40]

Between the opening conserving tears in the play and the ending reanimation of the dead, *All's Well* keeps seasoning on its audience's radar. Lafeu extrapolates one of its meanings when he figures men as raw, unspiced kitchen ingredients. Bertram's flaw, he notes, lies in being influenced by his lying friend Paroles "whose villainous saffron would have made all the unbaked and doughy youth of a nation in his colour" (4.5.2–3). The younger generation of men stands as temporally unfinished raw material, susceptible to a cook's malevolent touch. Eleven lines later, Lafeu, by contrast, describes Helena as "the sweet marjoram of the salad, or, rather the herb of grace" (4.5.14–15). As sweet marjoram and bitter rue, Helena is portrayed as the tempering, preservative, and medicinal element she formerly manipulated in her recipe remedy.[41] And, in fact, she first offers the titular proverbial message of the play by blending culinary taste and with temporality:

> The time will bring on summer,
> When briers shall have leaves as well as thorns
> And be as sweet as sharp. We must away,
> Our wagon is prepared, and time revives us.
> All's well that ends well; still the fine's the crown.
> Whate'er the course, the end is the renown. (4.4.31–36)

In evoking this seasonal mixed blessing, Helena uses the word "sharp" to refer to the tactile quality of thorns, yet its specific pairing with "sweet" links it to the moderating properties of the taste palate. The agential subject able to offset and temper the gripping losses of time seems now to be time itself, whose cycle forward and guarantee of renewal signify within flavor combinations. The play goes on to juxtapose tropes of seasoning with the conventional language of disease used to expose problems of individuals and the body politic. Bertram's "sick desires" are positioned alongside the social wrongs of the world and the losses of time, as characters mourn plaintively.[42] The plot drives toward an unspecified vague state of being "made well," which is figured as an interwoven culinary, seasonal, and medical product.

The play ends by reflecting on its conditional wellness, as the king declares shakily:

> All yet seems well; and if it end so meet,
> The bitter past, more welcome is the sweet. (5.3.329–30)

Now supersessionary and conditional, time is "sweetened" only through deceptions, bed tricks, and the falsification of death, with Bertram being dragged by others kicking and screaming into consummation. This tension produces for Helena a momentary ontological rupture: she declares herself a "shadow" of a wife, "the name and not the thing," although Bertram offers reassurance: "Both, both," he cries (5.3.305). The ingredients of this strained closure point to a relational flavor-time: a "bitter" past preserved as a trace within a "sweet" present. In noting the irony and qualifications of this distempered closure, however, we should not overlook its expression within redemptive acts of housewifery, and, by extension, its rich annotation of the meaning of domestic labor.

My argument has been that the rich lexical interplay of seasoning in *All's Well* exposes the philosophical and intellectual dimensions of practical labors as a crucial part of the play's framework. It offers an unusually full elaboration of the temporal problems and philosophical conundrums associated with seasoning in the early modern imagination. Over time, this discourse would become harder to recognize as its contours changed. The waning of humoral theory and consolidation of professional medicine in the seventeenth century differentiated cookery and medical care. When food-as-medicine gave way to food-as-cuisine, the link between food preparation and the managing of human bodies was attenuated.[43] Yet in the early seventeenth century, the connections between seasoning bodies and seasoning foods were deep structural. *All's Well* capitalizes on the paradoxes and problems of preservation circulating in popular printed recipes in the book market in England.

Distilling What Nature Has "Wrought"

Returning to the poetic manifesto introducing *Delightes for Ladies*, we see that Plat not only celebrated the triumph of domestic preservation, but also asked his readers to visualize this technique in the material book itself. Plat claimed, that is, that his published recipe collection executed the "arte" it describes. "Yet here behold the clusters fresh and faire, / Fed from the branch, or hanging on the line," he commanded readers when speaking of the fair fruit that has withered, for they are "here from yeere to yeere preserved, / And made by Arte" (A3). The act of reading, understood as a *beholding*, enacted the kitchen processes that the book recommended, for the "tender grape" was now etched in print for all eternity, spared from nature's consumption so as to reappear perpetually fresh on the dining table or in the library (the word "line" doubly referring to a drying device and the line of a poem). In beholding the revivified fruit, the reader was to "hold" the book in hand and apprehend its power. As frost devoured grapes and time consumed sweetness, domestic work (and its double, the printed recipe book) renourished organic materials. Two modes of consumption were thus interlocked and held in tension against the consuming pressure of time. Domestic work, and its medium, the purchasable recipe book, held out the promise of (house-)*keeping* the physical world, first in the instructions they offered for transforming foodstuffs and bodies, and then again in the occasion of being etched in print.

As Plat continued his meditation on domesticity's transfigurative power, he pointedly categorized human bodies as in need of keeping:

> For Ladies closets and their stillatories,
> Both waters, ointments, and sweet smelling bals.
> In easie termes without affected speech,
> I heere present most ready at their cals.
> And least with carelesse pen I should omit,
> The wrongs that nature on their persons wrought,
> Or parching sunne with his hot firie rayes,
> For these likewise relieving meanes I sought. (A3)

Just as they miraculously preserved the color, taste and smell of ripened fruits, housewives could fill their closets or "stillatories" with cosmetics that erased signs of aging. While it was common, as we have seen, for recipes to place human bodies within the economy of "preservation," Plat unusually described recipe workers and Nature as rival "writers." Both the actions of his "pen" and ladies' cosmetic tools could oppose what Nature had "wrought" (or written) on the body. Plat thus drew on a vocabulary that lodged *textual* production and consumption within the temporal problems that recipes addressed. Medical care and culinary preparation emerged as counterwriting to the cosmically meaningful labors of time. Given that this passage contextualized these contrasting modes of writing within the irony of an organic world kept "naturally" "by arte," it raised for the reader's scrutiny the paradox of maintaining the essence of the organic world precisely by extracting nature from itself.

It's difficult for a literary scholar to read Plat's preface and not recall the graphic depiction of human struggle with mortality depicted in Shakespeare's first group of nineteen sonnets. In poems that critics have dubbed "reproduction" sonnets, the speaker repeatedly grapples with the dilemma of mortality, as he tries to convince his beloved to multiply himself in order to preserve his idealized fairness. Vividly describing ways that tyrannical time can threaten the beauty and life of a creature, the sonnet speaker uses various conceits and vocabularies to suggest strategies that might be used to counter time: agrarian husbandry, music, accounting, investment, ethical obligation. Against the possibility of "bareness everywhere," the speaker seeks measures for insuring plenitude and duration (Sonnet 5, 1.8).

In Sonnets 5 and 6, the speaker draws specifically on the trope of distillation to portray the problem, and potentially the solution, of aging. After personifying summer as someone lured into the withering cold of winter, he states:

> Then were not summer's distillation left
> A liquid prisoner pent in walls of glass,
> Beauty's effect with beauty were bereft,
> Nor it nor no remembrance what it was.
> But flowers distilled, though they with winter meet,
> Lose but their show; their substance still lives sweet. (5.9–14)

In Chapter 2, we saw that this sonnet reflected on culinary practices that queried the distinction between forms and essences. Here we can turn to specifically to the dimension of time as imagined within those practices. Holding at bay death and decay, distilling provides a form of remembrance in which the flower's mere trappings—its "effect," "show," or, in the words of alchemists who describe distilling, its "body"—can be discarded so that its true substance might persevere without loss ("still" living "sweet"). Using characteristically complex double negatives, Shakespeare reintroduces the "rose" whose beauty the speaker declared himself so interested in increasing in the first sonnet ("From fairest creatures we desire increase / That thereby beauty's rose might never die" [ll. 1–2]). The sixth sonnet extends the distillation conceit, with the speaker urging the beloved to undertake the sexually suggestive action of *being distilled* so as to prevent himself from being deformed and defaced in time: "Then let not winter's ragged hand deface / In thee thy summer ere thou be distilled. / Make sweet some vial" (ll.1–3). The speaker calls forth sexualized images of bodily receptacles in pleading for a seasonal preservation, the "vial" that must be made "sweet." Distillation seems a metaphor for reproduction, with the "liquid prisoner" from Sonnet 5 now back-projected as semen that can reduplicate fathers into children who will bear the parents' memory. The beloved is asked to act as agent and object of an act of conservation; he must be the distiller and the distilled flower in order to refigure his summer "substance" and "still" live, like the rose: sweet, remembered, beautiful, and fair.[44]

Critics tend to see distillation, which creates the "pent" (or penned) essence, as figuring both biological reproduction and textual immortality, the two forces that are alternately complements and rivals in the first group of sonnets. As did Plat, the speaker imagines Time/Nature as a rival author whose "hand" can deface creations. When the speaker declares boldly in Sonnet 15, "all in war with time for love of you, / As he takes from you, I engraft you new," he points to a horticultural and textual process (graphing, engrafting) that moves away from the call to create biological progeny (ll. 13–14). If we draw from the sonnets' own language, we might say that the poems begin to self-declare their distillatory power to preserve the object of one's love for eternity. Indeed the speaker later assures the beloved that his "verse distils your truth" (Sonnet 54, l. 14). The sonnets thus show how readily distillation could be injected into the conventional claim that poetry could serve as a tool in a war against time.

As recipes so patently evidence, distillation was hardly an esoteric practice carried out solely by formally trained natural philosophers and alchemists. At home, women and servants freely distilled, a process that involved heating and cooling a substance so as to vaporize and concentrate the properties of a given entity.[45] Based on the principle that entities vaporize at different temperatures, it allowed for a separation of chemical substances, which were sometimes described as the extraction of the essence (the "spirit") from its waste matter or corporeal residue. As Plat explained in his recipe for "the spirit of spices," the reader is to seethe herbs or spices in a limbeck to separate "spirite" from body: "Distill with a gentle heat either in balneo [vessel of boiling water much like a double boiler today], or ashes, the strong and sweet water wherewith you have drawen oile of cloves, mace, nutmegs, juniper, Rosemarie, &c. after it hath stoode one moneth close stopt, and so you shall purchase a most delicate Spirite of each of the saide aromaticall bodies" (*Delightes*, E2). Imagined within the corporeal vocabulary of alchemy, distillation was to volatize substances so as to alter their nature and physical form. Plat's honey recipe, for instance, promised to make this gooey substance "yeelde his spirit by distillation" (E8). In the household, distillation was, like preserving, a chemical transformation that enabled a substance to take on a new and potentially more enduring incarnation. At stake was nothing short of the elimination and transcendence of elements that corrupted matter.

All major editions of Shakespeare's sonnets available to students gloss the "distillation" referenced in Sonnets 5 and 6 as a perfume made of flowers, and many suggest that the appropriate context for understanding the conceit is esoteric alchemy.[46] This assumption has the salutary effect of aestheticizing the preserved liquid described in the poem so as to render it a ready analogy for poetry itself. Yet distilled roses and flowers were commonly featured in household recipe collections, used by amateur practitioners undertaking daily work; and these recipes were not exclusively or even centrally concerned with cosmetics. Distilled roses were central ingredients in medicines and food seasonings as well as aromatics such as air fresheners, pomanders, and perfumes. Even when used as odor repellents, rosewater and oil of roses had the medicinal effect of voiding the bad vapors that were seen to produce fevers and distempers. Rosewater was not only a staple in extravagant confectionary dishes, but also a key ingredient in herbal medicines.[47] In *The English Housewife*, Markham listed numerous curative herbal distillation recipes, which featured sage, radishes, endive, sorrel, roses, rosemary, strawberries, cloves, and aluminum. He urged the housewife to "furnish herself of very good Stils, for the distillation of all kindes of Waters, which Stils would either bee of Tinne or sweet Earth, & in them shee shall distill all sorts of waters meete for the health of her Houshold" (1623; 129). In *Delightes for Ladies*, Plat included seven recipes for distilled roses alone. "Stampe the leaves, and first distill the juice being expressed, and after distil the leaves," he said of his rosewater, "and this water is everie way... medicinable..., serving in all sirrups, decoctions, &c. sufficiently" (E9). Other sources tell us that that rosewater "comfortheth and strengtheth and coleth the braynes the harte, the stomake and the pryncipall membres & defendeth them for dyssolvynge."[48]

Rather than as an elite arcane activity, distilling was widely recognized as a craft skill undertaken by housewives, ladies, and artisans working in domestic and commercial domains (Figure 45). It is one of the key tasks recommended by Thomas Tusser in his poetic agrarian handbook for farmers and their wives. In *Five Hundred Points of Good Husbandry* Tusser emphasized the pragmatic preservative value of distillation for families fairly low on the social scale.[49] In easily remembered tetrameter couplets, Tusser wrote:

> The knowledge of stilling is one pretty feat,
> The waters be wholesom, the charges not great.
> What timely thou gettest, while summer doth last
> Think winter will help thee to spend it as fast. (108)

Tusser specifically conceptualized this household task within the temporal circuit of getting and spending. "Getting," closely aligned semantically in early modern texts with "begetting," was driven by a seasonal imperative: the storing of bounty from summer's harvest provided for winter's expenditures. Tempering the triumphalist claims made by Plat and Shakespeare, Tusser acknowledged the limited power of domestic preservation, which ensured only that savings were carried from one season to another. Although Tusser emphasizes that winter will force the disbursement of resources generated in summer, he framed distillation in terms of the warring economy of seasons that Shakespeare's sonnets portray so richly. "For never-resting time leads summer on / To hideous winter, and confounds him there," the speaker laments, as we remember, in Sonnet 5, before offering distillation as a potential solution (ll. 5–6). Markham, whose pragmatic bent made him less willing to indulge in reveries about time, nevertheless used this same philosophical and meditative language when he contemplated the relative deficits of the seasons. A meal must "hold limitation with . . . provision, and the season of the yeere," he observed, "for summer affords what winter wants, and winter is master of that which summer can but with difficultie have" (1623; 128). In a preface to *The Queens Closet Opened*, W.M. more optimistically praised preservation as harmonious balancing an ecological economy: "though Summer gave those pleasant Fruits, yet that *Art* is able to make Winter richer than her self."[50] Can you replenish winter's scarcities? recipe writers asked. Can you alter the expenditures of the seasons? Balancing the deficiencies of nature involved recalibrating temporality, making winter and summer relational and interchangeable. Providing impoverished winter with what it lacked, in fact, was one of the most evident preoccupations of English recipe writing, where conserves and distillations took center stage.

The shared vocabulary of poetic and recipe writing brings to the fore the cerebral challenges of housewifery (or "husbandry") necessitated by the inexorable passing of time and the struggle to retard loss. The material forms of recipe

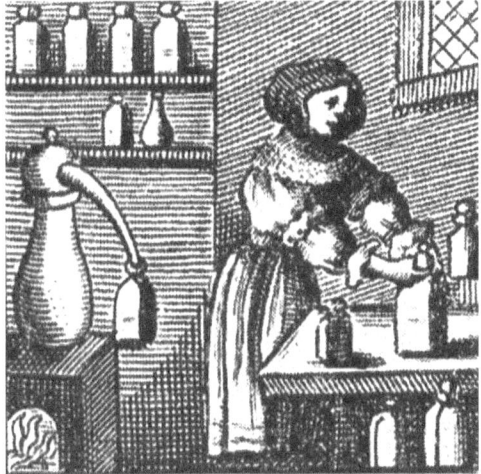

FIGURE 45. Woman distilling, detail from the title page to Hannah Woolley's *The Queen-Like Closet; or, Rich Cabinet* (1675). Reproduced by permission of the Folger Shakespeare Library.

writing took meaning from their location within this process. It is perhaps the dedicatory address prefixing Plat's all-purpose recipe book, *The Jewel House of Art and Nature* (a text not specifically addressed to women) that offers the most cogent articulation of this issue. In seeking a language to portray the relationship between recipe art and the material world that was its object, publisher D.B. employed the analogy of soul and body to make extremely bold claims. "Although Nature appears a most fair and fruitful Body," he stated, "yet the Art, here mentioned, is as a Soul to inform that Body to examine and refine her actions, and to teach her to understand those abilities of her own, which before lay undiscovered to her" (1653; A2v). The technical arts of seasoning, distilling, and preserving appeared to have monumental and grand ambitions: to inform and teach nature, so that an artfully reconceived nature could be revealed to herself. Such was the power of the seventeenth-century recipe fantasy.

Recipe Writing as Memorialization

And so we turn to the act of collecting and transmitting written recipes in a milieu where cooks were conceptualized as preservers combating a cosmic time bomb. In creating collections, compilers converted the fleeting experiences of cooking, healing, and eating into forms with personal and collective staying power. As such, they reengaged in the context of writing the temporal issues that already attached to their labors. This merging is perhaps most evident when recipe books acted as technologies of memory. The act of setting down methods for making foods and medicines in writing, creating what Woolley called a "memorandum," allowed an individual the luxury of forgetting.[51] But it also enabled a favorite cream mixture or meat pie to survive beyond an individual practitioner's life. The recipe collection could thus commemorate bonds of kinship, nation, region, or network "in the idiom of food," as it recorded the quince preserves and elder ales that bore the hallmark flavors of a community.[52] "As a form through which celebrated figures or the dead might be memorialized and re-encountered every time one read or made a dish or medicine, recipe collections exert a powerful associative and even psychic force," write Sara Pennell and Michelle DiMeo.[53] In consulting and using her collection, for instance, Dorothy Broughton could visualize her grandmother Broughton making currants, her aunt Lourham Broughton concocting sugar cakes, and her cousin Sickeravil rolling jumbals.[54] The Broughton repertoire of inventions and delicacies then became available to a later owner of the collection, Mary (Egerton) Puleston, who folded this earlier community of makers into her own. Similarly, Mary Hookes's recipe book allowed her to reenact childhood experiences by devising almond puddings and march beer just as her mother had done, or by experiencing the "courtt fritters" that her grandmother Hookes liked to prepare.[55] Later readers of Hookes's collection were invited to experience interactions among the Hookes, Carr, and Glanville families. As these examples attest, recipes materially formatted memory, with the written collection acting as a durable substitute for ephemeral food and dining occasions. What was left over—after death or after dinner—was often the commemorative recipe itself, a consumable index to histories of social bonds.

Culinary historian Priscilla Ferguson uses a theatrical analogy to articulate the tension that compilers felt between the weighty physicality of food and its seemingly endless repetition as a vanishing act. "As with the performing arts," she writes, "cuisine offers less a product than an *occasion* for a particular kind of consumption experience."[56] After "performing" everyday rituals, practitioners re-performed, in textual form, ways to transform materials so that they might endure in and through time. Writing, that is, enabled recipe workers to generate a new "consumption" experience: the moment of socially and emotionally saturated reading in which future selves or future practitioners could fantasize about accessing the past. Readers might enjoy the pie that, when prepared, called to mind a family occasion or an otherwise unknown ancestor. When writers took pains to hand down their texts to future generations, they conceived of recipes as material memory systems much like those that Ann Rosalind Jones and Peter Stallybrass have analyzed in relation to early modern clothing.[57] Recipes demanded that users place themselves, in various ways, in relation to time.

We have ample evidence that recipe manuscripts were routinely transmitted across and through generations—from mother to daughter, mother to son, father to daughter, aunt to niece, cousin to cousin. It is abundantly clear that compilers assumed that their recipes would not be discarded but would be reused over time. If only because of the price of paper, the recipe book was destined to outlive its creator. Sometimes, to be sure, collections were part of the general goods distributed after a person's death, but often compilers and inheritors consciously marked recipes as legacies and heartfelt gifts. When Mary Bromehead continued a recipe collection given by her aunt, one that probably housed her husband's family's recipes, she recorded the moment of giving on the opening page for later readers to contemplate.[58] Passing her recipes down to her daughter Katherine, Lady Ann Fanshawe enabled her to imagine three generations of women's practices in the family, including those undertaken by Katherine's sister (Margaret Grantham), mother, and grandmother Margaret.[59] The memory system was triggered by Katherine's simple inscription: "Given mee by my mother March the 23rd 1678."

Elinor (Poole) Fettiplace and Frances Catchmay commented on recipe commemoration from the perspective of the recipe giver. Fettiplace, daughter of Sir Henry Poole of Gloucestershire who married into the prestigious Fettiplace family, gathered recipes from friends and family, including those by her cousins Walter Raleigh and Gresham Thynne. In part because her two daughters had died as infants, Fettiplace bequeathed her recipe collection to her niece, Ann Poole, who had married George Horner.[60] Fettiplace clearly saw her book—dated 1604, bound in leather, and stamped with the Poole coat of arms—as a keepsake that might commemorate identities and worlds. "Thes bock I geve to my deare nees and goddutar Mrs Anne Hornar," she wrote, "desiring her to kepe it for my sake: 1647."[61] The sentiment binding compiler and recipient ("*for my sake*") and the family crest marked on the cover reveal personal and collective dimensions of commemoration. Extending the rhetoric of preservation that saturates recipe instructions (for instance, the quince conserve that will keep all year) to the book itself, Fettiplace urged her niece to "kepe" her memory textually.

Lady Catchmay felt so strongly about her collection that she left explicit instructions that it be delivered to her son after her death and that he offer to copy it for his surviving brothers and sisters. Edmund Bett, Catchmay's emissary, not only enacted her informal will and testament, but also marked the text with Catchmay's *desire* to have it serve as a legacy. "This Booke with the others of Medicins, preserves and Cookerye, My lady Catchmay lefte with me," he wrote in an inscription in the text, "to be delivered to her Sonne Sir William Catchmay Earnestly desiringe and Chardginge him to lett every one of his Brothers and Sisters to haue true Coppyes of the sayd Bookes, or such parte thereof as any of them doth desire. In witnes that this was her request, I haue hereunto sett my hand at the delivery of the sayd Bookes. Ed. Bett."[62] As Bett solemnly testified, he performed his duty as recipe scribe and executor, enabling Catchmay's voice to speak from the grave. The legalistic language that Bett used in his oath is telling ("witness," "sett my hand"), given that recipe books were not valuable enough to be named individually in household inventories or wills (they might have been referenced by the term "small books" that are mentioned in wills). Because they did not typically become visible in legal records as property, most genealogies of transmission that we can now reconstruct derive from inscriptions and attributions in the texts themselves.

We might scrutinize the workings of this memory system by considering the case of Mary (Westcombe) Granville from Dorset, who, in the seventeenth century, inherited a recipe book that had been in the Westcombe family for two generations. This collection included recipes gathered from friends and family in England as well as those acquired during the family's residence in Spain, where her father, Martin Westcombe, had served as English consul until 1685.[63] After her husband, Colonel Granville died, Mary settled in Gloucester with her younger daughter, Anne, where the two lived until Anne's marriage to John D'Ewes. Over the course of several decades, Granville added recipes to the book and then presented it, in 1740, as a wedding gift for Anne bearing this inscription: "Mrs Anne Granville's Book which I hope she will make a better use of then her mother. Mary Granville." The fact that Mary used Anne's maiden name on this momentous day, when Anne's name changed, seems noteworthy. Whatever the motive, it had the effect of preserving the affiliation between mother and daughter through the gift-artifact. Mary's decision to use the Granville name on the collection is especially noteworthy given later comments by her oldest daughter Mary (Granville) Delany, who became a famed court favorite and collage artist. In her memoir, Mary

Delany expressed delight that the heir to her father's estate, John Dewes, had gained permission from the king to change his name officially to "Granville," thus reinstalling someone bearing the maternal family name in the estate at Calwach.[64] While Mary Delany affirmed the family name, sister Anne, inheritor of the Granville recipe book, answered her mother's message by pointedly emending the inscription, with emphasis: "*Now* Anne Dewes," she wrote. The recipe collection, it seems, registered a contest of names.[65]

What Anne inherited was not only her mother and grandmother's ways of making remedies and dishes but also a record of the communities in which her maternal ancestors circulated. Composed by at least ten different hands, this compilation cemented a kinship system as it registered movements geographically, temporally, and socioeconomically.[66] Granville's collection introduced readers to family acquaintances: the wife of a baronet and politician (Lady Katherine Windham, likely wife of Sir William Wyndham) as well as captains, soldiers, midwives, and local women. We meet Granville's sister (Margaret) Melbourne of Essex, who advised that cake batter should be "baked in a quick oven and Eaten New" (92). Granville chronicled her husband's family through reference to her socially prominent brother-in-law, Lord Lansdowne, whose wife provided a recipe for French bread (201). We encounter other (mysterious) people: Ann Melcomb, who donated Mrs. Lake's liquorish cough syrup to the Granvilles; Mrs. Pain of Gloucester, who had a flair for making raisin elder wine; Mrs. Rebecca Ashan, who was famed for an eye remedy; and Mrs. Taverner and Mrs. Berker, who offered competing techniques for making seed cake.

In addition to commemorating neighbors, acquaintances, and locations in England, the Granville recipe book preserved the spatial and social networks in which the family operated during their stay in Spain. Inheriting this collection gave Mary and her daughter Anne a family history lesson as they cooked or made medicines: they discovered that Colonel John Belasye visited the family in Cadiz on October 4, 1665, and gave them Mr. Leonard Wilke's recipe for exotic New World hot chocolate. This entry might well have reminded readers of Westcombe's role in providing intelligence to the English military about Dutch and Portuguese political and commercial operations in the area. (Westcombe was even briefly imprisoned for suspected involvement in espionage and/or piracy, something common in this contentious site, where the Mediterranean opened onto the Atlantic.) In reading the collection, Mary discovered that her relatives in Malaga in 1646 had met Mr. William Fens, who provided them a good ink recipe, and that her mother visited her brother in law in 1671. She would have seen that Captain Francisco del Poço de Rota gave Mary's father a recipe for "Picadillo of Leg of Lamb" in Cadiz on August 22, 1682 (which her mother improved by noting that one should use pork grease or butter from Flanders). Mary read that a one-eyed sergeant from Xeres (now Jerez, Spain) arrived in the flotilla with a very good recipe for preserving vanilla (121). The text brims over with the names of Spanish, Portuguese, and English soldiers and diplomats, who engaged in war, commerce, and diplomacy. As recipe books do today, the Granville collection served as a community diary or memento of place, relationship, and wealth. When Anne inherited the collection, she reexperienced the family lore, now supplemented with her mother's voice: "I Thinke that leamon wilbe better then Vinegre," Mary had written tentatively about a fricassee (25).

Because Anne's sister Mary preserved her correspondence and penned an autobiography, we have access to other evidence about the family's domestic concerns. The scholars who have read Mary (Granville) Delany's letters and writings have not gravitated to her comments on housework but instead have mined the text for information about fashionable social, artistic, and cosmopolitan circles of the day. Delany hobnobbed with Swift and Hogarth, gossiped about King George and Queen Charlotte, and recorded her interest in collage art (her works are now housed in the British Museum). Delany's letters also, however, help us to contextualize the family recipe book. They show us, for instance, that matriarch Mary Granville created eye water remedies so popular that her daughters' acquaintances requested them (evidence, to my mind, that Granville's inscription to her daughter proclaiming her limited use of the recipes expressed humility rather than ignorance).[67] Delany's correspondence also tells us that Anne Granville (deemed a good economist by her sister) exchanged recipes with Delany, which provide comments on prescriptions for smallpox, cures for the ague, and a balsam and elderberry water (3:358; 1:366). Perhaps using the recipe in the collection, Anne made a plum cake, which she sent to her sister and to friends (1:124). At a young age, Delany had been sent to live with socially connected relatives in hopes of advancing her social standing. She inherited an education to be a lady-in-waiting at court; Anne inherited the family recipe book instead.

We do not know what happened to the Granville recipe book after it passed through Anne's hands. We do know that one of Anne's later descendants, Augusta Hall, Baroness Llanover, reconstructed her family history by publishing the memoirs of her distant aunt, *The Autobiography and Correspondence of Mary Granville, Mrs. Delany* (1861). In a separate venture six years later, she published *Good Cookery Illustrated*, which appears to incorporate a recipe for fish served in anchovy and wine sauce from her ancestor's seventeenth-century collection.[68] The fictional character who introduces the recipes states that "Granville Fish Sauce" was a family recipe, found among old papers, imperfect because "hereditary and traditional in his family, and handed from mother to daughter" (176).[69]

To get a sense of how recipients of collections might have understood their commemorative functions, we might consider the case of a nineteenth-century man named Robert Ainsly, who inherited a beautifully bound seventeenth-century manuscript recipe collection. This compilation of over three hundred pages, now housed in the Szathmary Collection at the University of Iowa, includes advice about remedies, foods, and confections. As the original collection circulated, family and friends made emendations and additions, sometimes murmuring approving comments ("this is wrot perfect" or "very pretty"). Mr. Riggs (whom we know nothing about), for instance, pinned a piece of paper to a page specifying precise ingredients and boiling times for a red clear cake recipe (46). Initially signed by Anne Bayne, the collection functioned as a working document for over a century before it was handed down as a quaint family heirloom.[70]

On the opening page, beside a visible kitchen smudge, Ainsly speculated about the artifact he had inherited. "This receipt book belonged to my Great Aunt Rachel Bayne daughter I believe, of the above Anne Bayne. Rachel Bayne died in 1799 above seventy years of age," he wrote (Figure 46). Ainsly desires to affiliate over and across time and space through the imagined world of kitchen work. Ainsly "believes"—he admittedly conjectures—that he has discovered the textual footprint of his great aunt's mother. In reconstructing the past, Ainsly identified the possession of his aunt Rachel (whose year of death and age he knows and whose connection to him is already firmly established) as a possible link to a mother named Anne, someone who materializes for him through advice on gingerbread and puddings. As was often the case, the recipe artifact served as one of the few traces remaining of a person's existence. Ainsly's genealogical detective work led to his poignant statement, "I believe," the conjecture that allowed him to connect his great aunt to a named mother whose characteristics he then could imagine concretely. He learned that Anne Bayne saw it expedient to save the blood of the pig she had killed so as to strain it with oatmeal. He learned that she was interested in comparing her pickled walnuts with those of her acquaintances Madam Best and Mrs. Clay (1v; 2v). He could picture the scenario in which Anne graciously invited Mrs. Ascough to write her recipe for preserved oranges in the collection. He could register

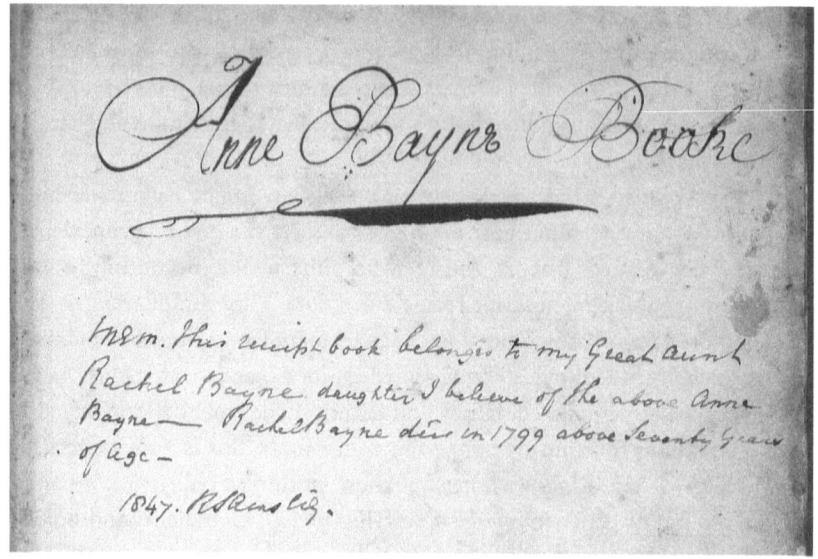

FIGURE 46. Ainsly's inscription on the title page to Anne Bayne's *Book of Recipes*, c. 1700, Szathmary Culinary Manuscripts Collection, MsC0533, University of Iowa Library, series 4. En13, 9.

Anne's appreciation for the aesthetic appearance of her food, as she experimented with food dyes and mused of her candied flowers: "They are very pretty" (24). He learned that Anne enjoyed preparing exotic chocolate (36) and "East Inde" spiced punch (2v), as well as old-fashioned meat pies and pastries. Ainsly, that is, found a means of conjuring up a woman of means who entertained guests with elegant liquors, decorative cakes, and fashionable consumer goods.

As we've seen in the case of other collections, the ghostly Anne would have herself been involved in physical commemorative work when she converted the actions of grinding, roasting, and stirring into home rituals attributed to a circle of friends and acquaintances. Conventionally marking her recipes with donors' names—such as Madam Best, Mrs. Clay, Mrs. Ascough, Aunt Kingsley—Anne created a personal memory book. In producing a "fair copy" collection with all two hundred recipes written in the same hand and ink, Bayne enhanced the possibility that her congealed domestic world would travel across time. For Ainsly, the collection served, in part, as a culinary-genealogical document. Reading his fantasized link to Anne Bayne in proximity to the tasks of preservation described in the collection offers a tantalizing hint about the conceptual and intellectual issues bound up with early modern recipe work: its engagement with managing a mutable and ephemeral world and its energetic concern with relating past to present.[71]

The word "preserve" does not do justice, however, to the temporal transport that recipes enabled in their production, bequeathal, and consumption. Preserved fruits were not, that is, accurate analogues for written records. Rather than attempting to fix a static past in time, written recipes, as we have seen, provided methods for readers to relate past and present worlds and to think through strategies for processing the passing of time. When anthropologist Janet Theophano analyzes recipes as providing historical access to the lives of past women, she rightly understand those "lives" to be an aggregate of lived practices. But what recipes also unearth, contrary to the sentimentalized fantasies that sometimes fueled their making and their recovery, are worlds in flux and in sharp contest. While recipe writers blended material and abstract acts of preservation, they also often acknowledged how difficult or futile it was to consider material lived practices as static entities. When Hopestill Brett recorded recipes for quince cake, pickled cucumbers, wild duck sauce, possets in jelly, puff paste, violet syrup, dried fish, Naples biscuits, "ragoo," and "puddings in guts," she registered variation and disagreement among family members and friends. Her collection includes "my sister Knowles way to white cloth" followed by "my owne way." A competing recipe for pickled oysters made by Cousin Betty follows how "to pickle oysters my sister Higgins way." When we compare "my owne mothers way for hogspudding" to the recipe that follows ten pages later, "To Make My Hogspudding," we see that Brett modified her mother's recipe by using sack and a different type of bread. As was common, "the" family dish was not a stable entity, but a script subject to revision, even in its seemingly original incarnation. The signs of variation that Brett records provide another reminder that recipes do not function as a transparent window onto a readily determinable historical past ("what people did"). In addition to constituting particular forms that offset their documentary status, they represent heterogeneous practices continually in flux and subject to adaptation. Brett stages a competition when she records Mrs. Hasting's way of making violet syrup with this note: "my sister don't sett it in watter."[72] When she observes that Mrs. Knowles alters Mr. Moting's currant wine, she makes clear that she is not distilling one identifiable method but presenting an historical conversation. Her recipes open an animated world of dynamic exchange and disagreement among personalities. Cousin Betty, Sister Whits,

Sister Higgins, Sister Knowles, and Brett's mother become part of a chorus of sometimes dissenting voices shaping the later experience of domestic reading.[73] The metaphor of preservation, which implies a kept "essence" distilled for duration, breaks down as a conceit for understanding the written recipe as it was imagined to travel through time. The rituals and practices recorded in recipes were not as static as they might sometimes seem when viewed through a nostalgic lens.

The sentimentality that can saturate desires to use the recipe book as a window onto a perpetually re-animable past is additionally undercut in early modern collections where compilers created self-conscious and sometimes self-critical memorials.[74] Hopestill Brett, Frances Springatt Ayshford, Grace Blome Randolph, and Ann Glydd used the occasion of their collections to record other types of commemorative writing within their recipe collections. It was common, as we have seen, for writers to view their collections as all-purpose textual storage sites where they inventory household items, list debts, and recount favorite maxims. In addition to itemizing household goods, Brett documents favorite Bible verses for some members of her family. Yet the *content* of the selected verses she names tilts against any reassurance about endurance. She writes:

My mothers texx Ecclesiastes the thurde Chapter and the 2 verse
A Time to be born and a time to die

My Uncle Goddard texxe the 39 psalme and 5 verse
verily every man at his best state is alltogether vanity

Mr Sheppeards texx Eccesiastes the 11 Chapter and the 8 verse
But if a man live many years and reioyce in them all: yet let him remember the days of darkness: for thay shall be many: all that Cometh is vanity

My own tex Jobe the 7 [Chap] and the 8 and 9 verce
the eyes of him that hath seen mee shall see noe more; thine eyes are upon mee and I am not as the Cloud is consumed: and vanished a way: soe he that goeth down to the grave shall Com ye no more

Eccliastees the 12 chapter and the 7 vears—my father's texx:

Then shall the dust return to the earth as it wase: and the spirit shall return unto god who gave it

My sister Knowls texx: provarbs the 31 Chapt and 30 & 31 vers: she dyed April the 24 daye 1690

Mary Gillburd dyed the 13 of July 1690 her tex of Jobe the 14 verse. (141v–42)

The cast of characters who have disagreed about ways to make white cloth and hogspudding reemerge in this differently formatted family history. While these biblical verses cover a vast terrain of spiritual issues, they have the culminating effect of drawing the reader into consideration of the finality of mortality and the vanity of physical life, common topics in the period, to be sure. Given that preachers encouraged people to use visual symbolic icons as *memento mori* (remembrances of death), the image of Hamlet with Yorick's skull in hand appropriately emblemizes the medieval and Renaissance world. When Brett lodges these commonplace meditations within instructions for domestic labor, she loosely associates the lifecycles of individuals with the seasonal imperatives of housework. Brett's mother's choice of verse, the famous passage in Ecclesiastes 3:2, for instance, suggests a cyclical timeliness that is both the object and nemesis of housewifery: the world of determined temporality that must be accepted rather than triumphantly rearranged. Brett's own verse beckons no hopeful vision of the soul returning to God at the moment of passing but instead emphasizes that the grave consumes all. As if translating abstractions into particularities, Brett glosses her sister's and Mary Gillburd's verses with the time of their deaths. The relative devaluation of material practices and entities in these verses (with their celebration of the spirit) undermines recipe confidence in managing the physical world. Rather than lauding the power of keeping—the grand act of suffering nothing to be lost in time—the text ends with a reminder of materiality's ultimate vanity.

Although we cannot say that most recipe writers gravitated toward biblical mediations on earthly limitations, Brett's transition from puff pastes to family memento was not atypical. Recipe collections, like Bibles and devotional books of hours, often lodged family histories of births and deaths on opening or closing pages.[75] In serving as the repository for genealogical information, the recipe collection was deemed to be a significant artifact that should and would be *kept*. In a collection of recipes written over the course of over one hundred years and signed by Frances Springatt (Ayshford), someone recorded birthdates for Frances and Daniel Ayshford's nine children, inscribed beneath a recipe for sticking cherries together with egg whites (Figure 47).[76]

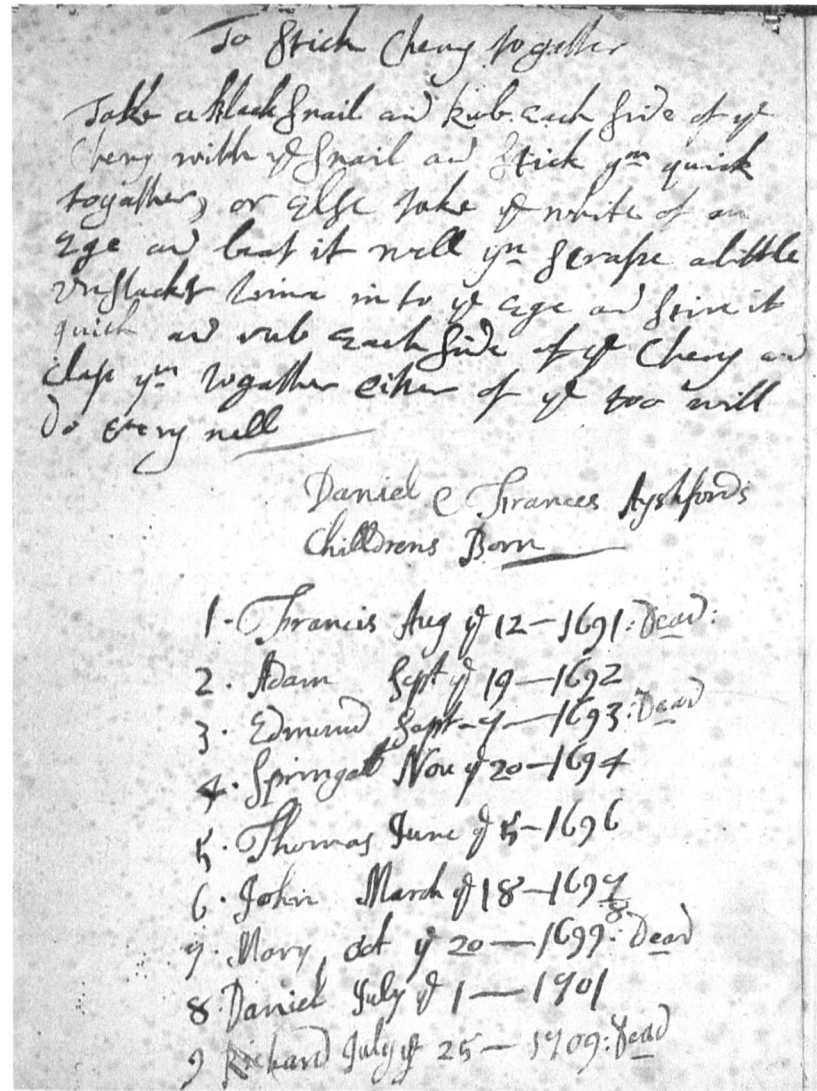

FIGURE 47. Family record in Frances Springatt's *Collection of Cookery and Medical Receipts*, 1686–1824, Wellcome Library, MS 4683.

Frances would have found a convenient reminder of her children's birthdays as she consulted her kitchen recipes, many of which show signs of use: the collection inscribes birthdates for Francis, Adam, Edmund, Springatt, Thomas, John, Mary, Daniel, and Richard. Frances signed this book, bound with leaves from a black-letter Bible, with her maiden name in 1689 and again with her married name in 1694. Noting life events while cooking or making medicines, Frances (and later readers) engaged a composite picture of the culinary life of the family. A later hand (perhaps that of Frances?) has updated the listing of children's birthdates, scrawling the word "dead" beside the names of Frances, Mary, Richard, and Edmund. Of nine children born within eighteen years, four died in their early years.

Poignant family memorials, each of which embeds a reminder of loss, frame Springatt's book. After one hundred pages of recipes, the text concludes with an inverted section recording two medical remedies, a description of where a rheumatic tincture can be bought, and a section titled "Children Dead of Dan & Fran Ayshford," which reads: "Mary feb 28 1700. Frances: Oct 25 1709. Richard Feb 12 1710. Edmund at sea 1713." The recipes are bookended, that is, by lists of children, but these inventories do not simply designate family heirs. As if to insist on the fragility of the lives that the recipe collection commemorates in other ways, the book unusually repeats, at its end, only the offspring who did *not* survive and the dates for their respective deaths. Recipes for puddings, pies, potted swans, collared eel, boiled pigeons, and clear jelly mingle with the commemoration of live and dead children. What type of memory work did this recipe book feature provide? The writers have inflected the conventions of the genealogical record so as to emphasize and preserve collective *loss* as well as to tell the story of generational renewal and continuity.[77]

Grace Blome's collection similarly modified the typical commemorative functions of the recipe book. This hefty collection was begun when Grace Blome was twenty-four years old and living in Sevenoaks, Kent (three years before her marriage to William Randolph). Neither she nor the later compilers who continued the assemblage chose to record the names of recipe donors and thus the collection does not create a populated community. Yet the collection concludes with two graphically distinct pages listing family births and deaths in a single, neat hand. By inscribing names in blocked lettering with dark ink capitals and by separating each "entry" with double lines, the inscriber creates a spatially demarcated textual cemetery within the recipe collection (Figure 48). Beginning with Grace's parents—John and Jane Blome—and then turning to their seven children, the writer records birthdates, death dates, and causes of

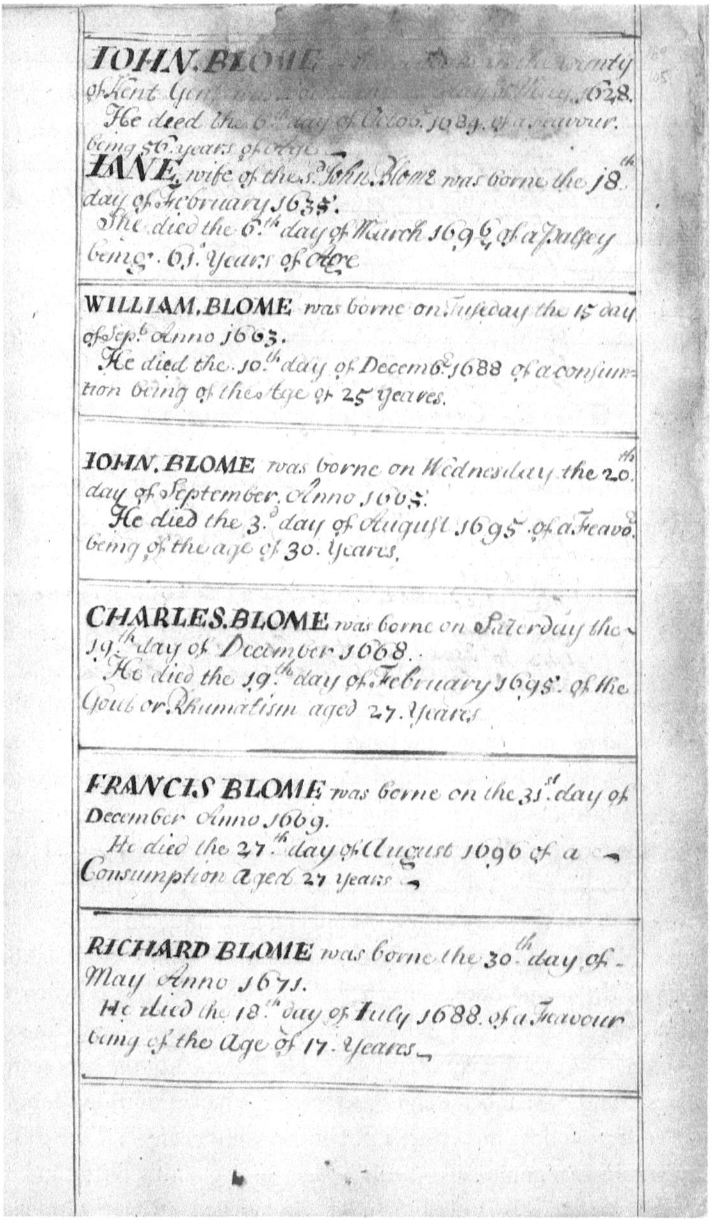

> **JOHN BLOME** [...illegible...] 1628.
> He died the 6[th] day of Octob[er] 1689 of a [f]eavour
> being 56 years of [age]
>
> **JANE**, wife of the s[ai]d John Blome was borne the 18[th]
> day of February 1635.
> She died the 6.[th] day of March 1696 of a Palsey
> being 61 years of age
>
> **WILLIAM BLOME** was borne on Tuesday the 15 day
> of Sep[tember] Anno 1663.
> He died the 10.[th] day of Decemb[er] 1688 of a consump-
> tion being of the age of 25 yeares.
>
> **JOHN BLOME** was borne on Wednesday the 20th
> day of September Anno 1665.
> He died the 3.[d] day of August 1695 of a Feavo[ur]
> being of the age of 30 yeares.
>
> **CHARLES BLOME** was borne on Saturday the
> 19th day of December 1668.
> He died the 19.th day of February 1695. of the
> Gout or Rhumatism aged 27 yeares
>
> **FRANCIS BLOME** was borne on the 31st day of
> December Anno 1669.
> He died the 27th day of August 1696 of a
> Consumption aged 27 years
>
> **RICHARD BLOME** was borne the 30th day of
> May Anno 1671.
> He died the 18.th day of July 1688. of a Feavour
> being of the age of 17 yeares

FIGURE 48. Family records in Grace Randolph Blome's *Cookbook*, 1697, Folger Shakespeare Library, MS V.b.301, fol. 105. Reproduced by permission of the Folger Shakespeare Library.

death.[78] The care with which the genealogy is stylized and formatted suggests that it was to serve as an heirloom, an artifact to be displayed to future generations. By detailing the diseases that family members suffered—palsy, consumption, fever, and gout—the writer converts what might be an impersonal family registry into an account emphasizing the individuals' physicality. When a later compiler enters the last two daughter's names, Grace and Judith Blome, s/he returns to the more conventional format and does not mention causes of death.

The Blome collection closes with two unusual and unusually different genres of textual memorial. First, Grace opts to include an exceptionally detailed medical description of the chronology of the illness, death, and autopsy of her father John Blome. This narrative seems to have been written in 1684 partially by a doctor (presumably to be sent to another physician for advice) and partially by Grace. The recipe collection, which has circled near bodies eating, tasting, and consuming foods, concludes with a vivid narrative of John's symptoms, treatments, and physical responses. Taken with a cough, fever, difficulty in swallowing, and hemorrhoids, John was given, the writer explains, a series of failed courses of physic: purging pills, vomits, powders, and purgatives. The account describes John's vomiting of phlegm "the consistency of frogs Spawn," bits of "glandulous flesh about an inch long," and blood-colored phlegm "as big as a hens egg." When Grace takes over the narrative, she clinically describes how they subjected the vomited fleshly gobs to examination by submerging them in water. She also dispassionately registers, without any commentary about the providential nature of suffering, her father's anguish with fever, shaking, and aches until his eventual death. The text then takes an even more peculiar turn, by reporting, in detached fashion, the findings of the autopsy that the physician undertook. Numbered as a checklist, this account documents the healthy state of John's lungs and spleen as well as the presumable cancer that riddled his esophagus and stomach. The family and doctor interpret as "miraculous" the fact that the body bears no "Relique or sign" of the black fleshy pieces that John had excreted for months. We cannot know why a young Grace Blome would include this morbid account of suffering and death as a remembrance of her father among her recipes, nor can we understand the nature of the interpretive quandary that the autopsy raised for the family. However, it is clear that that their inclusion had the effect of lodging the everyday tasks of the domestic world within a broader context in which pathologies conquer flesh despite attempts to safeguard health. In ending not simply with a record of family births and deaths but also with this stark portrayal of the anatomized corpse, the recipe "commemorates" a mortal world that cannot be preserved or explained materially.[79]

Blome's recipe collection concludes with an inscription of the poem "On the Much Lamented Death of That Incomparable Lady, the Honorable the Lady Oxendon. A Pindarique Ode by Mrs. Randolph," which eulogizes Lady Oxendon, wife to the baronet George Oxenden. This ode, added to the recipe collection at some unknown date, was also printed separately as a stand-alone poem. A female member of the Randolph family, either Grace Blome, or, more likely, Mary Castillion Randolph, was its author.[80] Her identity has not been definitively determined by scholars, who nevertheless acknowledge that the otherwise unknown "Mrs. Randolph" was a passionate participant in female poetic manuscript circles of the day. Her poem in praise of Anne Finch as the next Katherine Phillips prompted an appreciative response poem, "An Epistle from Ardelia to Mrs. Randolph," which celebrated the intimacy of female friendship and Randolph's superlative poetic talent.[81] In her elegiac ode on Lady Oxenden, Randolph meditated on the ethics of memory, the injuries of bereavement, and the virtues that lifted Lady Oxenden rightfully out of a physical world and made her divine—all subjects conventional in the elegy, a genre that contemplates the operations and vocabularies of commemoration. Regardless of whether Blome herself recorded the family "cemetery" or added this family-identified poetic eulogy to her compilation (and we cannot determine this with any certitude), readers using the collection later would have encountered strikingly different modalities of commemoration—culinary, classically elegiac, genealogical—as they preserved food, cooked, and made remedies. When a later hand poignantly added Grace's own marriage, descendants, and death to the history, the collection further projected its commemorative reflexes. It incorporated the owner of the collection into its memorial domain, along with the family's favorite almond cakes, scotch collops, pickled nasturtium seeds, jellied partridge, mutton with cauliflower, and potted hare.

Finally, we might turn to the case of Ann Glyd, who consciously converted her recipe book into a "mother's advice book" for her children. In her collection begun in the 1650s, Glyd presented culinary and medical recipes that named acquaintances and family members. She added on the flyleaf a family history entitled, "A Memorial of Our Childrens Births: Sept 23: 1650," which listed seven of her children's birthdates and the day of the week in which they were born.

> John Glyd born . . . 1650
> Elizabeth Glyd born 1651 who lived no longer than til she was
>   7 weeks old
> Anne Glyd, 1652 who lived no longer than she was just 6 weeks old
> Richard Blyd born . . . 1653
> Martha Glyd . . . 1654
> Lawrence Gllyd 1655
> Elizabeth Glyd 1657
> Anne Glyd 1658 (fol. 84)

In 1689, Glyd added the subsequent deaths and marriages of her children as well as the births of her grandchildren (many named in remembrance of various family members). She details the deaths of three children who did not survive infancy:

> Lawrence Glyd Departed this life May 1659 at night being 3 years
>   2 months and one day old
> Richard Glyd departed this life 1662 . . . being 8 years 7 months and
>   3 weeks old
> Elizabeth Glyd Departed this Life the 7 of November 1681 . . . she
> was twenty four years and nine weeks lack a day old. A good and
> gratious child, praised be thy name. O my gratious god for making
> her such a one. (82v)

Glyd, as we see, has an interest in recording the precise time of day and day of the week for significant events. As she supplements the record over the years, she expands her genealogy to include prayers for her descendants' continued virtue and happiness. When she commemorates the births of grandsons William and James Brockman, for instance, she asks God to bless their lives on earth before imagining, in more detail, their eventual fortunate deaths and happy ascendances to heaven. The moment of their birth, that is, is yoked to a future non-mortal state. In her writing, Glyd alternates between detailed accounts of times and dates, on the one hand, and the "everlasting," eternal world, on the other. Her family memorialization progressively becomes a study in contrasting modes of temporality.

What is unusual about Glyd's entries is not only the length of the family record, which extends to twenty-one paragraphs, but also the protracted narrative she offers her children about their father's illness and death. It is here that Glyd uses the recipe collection most directly as a teaching moment for her descendants. She praises her virtuous husband for giving her grace that will enable her to enter the pearly gates eventually, and she celebrates God's mercy in taking her husband and becoming a substitute "Father" to her children. Her husband's shining example, she observes, can instill true belief in his "seed" (83). Glyd interrupts this eulogy to issue her children a stern warning about the dangers of abandoning spiritual belief. To underscore the seriousness of her exhortation, she conjures up a vivid image of her own body dissolving into dust and of her dead husband cursing his children to damnation from the grave. Imagining her children as readers of the recipe collection after her death, she urges this remembrance:

> My dear children Let these things be remembered by you when my body shall be desouled into Dust that you had a Father whome if he should have lived to have seen you Children of unbelieve wold have as much as in him Lay have hindered you of the good things of this Life and shall at the day of Judgment rejoice in your Just condemnation if you should be wicked wretches. O my dear children fear and trambell and beg of god one your knees that he would give you grace to hear him that god your maker and man your father may not pronounce that sentence against you Depart you cursed into hell fire prepared for the Divill and his angels. (83)

Let these things be remembered by you. Glyd asks her children to visualize their dead father rejoicing as the deity sentences them to damnation on Judgment Day. Her testimony of her husband's righteousness projects her family imaginatively into two temporal spheres—the moment when she is dead and the moment when her children will die. Projecting her voice from the grave and lodging it in a practical book that the children will need to consult if they want to know how to make a gammon of bacon that masquerades as a Westphalia ham, Glyd uses a memorial to threaten and/or instruct her children. Glyd's sober sermonizing contrasts sharply with the faith in material making that sustains the recipe ethos. Preserving culinary traditions (and implicitly memorializing her own capacities as healer, cook, and spiritual guide), her text strategically uses commemoration as a means to shape the future.

We might return to the basic assumption that recipes are artifacts that will be *kept*. Glyd's book is to be her proxy after death, one that will continue her children's religious instruction. In another seventeenth-century collection, an anonymous inscriber made this function clear on the flyleaf:

Remember man
as thou goes by
[as] thou art now
so once was I
as I am now
So thou must be
remember man that thou must die.[82]

"Going by," in this textual location, signifies the act of reading, as the absent "dead" voice speaks from the afterlife to remind the reader of death's inevitability. The "I" that speaks through recipes generally urges a particular form of remembrance that weights the pragmatic resourcefulness of domestic life, but this inscription creates a nihilistic tension. In using recipe collections to contemplate the power and limits of different modes and objects of commemoration, compilers invest in the recipe book as a durable medium, even as they often acknowledge the shortsightedness of believing in any lasting material preservation.

We have come far from Shakespeare's depiction of seasoning as disclosing domestic dreams of redeeming time. And yet, my selection of Shakespeare's works as the entry point to this investigation should not suggest an implied chronology in which faith in domestic preservation was gradually undercut as the decades went by. Instead my point is that seventeenth-century recipe collections register different ways that domestic workers placed themselves, their labors, and their written texts in relation to time. Recipes in the eighteenth century continued to play a role in articulating family histories and in promoting the pragmatic tasks of preserving fruits, vegetables, and meats. But the early recipe's stake in "preserving" the human body shrunk as culinary and medical paradigms gradually segregated.

The seventeenth-century recipe collection offers a delimited archive where human life figured prominently at the three-way intersection of temporality, domestic work, and writing. *All's Well That Ends Well*, read alongside recipe collections, trades on the discourses, lexicons, and conceptual frameworks of "preservation" that made domestic work meaningful. It allows us to understand the far-reaching implications of one woman's recipe inscription: "Sarah Hudson her book February the 15th day in the year of our Lord and

Savior Jesus Christ 1678. Sarah Hudson god preserve her in all her [voyages] wheathersoeuer she goeth god preserve & keep her in all parts of *th*e world whear so ever she goeth & whith whosoever she goeth."[83] Positioned as the first words that the reader encounters in consulting a book that was meant to be practically used, Hudson's desire to be "preserved" reverberates against the opening thirty recipes, all of which turn out to be for preserves—"To Preserve Red quinces," "How to preserve cherries without stones," "How to preserve cherryes the best way without stones," "How to preserve gooseberries," "How to preserve Raspberries white or red," and so on. In Hudson's evocation, the mortal human body moving in time and space emerges as part of a gross world in need of spiritual safekeeping. Her prayer for divine protection and her concern for preserving food no longer seem to me to be distinct and unrelated, but instead parts of what I think of as "the imaginary of domestic preservation." The linkage between the erosion of flesh and the reparative work of food technologies was not just evident in Hudson's practices, but also in the textual incarnation of those labors, which aired the dream of transcending the life of any particular human being or of the material world itself. "Remember this," recipes instruct temporally distant readers, even as they show the limitations of that fantasy. As they taught practical methods for how to season, keep, and transform the organic world, recipe texts queried the frameworks humans used to make sense of time itself. Their capacity for reflection also extended, as we will see in the next chapter, to the question of what constitutes knowledge.

CHAPTER 5

Knowledge: Recipes and Experimental Cultures

> They who *do* (though empirically) are to be preferred before those who dispute and talk. All which hath been said in order to justifie the sedulous observations and collections of these ensuing receipts, which are commended because they have *done* upon many, and do carry their reason of *doing* upon most.
> —*Natura Exenterata* . . . *Wherein are contained, Her choicest Secrets digested into Receipts*

"Lerning I would d[e]sire and knowledg crave If I weare halfe sepulcered in my grave": so reads the opening inscription to *Mrs Anne Brumwich Her Booke of Receipts or Medicines*.[1] Although our knowledge about the compilers of this seventeenth-century recipe collection remains conjectural, it was likely begun by Anne Brumwich, the daughter of a Gloucester lawyer, and continued a few decades later by Rhoda Hussey. Hussey, daughter of Thomas Chapman of London, moved up in the world when she married Baron Ferdinando Fairfax of Cameron II.[2] This lavish artifact, complete with gilt-stamped calf binding and clasps, traveled to Rhoda's daughter, Ursula, as well as to her granddaughter, Dorothy. For years, the Fairfax family consulted a recipe collection whose opening page conjured up the image of a half-buried person who nevertheless remained animated by an intense longing for knowledge.[3]

It might be sheer coincidence (or mere expediency) that this inscriber declared a thirst for knowledge in this particular location. After all, it might have been the only piece of paper available when the writer wanted, for whatever reason, to craft iambic pentameter couplets validating intellectualism. As an economizing gesture it might have had little to do with the book's content.

Yet the relationship between knowledge and mundane labor that the inscription raises is worth serious consideration; for regardless of the writer's intentions, the collection and its inscription were read in tandem by later users, who might have wondered what knowledge was imagined to exist in, and around, the recipe world. For the recipe consumer who craved knowledge, what would such a book deliver? How might a person using a recipe have understood the criteria for producing "knowledge"?

The learning that the annotator sought might have referred to the matrix of recipe skills that we have seen in previous chapters: "literacy," broadly construed, with its attendant social status, commercial value, bodily disposition, and expressive potential. Yet my analysis of the intellectual world of the recipe thus far has not yet addressed one of its key functions—its role in producing and theorizing knowledge. The annotation in Brumwich's book invites us to consider ways in which the compiler's translation of labor into writing edged into an articulation of the vocabularies and evidentiary bases for seventeenth-century knowledge practices.

In the most common narrative told by historians of science, the seventeenth century marks a watershed moment for Western knowledge paradigms. As virtuosi such as Robert Boyle, Robert Hooke, John Evelyn, Samuel Hartlib, and John Dee reconceived dimensions of what was then called natural philosophy, their collective efforts both instituted and marked significant changes in how knowledge itself was understood in institutional settings. Because reformers claimed that Francis Bacon had earlier theorized their disparate practices, the name "Bacon" began to stand in for a host of ideas, some of which were not actually advocated by Bacon or put into practice by him. This story of the "rise of Baconian science" is one whose specific contours has been subject to revision, refinement, and critique from numerous vantage points. Some scholars contest any account of historical and intellectual change that isolates and/or heroicizes the actions of a few individual men. Others argue that the term "scientific revolution," often used to describe this shift, obscures gradual changes in intellectual modalities carried out earlier and after this period. Still others skeptically wonder whether there were truly points of commonality among reformers' thinking that qualified their practices as a shared enterprise. And some doubt that the experiments undertaken by those in the Royal Society were truly inductive or empirical in the way that standard histories, colored by developments later in modern science, imply. While the term "scientific revolution" has been discredited as overly sensational and inaccurate, the "rise of experimental science" is a story that, in its broadest strokes, still stands despite nuance and refinement.[4]

In injecting the home labors of food preparation, preservation, and health care into histories of science, I build on a robust body of recent scholarship. William Eamon has identified books of secrets and their heir, the recipe, as helping to reconceptualize natural knowledge and experience in precisely the way that Peter Dear and Lorraine Daston have shown to be critical to the basis of experimental science.[5] This insight allows us to assimilate women's labor to the craft practices of artisans, brewers, tradesmen, and mechanical artists, work that Deborah Harkness, Pamela Long, and Pamela Smith interpret as a popular basis for experimental science.[6] Lynette Hunter, Doreen Nagy, and Rebecca Laroche have made us aware of analogous chemical, herbal, and physiological inquiries undertaken across domestic and scientific domains.[7] The tasks of making cordial waters, omelets, and preserved fruits required a foray, these critics demonstrate, into botanical, herbal, medicinal, anatomical, and chemical knowledges. Domestic work also involved techniques, equipment, and objects of study that overlapped with those engaged in the more recognizable experimentation conducted by members of the Royal Society. We are now in a position to recognize and theorize ways in which recipes *as written forms* might refine these histories. It is precisely this issue that Sara Pennell and Elizabeth Spiller take up in their treatments of the household recipe as a situated knowledge form in this historical matrix; their work opens the door for a more gender-inclusive investigation of seventeenth-century English cultures of knowledge.[8] Scholars may now take seriously the fact that scientific and domestic communities were not just analogous but *overlapping* communities, with recipes providing a shared medium of communication among reformers, ladies, gentry, tradesmen, housewives, and servants. Recipes thus can provide an entry point for considering how people across the social spectrum conceptualized knowledge as they experimented with natural phenomena in their manufacturing of household products, foods, and medicines.

In this chapter I argue that a seemingly mundane form of writing attached to domesticity (though extending beyond its domain) participated in and broadened cultures of experimentation in the period, precisely in its status as a circulating textual form that invited people to reflect on standards of verification. The recent retrieval and availability of manuscript sources is crucial in evidencing this claim, for these sources show that individual labors in the home provided the basis for a textual community of practitioners. When people such as Susanna Packe, Elizabeth Okeover, Ann Glyd, Elizabeth Freke, Philip Chesterfield, and Elizabeth Hirst devised strategies of authorization in their exchange of recipes with others, they generated a collective of knowers who could collaboratively grapple with the relationship of information to "knowledge." The recipe's status as *writing* is thus central to its epistemological mode and its place in a culture of experimentation.

While attention to the recipe archive does not significantly alter the broad contours of the "rise of science" story, it importantly expands our understanding of the popular domains of knowledge production that enabled it. Recipes offer a somewhat unexplored avenue for seeing how people other than a handful of individual reformers thought about modes of knowing through their own created vocabularies and networks of trust. Their working practices formed corollary, analogous, and sometimes intersecting communities with those inhabited by the "new philosophers" of the late seventeenth century. As such, literate domestic work was not outside the cultures of knowledge that were being reshaped on many fronts in seventeenth-century England. Recipes presented routes of truth making.

Probatum Est; or, the Proof of the Pudding

"The proof of the pudding is in the eating": this proverbial saying, operative at least from 1600 on, seems transparent in meaning: a truth can be evidenced by putting it to a test. But what condition of proof rests in eating, or in a pudding? Isn't there a patently faulty analogy between the demonstrable realm of knowledge making and the subjective domain of gastronomy? An otherwise unknown woman named Susanna Packe did not think so. In 1674, she created a collection with recipes for over three hundred products: pickled herring, cheesecakes, preserves, wines, eye ointments, calves head hash, hair stimulant, puff pastes, veal pies, harts horn jelly, anticonvulsants, snail water, and headache remedies. Packe's recipes form a neat presentation copy—written in a fair hand, blocked with justified margins, carefully categorized, and ornamented with flourishes.[9] While we do not have certain information about the compiler, we can surmise that Packe was a woman of means, because the recipes show little concern for economizing paper. (It fell to later writers to scrawl recipes on verso pages and in the margins.) Packe's voice also rings out in the prescriptions through repeated references to her experience in the kitchen and stillroom.

Packe finished her recipe "To Preserve Apricocks Green" by using a phrase that might seem to be out of place in a homey genre of writing. After instructing her reader on the time-sensitive operation of alternately scalding apricots with sugar and letting them rest at intervals, she concluded with the Latin tagline *probatum est* ("it has been tested/proved"). This academic-sounding claim appears sixteen times in Packe's collection, reverberating with similarly authorizing notations, such as "proved" or "approved." It is easy to read *through* this phrase, because it was a conventional "efficacy tag" in medieval and Renaissance medical treatises and books of secrets, sometimes applied to patently impossible formulas and acts. Critics largely dismiss *probatums* as phrases that writers unthinkingly copied by rote from sources or wielded in bad faith to make a sale.[10] But manuscript recipe sources, as I will show, do not allow such a sweeping dismissal; they lead us instead to assess individual claims to proof on a case-by-case basis.

Interpreting recipe claims of proof takes us to the more basic question of how recipe books were conceptualized and used in the early modern period. Until recently, scholars have been unconvinced that early modern recipes had much to do with actual practice. They have been skeptical that women employed recipes to undertake work, because it was assumed that people who actually performed manual labor were illiterate. As such, handwritten recipe collections have been assumed to be presentation copies exchanged in patronage-gift economies and/or proudly displayed, the equivalent of modern-day coffee-table books. This perspective has been reinforced by general skepticism about whether prescriptive texts of any kind connected to genuine historical practice. Even if one concedes that workers read recipes, how do we know that these writings bore any resemblance to what went on in the kitchen?[11]

Yet, as Sara Pennell has instructed us to see, manuscript recipe collections provide invaluable evidence of firsthand practice, particularly when contextualized by sources such as household accounts and diaries. Elizabeth Hirst's collection becomes a case in point. Housed in a worn calf binding sealed with leather clasps, *Mrs. Elizabeth Hirst Her Book* is alphabetically organized as a recipe encyclopedia, with space left under elegant header letters for future readers to supplement. We have no definitive evidence about who lettered this collection or any means for identifying its historical context, though we do know that Hirst was from a Yorkshire family and that recipes in the collection mention nonaristocratic sources. As the compiling agent, Hirst peppered the margins with comments, many of which registered her personal evaluation of remedies. She assured readers that she "often & effectually experimented" with the ubiquitous mad dog bite cure (6), that she was "certaine" that her appetite stimulant would "take away the loathsomeness of meate" (2), and that her pimple cream "will infallibly cuer without danger" (38).[12] Dozens of recipes are marked "probatum," "try'd and approved," and/or "excellent."

Hirst's collection provides insight into her concerns and thought processes. In weighing the benefits and pitfalls of two remedies, for instance, she declared that her "balsom is equivolently vertuous to the Pretious great Balsome, only it lasts but 3 yeers" (6). While she sometimes exaggerated (e.g., her cure for shortness of breath, "is the best remedy for this distemper known" [9]), she also scrupulously used marginal commentary to translate all-purpose panaceas into curatives for specific ailments (24). In short, Hirst claimed direct knowledge of the fine points of treating illnesses and manufacturing confections while using her collection to assert her learning. "This watter to my own knowleg hath dun great cures," she proclaimed of her remedy for a kidney stone (65).

Elizabeth Okeover similarly testified in her collection to her involvement with culinary and medical work. Okeover, who helpfully signed several recipes and volunteered her married name (Adderly), inherited a family recipe book within the Okeover family of Staffordshire that she then continued.[13] In a running commentary carried out largely in the margins, Okeover amended and improved recipes for ointments, salves, cordials, cheesecakes, biscuits, and stews, while singling out treatments favored by particular aunts and cousins. She cross-referenced information, provided an extensive index, and cited a wide array of family members, friends, famous elite women, printed sources, and doctors (including, in one case, her nurse). Her annotations are chatty and personal.

An earlier compiler modeled for Okeover the value of personal experimentation. A balsam remedy, not in Okeover's handwriting, concludes with testimony to a sensational, if gruesome, medical success: "I: pr: this cured a head that was burned to the very skull" (88). The "I" that "proved" the remedy provided a template of practical engagement that Okeover took to heart; after inheriting the collection, she tested already-gathered recipes, added her own, and repeatedly backtracked through her contributions to update methods. As in Hirst's text, Okeover's notations have different goals—to promise effectiveness; clarify, emend, or elaborate instructions; and sort information efficiently. She could not praise highly enough, for instance, a "blast salve" treatment, a diagnostic and palliative ointment for "blasted" or infected sores. Okeover endorsed her ointment made of cream, marigolds, chamomile, and hyssop no fewer than five times. She underscored her titular endorsement, "Blast Salve

Most Exelent," with the further notation—"good" (229). In the margin, Okeover reinforced her enthusiasm by staking her (shifting) identity and labor on its worth: "this I make Eliz: Okeover now am Eliz. Adderley." As if this were not enough, she reiterated her zeal for this salve in a note in the index: "tried & is good" (185v). While the collection includes generic markers of approval, these idiosyncratic bits of testimony persuasively document a hands-on knowledge tied to the assertion of her identity.

Okeover also presented herself as a curious researcher with a clear interest in tinkering with processes and sifting information. It was somewhat orthodox for her to note that she innovated her mother's method for making "Flose Unguentorum" ("ointment of flowers") by altering the proportions. "This is the salve I allwais make," she wrote, "putting in half a pound of each sort of rasin and a pinte less of wine" (219). In other recipes, she went beyond an account of how she altered existing formulas. Beside a remedy for scrofula or the "kings evill," Okeover documented ways to identify a key ingredient, "green flag," which, she notes, resembles the "sword flagg and growes in the water" (Figure 49). "The root," she observed, "may be knowne in being of a red or flesh couler" (20). (Though now classified within the Iris family, "flag" in the seventeenth century referred to any plant with a bladed leaf, such as a rush or reed.) Okeover's skill as amateur botanist cropped up again in her commentary on a rickets remedy that required fox fern, a term that she obligingly glossed as a "male fern" (230). She provided helpful tidbits on many fronts: how to understand weights for cherries (inverted 10); how to choose the best sugar candy for a cockwater (76); and how to economize when stewing a rabbit (inverted 2). Her expertise included seasonal advice: "the cure is best in the spring if it be not very cold in Aprill," she said of a rickets remedy (231). Finally, she confidently assessed the relative merits of recipes and directed her readers to see similarities between curatives scattered throughout the collection. Of an herbal garlic-and-sage cordial, for instance, she observed, "it is good for the same things that Mrs. Roes yallow salve is and is called the flowre of oyntments because it is good for so many thing[s]" (42). Like Hirst, Okeover left abundant traces of her activities as a cook, herbalist, researcher, and writer. The cumulative effect of Okeover's additions, however, is to display not merely herbal and culinary knowledge, but also her active and sensory involvement in the process of managing information. In its construction of a writing persona, her collection calls forth a vivid sense of lived experience: the head wound burned to the very skull, the person suffering back pain who nevertheless searched ponds for red-rooted ferns, the observer who tested the orange har-

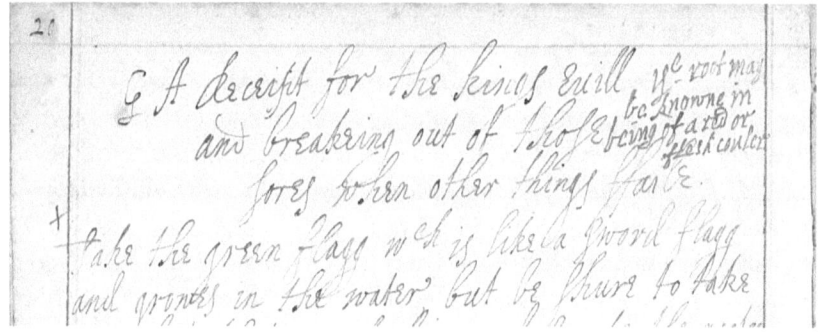

FIGURE 49. Elizabeth Okeover's herbalist marginal notes in *Collection of Medical Receipts*, ca. 1675–ca. 1725, Wellcome Library, MS 3712.

vest in different months, the vernacular intellectual eager to know how to gender plants.

Given the signs of practice evident in manuscripts, it seems wrongheaded to disregard claims to verification made by recipe compilers as mere convention. Yet the question still remains: when compilers used phrases such as *probatum est*, what did they imagine their recipes to have proven or "tried"? In marking recipes for stewed carps, pigeons, and fricassee with "probatum est," Susanna Packe seemed to judge success in terms of taste. In these cases, she used the phrase, in short, as a subjective valuation akin to her other expressions of enthusiasm ("very good," "most excellent"). Recipe users, then as now, signaled disapproval by cancelling the text with dark slashes or denouncing it in the margins. A sausage recipe in a collection that went through the hands of Elizabeth Browne, Penelope Humphreys, Sarah Studman, and Mary Dawes was mildly valued as "not very good," while a limeade recipe in a compilation by Mary Ann Anstey and Diana Matilda Fenwick suffered harsher judgment: "by no means good."[14] You can almost hear Elizabeth Godfrey's snort of exasperation as she crossed out a recipe for candied angelica and proclaimed: "this is the worst way to doe them" (11) or Lettice Pudsey's frustration when she struck out her own recipe for preserved cucumbers and protested, "This receipt is good for nothing" (fol. 57). The recipe collection was, we might expect, a site for asserting individual preference.

Yet more often than not Packe used the term "probatum" to launch one of three different types of truth claims. Her phrase implied, first, that a medical remedy, despite modern skepticism to the contrary, had been proven to be effective in curing a particular ailment.[15] When Packe marked her recipe for surfeit water, which promised to "clear the stomach of what offends it," as "probatum est," she testified to the "proven" quality of the knowledge. This notation thus chimed with other claims to verifiability, as when she indicated that a scurvy remedy "cured G.P. when his head was all of A whit scourse which caused his hare to com ofe" (63), or when she observed that an eyewash "restored the sight of one Blind 3 years" (76). Second, Packe used "probatum" to guarantee that some foodstuffs and concoctions would effectively last in preserved form and not mold or sour for a given number of months or years (Figure 50). Her instructions for making raspberry paste, currant wine, pickled marigolds, damson, and cherry gum were tested with this understanding of proof in mind. When she marked candied angelica (a commonly used medicinal plant with long, thick, fragrant roots) as "probatum est," she pledged that the processed plant would remain moist and durable for two years, with "proven" being a quality of the material in question—like steel that has been

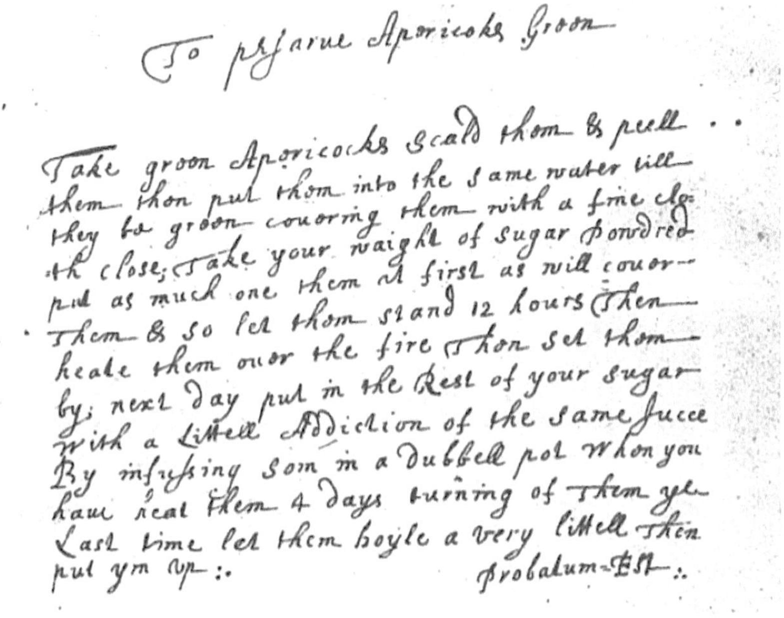
To preserue Apericoks Groon

Take groon Apericocks scald thom & peell
them thon put thom into the same water till
they be groon couering them with a fine clo
th close; Take your waight of sugar powdred
put as much one them at first as will couer
Them & so let thom stand 12 hours Then
heate them ouer the fire Thon set thom
by; next day put in the Rest of your sugar
with a Littell Addicion of the same Jucce
By infusing som in a Dubbell pot when you
haue heat them 4 days turning of them ye
Last time let them boyle a very littell then
put ym vp:. Probatum Est:.

FIGURE 50. "Probatum est," in Susannah Packe's *Her Book Anno Dom 1674*, Folger Shakespeare Library, MS V.a.215, p. 11, fol. 5. Photograph by Wendy Wall, from the collection of the Folger Shakespeare Library.

"tempered." Properly pickled orange and lemon peels, she stated, would last half a year if seethed in a vinegar and sugar based syrup: "Only if you see any defect as to mould, then . . . heate them over the fire or set them in a warme oven," she warned, an operation that she deemed as "approved" (177). What she saw as "proven" in pickled marigolds was their durability: "these will be as fresh all yeare as new got," she promised (175).

Finally, Packe offered assurance that one could reliably predict how a substance would be altered by a technical operation such as heating or cooling, processes that might congeal, purify, or liquefy substances. In this case, "proven" was a quality of the broader material environment beyond the case of a particular recipe. With this definition in play, Packe asserted that changing what we now think of as the pH balance of a concoction would vary a substance's color.[16] Her syrup of violets and preserved green plums required precise manipulation and seasonal timing in order to create the proper color, a reliable indicator of taste and durability (117; 244); her "experience" led her to see that adding egg to puff paste decreased its firm texture (166). Occasionally it is not clear what is being "proven" in a given recipe, for two main reasons: (1) recipes assumed this information as self-evident, and (2) some claims fit multiple and overlapping categories. To take one example: Packe promised that her cowslip wine, which could be ready in a month's time, "will drink Excelent brisk & clear." "I have experienced it," she added (81). The reader might wonder whether Packe meant to bear witness to the wine's flavor, its timeline for fermentation, or its clarity, which elsewhere marked durability. When she declared her harts horn jelly "proven," it's not evident whether she meant to refer to the success of her dyes, her method for creating viscosity, or the jelly's benefits in preventing fatigue (241). While the scope of some truth claims are difficult to delimit with precision, and while numerous manuscript and printed recipes, medical treatises, and books of secrets conventionally included the all-purpose "approved" in their titles, some recipe writers nevertheless couched specific assertions of proof amid their commentary. The *probatum ests* that saturate manuscript recipe writing thus have to be assessed within their individual contexts.

In what follows, I address ways in which recipes constituted knowledge practices and participated in general experimental cultures of the seventeenth century. I first examine the experimental work that recipes describe and then look to the rhetorical and syntactical ways that the recipe world of letters explored the grounds of legitimate knowledge.

The Home Lab

Does the work undertaken by recipe users have any bearing on experimental science in terms of questions and methods? At first glance, the answer seems to be a decided "no." When we read Thomas Dawson's late sixteenth-century recipe for spiced salmon balls, we are struck by his lack of specificity as well as the inexact manner in which he couches his instructions:

> Take your Salmon and cut him small in peeces of th[r]ee fingers breadth, and when you have cut so many slices as you will have, let them be of the length of a womans hand, then take more of the salmon, as much as you thinke good, & mince it rawe with six yolkes of hard Egges very fine, and then two or three dishes of Butter with small raisons, and so worke them together with cloves, Mace, Pepper, and Salt, then lay your minced meat in your sliced Aloes, every one being rolled and pricked with a feather, full closed, then put your aloes, into an Earthen pot, and put to it a pinte of water, and another pint of Claret wine, and so let them boile til they be enough.[17]

While Dawson was precise about the number of eggs to be used, he left the seasoning of the dish and cooking time entirely at the reader's discretion. To the modern eye, the recipe appears quaintly folksy in its inexactitude: Dawson's reader was called to use her fingers to measure salmon strips and was asked to approximate the median size of a woman's hand. How much fish to use? "As much as you thinke good," Dawson directed. How long do you boil the ingredients? "Til they be enough," was the answer. Dawson either assumed the practitioner's experience or aimed to encourage invention. Rather than inviting users to reconstruct particular techniques within a fixed stable environment, recipes such as this one encouraged the reader's exercise of skill and taste. While the recipe genre did establish and calibrate units of measurement over the course of the seventeenth century, it was only later that it sought to establish the standards of precision necessary for modern scientific trials.[18] As such, domestic experiments hardly resembled those that we imagine the Royal Society to have conducted, especially when we take as our point of reference the instances that historians foreground when describing the development of modern science.

Scientific reformers were ambivalent about recipes and the utilitarian culture of which recipes were a part. On the one hand, recipes offered valuable information about materials and methods. "New philosophers" sought to cultivate any sources that recorded observations about natural specimens because they aimed to enhance their stock of information about the natural world. They also depended on craft knowledge for some experimental techniques. On the other hand, they adopted Bacon's claim that "light-bearing," or pure knowledges, were superior to "fruit-bearing" ones (practical know-how).[19] Although the technical acts of making recorded by recipes often relied on the inductive mode that Bacon admired in artisanal crafts, Bacon saw them as an insufficient basis for a reformation of knowledge. Recipes failed to meet the criteria for knowledge laid out by Thomas Sprat in *The History of the Royal Society*; he insisted that miscellaneous observations had to be converted into systemic theories of causation and that rules needed to be extrapolated from the accumulation of particular instances.

Pamela Smith persuasively demonstrates, however, that artisanal knowledge played an important role in early modern cultures of knowledge, despite its overtly pragmatic aims and lack of theorization. When goldsmiths, painters, artists, and locksmiths developed techniques for manipulating natural materials, they formed a body of inquiry adopted by later reformers. Smith further contends that the empirical work of craftsmen constituted an experimental methodology in and of itself. In writings by artists and metal casters (who left detailed descriptions of how to forge enamels, cast metals, and create pigments), Smith identifies the seeds of a "vernacular science of matter" produced through embodied experience.[20] Antonio Pérez-Ramos's analysis of "maker's knowledge" provides a framework for understanding the theoretical framework underpinning vernacular science. Maker's knowledge, according to Pérez-Ramos, "postulates an intimate relationship between objects of cognition and objects of construction and regards knowing as a kind of making or as a capacity to make (*verum factum*)."[21] He explains: "Pictorially speaking, the sort of knowledge that results from making or doing something may be described as a kind of net which the prospective knower can impose on certain things in so far as they are potential objects of technical (re)production. So the idea-type of maker's knowledge can be first conceived as an internalization of operational skills in the most disparate fields of activity" (48). As craftsmen created and manipulated material substances, they demonstrated "the capacity to understand a reliable procedure for making" (50). Artisanal tasks involved an epistemology.

Recent revisionary assessments of early modern science and of its attendant epistemologies are beginning to acknowledge the importance of artisanal craft and recipe work. Deborah Harkness maintains that Bacon's visionary model of scientific experimental collective had its proper context in the social networks, urban workshops, and trades of London. Scholars have used the wrong metrics, she contends, to assess the contributions that manual workers made to scientific change. Artisans' "significance lies not in the elucidation of new formulas or the construction of new cosmological systems," Harkness writes, "but in the ways that they organized their communities and settled disputes; the value that they placed on the acquisition of various literacies (including mathematical, technical, and instrumental literacies); and the practices that they developed that led to an increasingly sophisticated hands-on exploration of the natural world" (10). According to Harkness, Lime Street botanists, apothecaries, barber surgeons, merchants, millers, grocers, and tradesmen laid the foundation for scientific development in England. In fact, she positions none other than recipe writer Hugh Plat as the unacknowledged leader of scientific experimentation at the turn of the century. It is vital to her conception of science that Plat filled his notebooks with lore that he gleaned from goldsmiths, clock workers, gardeners, wine coopers, haberdashers, soap boilers, schoolmasters, glassmakers, fruit sellers, salt makers, surgeons, preachers, vendors, female traders, ladies, and housewives. Gardening discourse, as Rebecca Bushnell has demonstrated, also constituted a nonobvious site of intellectual production and marked shifts in knowledge cultures over the course of the seventeenth century. Bushnell points out that recipe writer Gervase Markham grappled with issues fundamental to a Baconian project: empiricism, experience, and method.[22]

Expanding the term "science" to include the labors of a wider spectrum of the population in its rise has enabled scholars to make visible the contributions that specific and exceptional early modern women played in vernacular knowledge making. Witness Linda Pollock's work on Margaret Hoby's life and diary; Elizabeth Spiller's facsimile editions of recipe collections by Aletheia Talbot (Countess of Arundel) and her sister, Elizabeth Grey (Countess of Kent); and Lynette Hunter's research on "sisters of the Royal Society," including John Evelyn's sister, Mary, who described herself as "under the roof of the learned and in the neighbourhood of science," and Robert Boyle's sister, Katherine Jones (Lady Ranelagh), who housed her brother's lab, exchanged recipes with reformers, and ran a salon for the Hartlib Scriptorium.[23] Recipes were the *lingua franca* used by reformers (such as Hartlib, Boyle,

Oldenberg, and Digby) for conversations about natural matters throughout the 1640s and 1650s.[24]

These conversations extended beyond elite circles and the public limelight to the home front. In her 1655 commonplace notebook, for instance, an otherwise unknown woman named Sarah Horsington cited Boyle's published medical and experimental work. As Lynette Hunter has shown, Horsington tested Boyle's "Salis Armoniack" (a complex chemical distillation that she describes as having the same "nature" as "ruine & soot") as she concocted a curative for headaches, epileptic seizures, and water retention.[25] Jane Lowdham and her husband, Caleb, a surgeon in Exeter, similarly distilled medical, botanical, and craft knowledge from Boyle's writings.[26] The Horsington and Lowdham recipe collections prove that women who were not in inner circles of intellectual or social power engaged in now recognizably "scientific" knowledges as part of their domestic preparations.

Yet the extant recipe archive chiefly provides a way to place individual women and unusually educated readers on a continuum with women who were *not* physically in the neighborhood of science; that is, recipes allow us to consider the acts of women who had not read written records of experimentation by reformers and were not specifically seeking to apply that information to their tasks. It was not just a handful of extraordinary intellectuals that explored early modern natural knowledge, but also those performing the everyday culinary and medical experiments that we now categorize as domestic labor. The intellectual pursuits that people undertook in their domestic life overlapped, in this particular historical moment, with the processes that scholars recognize as "science" when practiced within a certain set of parameters and institutions. Harkness's research places women just on the horizon of vernacular knowledge. She unearths evidence that Plat used women as intellectual sources: Mrs. Carlton taught him how to store apples for winter; his children's nurse provided advice about how to provoke menstruation; and Lady St. John of Battersea shared tips about effective ways to use milk in making bread (220). Plat, according to Harkness, saw his central role as extending, recording, and testing experiments he witnessed throughout London. While Plat's journals document the methods he absorbed from heterogeneous sources, we have only hints about the activities of these "sources." But we *do* have extant recipe collections, texts around which readers formed non-site-specific intellectual communities.

The collaborative nature of domestic experimentation is evident in one of the most common recipes in seventeenth-century collections, books of secrets, and technical manuals: how to make ink. In collections claimed by Jane Newton, John Partridge, Lady Barrett, Elizabeth Hirst, Lady Dorset, Archdale Palmer, Mary Granville, and the Boyle family, compilers weighed in on how to modify a basic formula that depended on the interaction of galls with iron sulfate in a liquid. When oak galls (growths on oak trees caused by insects) are mixed with iron sulfate and exposed to air, they produce a black pigmentation.[27] That oak gall growths contained corrosive tannic acid was widely known. Sir Toby Belch, in Shakespeare's *Twelfth Night*, puns on the bitter sentiment etched in its galling medium when he urges Andrew Aguecheek to write a "martial" letter urging Cesario to fight a duel: "Taunt him with the license of ink. . . . Let there be gall enough in thy ink; though thou write with a goose-pen," he declares, pitting the cowardice of a goose against the perceived aggressiveness of ink (3.2.37; 40–41).[28] The trick to making ink involved getting the vitriol/gall mixture to form the proper texture, so that the product would stick to a quill but not run too readily or blot.

In a basic ink recipe, Partridge recommended that the gall and vitriol solute be suspended in wine; that gum arabic (the hardened sap of the acacia tree prized for its solubility in water and lack of taste) serve as the most effective thickening, stabilizing, and binding agent; and that sunlight be used as the best heat source.[29] Gum arabic played a role in embalming in ancient Egypt, illustration in medieval times, lithography in the modern period, and, as we have seen, confectionery in the early modern period. Over the course of the seventeenth century, recipe users from different regions and social circles identified and broadcasted particular problems raised by the basic ink formula. In recipe writing, they identified common elements among diverse formulas and positioned this repertoire as the basis for innovation and experimentation.[30] Making ink invited practitioners, for instance, to tinker with additives that might enhance viscosity and/or prevent deterioration. In an "aproved" ink recipe Jane Newton added bay salt to the standard mixture of galls, gum, and copperas, presumably as a preservative to prevent molding (209). The preservative nature of salt was, of course, well known, but Newton had hands-on experience in testing saline mixtures, as her recipes attest, when she brined and salted meats and fish. Newton also joined a debate about what container best facilitated pigmentation (she recommended an earthen pot so as to withstand acids); she also tweaked a basic formula by declaring it possible to create serviceable ink without applying sunlight or heat (209). When Newton recommended setting the galls and green copperas for three days before adding gum, she addressed the problem of how to maintain the consistency and color of the ink over time. A writer known only as R.W., on the other hand, resolved this problem by soaking galls in double-refined sugar water, a process that subjected ink to what we now see as fermentation. Newton and R.S. did not comment on the chemical properties underwriting their experiments with ink making. Yet the Lowdham recipe book suggested that tidbits of general natural knowledge could be abstracted from the particular process of making ink. "Vitriol placed near to Amber," the writer scribbled on the flyleaf, "loseth its colour & pungency."

Recipe compilers queried which liquid might best express the corrosive aspects of iron sulfate. Four different ink recipes in Lady Marquess Dorset's collection explored the benefits of alternative liquid bases—ale, wine, rainwater, or water mixed with vinegar.[31] The Granville collection advocated using vinegar or beer as the solvent, presumably to rid the substance of impurities and render pigmentation consistent (42). Elizabeth Hirst proclaimed beer to be a more effective thinning agent than rainwater (49). In an ink recipe that he attributed to his son, Archdale Palmer (landholder and High Sheriff in Wanlip) claimed that strong white wine "fetcheth out the substance & the life of the galls which water cannot doe."[32] Dorset appeared to favor this solution as well, for in her final ink recipe, she concluded that a nonalcoholic base could work effectively if one was willing to perform additional labors—stirring the mixture daily, housing it in an earthen pot lined with a lead base, and mincing galls and gum into "little gobbitts" (53). Lady Barrett experimented with using beer, rainwater, and vinegar in the four ink recipes she gathered from friends and family. "Rich malaga wine is best "if you have it," she concluded. The Boyle family collection advised mixing rain water with white wine vinegar, in order, we might surmise, to leach iron from green copperas.

What do we see from these competing ink-making techniques? In a practical task of home manufacture, recipe writers identified and attempted to resolve practical problems. Could ink set properly at room temperature or did it require a heat source? Could crushing galls in water achieve the same technical goals as boiling? Did alcohol act as an antifreeze? What substance enhanced ink's absorptive ability? In devising solutions (in both senses of the term), recipe collectors innovated the formulas they inherited. Identifying gum as the element that made ink shine, Lady Dorset, for instance, found that she could substitute ale wort to achieve the same level of glossiness. The Boyle family compiler (Katherine Jones, perhaps) elected to use pomegranate peels, which we now know contain tannins that intensify pigmentation. In seeking to unlock the mystery of ink, compilers enacted Baconian processes: they identified shared properties inhering in classes of natural substances by subjecting them to artificial manipulation; proceeded by analogy from one result to an unknown situation; and generated knowledge that extended beyond the purview of a single product. Domestic testers performed what Thomas Vaughan called, in 1650, "the Chimistrie of Sack-possets," to which, he noted, women were especially suited.[33]

Determining the precise ways that particular individuals experimented with recipe formulas is made difficult by our inability to map recipe routes of transmission with any certainty. Attributions and signatures are little help in this regard: ownership marks typically applied to only a fraction of the recipes in a given compilation and individual attributions often did not indicate personal associations.[34] Yet, in some instances, it is possible to identify a temporal line of transit and to determine how a particular recipe user customized a formula.[35] When Lettice Pudsey recorded "Mrs. Okeover's Recipe for Balsom," for instance, she was not simply repeating a well-known curative but reproducing a formula that exists verbatim in Elizabeth Okeover's collection. After copying the recipe, Pudsey supplemented the curative with new applications that she discovered: in addition to being able to "cure a head that was burned to the very skull" (88), it could treat venereal disease, convulsions, headaches, sores, gas, and burns. "I have allso found it most excellent for sore breasts & for swellings: & stopings in the stomach," Pudsey wrote. Have "noe fear of tacking to much," she assured readers, adding advice that the medicine would go down better if accompanied by a good stiff drink. Pudsey envisioned her source as proposing a hypothesis that she subjected to multiple tests over time.

Through their testing and their accumulation of data, recipe users formed diffuse research cooperatives that reflected on questions at the heart of natural philosophy. Reformers in the mid-seventeenth century looked back to Bacon's outline of inductive method in *The Novum Organum* as the foundation for a new natural philosophy. Bacon famously proposed to create a natural history that was "not only of nature free and at large . . . but much more of nature under constraint and vexed; that is to say, when by art and the hand of man she is forced out of her natural state, and squeezed and moulded."[36] The sexual politics of conceiving nature as a tortured and feminized entity have not gone unnoticed in feminist critiques of the history of science.[37] But there are other implications for women's labor vested in gaining knowledge of nature through artificial accommodations and mechanical actions (such as molding or squeezing).[38] Making the natural properties of flowers, minerals, and vegetables legible required what Howard Marchitello calls the "artifaction of nature" (177). Practical work in the kitchen was predicated on the assumption that artificial constructs *produced* "truth" about living matter.[39] The task of preventing fruits from putrefaction or making ink shine required workers not only to gather information about organic substances but to position natural knowledge specifically in relation to human intervention.[40] Such was Baconian experimentation shot through with the paradoxes that fueled humanist literary writing, chiefly issues revolving around the ever-perplexing relationship of art and nature.[41]

The ethos of experimentation was not confined to medical or preservative work but extended to cooking, as seventeenth-century Mexican writer, intellectual, and courtier-turned-nun Sor Juana Inés de la Cruz testified. In an epistolary response to Sor Philothea, which offered a defense of female education, Sor Juana wrote:

> What could I not tell you, my lady, of the secrets of Nature, which I have discovered in cooking? That an egg hangs together and fries in fat or oil, and that, on the contrary, it disintegrates in syrup. That, to keep sugar liquid, it suffices to add the tiniest part of water in which a quince or some other fruit tart has been. That the yolk and the white of the same egg are so different in nature, that when eggs are used with sugar, the whites must be used separately from them, never together with them. . . . What is there for us women to know, if not bits of kitchen philosophy? . . . If Aristotle had been a cook, he would have written much more.[42]

We might wonder as well if Aristotle's taxonomies of knowledge might have altered had he exchanged recipes and become part of this collective experimenting with the production of knowledges. It is to the transmission of home experimentations that I turn now.

Proof in Transit

Beyond the technical proficiency aired in the content of recipes—which included expertise about methods, the qualities of substances, and the laws governing the material world—their very form conscripted experimenters as stakeholders in epistemological questions. In what ways did recipes incite consideration of evidentiary standards? Answering this question involves seeing recipes not just as registering signs of practice (which remains an important element in recovering women's history) or as aide-mémoires for housewives and ladies, but also as literate forms that modeled and initiated processes of collecting, testing, altering, and emending.[43] Historical evidence of their circulation geographically and temporally makes it hard to imagine anyone crafting a recipe collection without *assuming* that it would be read by others.

In claiming to have proved the truth of a recipe, compilers might seem, at first glance, to be asserting and bequeathing definitive knowledge. Yet traces of recipe use show that readers often took *probatums* as starting points for customizing prescriptions and generating new knowledge. The recipe's grammatical formulation as a command is important in this regard. Opening with an imperative such as "take," "make," "distill," or "boil," recipes syntactically ordered readers to "actualize" knowledge by undertaking action. Even though recipes were written in the imperative voice, their second-person address acknowledged that readers had the option of refusing command as part of the condition of proving. Because they were codified syntactically as contractual forms, recipes were, by no stretch of the imagination, finished products but forms that asked to be received, tested, validated, or refused.[44] As its name indicated, the *receipt* ethos initiated a transaction with an active *receiver*, the implicit *you* who must take, boil, or distill as a relay point in the equation (the Latin *recipere*, "take," resonates strongly). The imperial command exuded by the recipe writer remained in tension with the prerogative of the implied "you" carried by the second-person imperative, a tension that exposed the conditional credibility they offered.

The recipe's syntactical form becomes meaningful when read through the history of its exchange. Even individual recipes marked "proven" reverted into untried sources subject to a second level of review when traveling to new audiences. As friends and family copied bits of collections, added recipes, tucked recipes into letters, and/or passed their "core" collections to others, they sought to re-prove information. Pennell labels the process by which the reader authenticates information as "perfecting practice," by which she means that recipes posit a "truth" that can never be identified in a stable point in time but instead exists as mobile information. In recipe work, "the reproduction of actions can never be perfected" (239).

From a modern viewpoint, it might seem unremarkable that domestic laborers would think of their sensory experience in manipulating nature as the grounds for establishing contingent truths. Yet this epistemology was somewhat at odds with more official paradigms taught in early seventeenth-century centers of learning, which continued to view *praxis* as offering a limited, lesser form of knowledge. In the Neo-Aristotelian models saturating universities, certainty flowed from the citation of ancient sources, deductive paradigms, and logic. As Peter Dear summarizes, scholasticism treated "experiments" as mere heuristic demonstrations confirming the truth of a world constituted by abstract first principles. "A statement of experience," Dear writes, "was acceptable because, at least ideally, it was what everyone knew. It was a universal statement of common experience, and could therefore be used as a premise in a scientific, syllogistic demonstration: just like the axioms of geometry, it was evident, and so required no formal proof."[45]

It's commonly accepted that seventeenth-century thinkers such as Robert Boyle, Robert Hooke, Samuel Hartlib, and John Evelyn challenged Aristotelian-based assertions by promoting inductive modes of inquiry and empirical engagement with nature. While some reformers turned to the mission of discovering the mathematical laws that governed the universe, others trumpeted the importance of firsthand observation of nature as a means of establishing new paradigms for natural history and philosophy. Knowledge of nature converted into a proliferating body of "facts."[46] Adopting Bacon as a rallying cry and theoretical nexus, reformers at midcentury sought to prove the characteristics of a natural object or system in a moment isolated in time and dependent on the production of human effects.[47] As Spiller, Eamon, Dear, and Daston have outlined so lucidly, the Baconian-identified scientific movement replaced the Aristotelian notion of experience as what is *generally* true with a modern idea of experience as a "singular, repeatable act that follows determinable physical laws."[48] What the Greeks called *metis* (practical intelligence based on acquired skill) was considered a lesser form of knowledge than *episteme* or *scientia* (certain knowledge). *Metis* divided into *praxis* (the study of particular experiences) and *techne* (which involved bodily labor): all were gradually recategorized in the early modern period as paths to valid philosophical knowledge.[49] Within the emerging model, Smith writes "a man, learned in the sciences, had to escape out of the library into the laboratory, field, or shop to undertake a knowledge-making process that included the production of effects" (17–18). The formerly distinct domains of *episteme*, *praxis*, and *techne* were newly interconnected in the paradigm that would later become known as "science."

As Spiller has argued, recipes participated in the redefinition of knowledge and experience in the seventeenth century. Published recipe writing occasionally brings this point home when positioning readers as skeptical experimenters. The title page to Plat's *Delightes for Ladies* commands "Read, Practice, and Censure," pointedly emphasizing the need for readers to subject information to judgment and testing.[50] Later in the century, collections attributed to Hannah Woolley and Aletheia Talbot insisted (ironically, perhaps, given their status as textual advice) that experience trumped attributed information. Talbot's *Natura Exenterata* included a preface signed by "Philastros," which made a bid for the recipe's place in an empirical rather than theoretical environment. "They who *do* (though emperically) are to be preferred before those who dispute and talk," Philastros declared. Spiller observes that this preface made "fundamentally the same case for recipes that the Royal Society would make for its experiments"; it explicitly engaged the "premises of Aristotelain scholasticism in order to present recipes as a meaningful and appropriate form of knowledge."[51] Recipe writing claimed a role for *praxis* and *techne*.

Household manuscript collections may appear to contradict the impersonal ethos of emerging empiricism, however, and instead hearken back to an older scholastic model resting on cited authority. After all, compilers freely credited their prescriptions to friends, family, and experts, citing Lady Allen's water, Mrs. Kirby's pickled walnuts, Dr. Willis's kidney stone drink, Robert Boyle's spirit of roses. If personal experience was so critical to domestic workers, why did they persist in attributing recipes to others? Did the recipe's generous citational structure work, that is, to contradict the *probatums* that were also a hallmark of the genre? One way to resolve this apparent contradiction is to recognize that there were discrete and compartmentalized modes of citation in recipes, some of which, as I have discussed in previous chapters, largely concerned community building, social aspiration, and commemoration. Entries marking a grandmother's treasured recipe for pudding, for instance, marked a concern for identity and affiliation that had little to do with crediting experimental methods.[52] The donor's name, in these cases, read less like a scholarly footnote and more like a diary entry. *I remember this act/event this way.*

Yet in addition to their social and personal utility, recipes referenced informants to establish credibility. Eschewing direct experience in favor of inherited expertise, the recipe compiler appeared, in these instances, to rely on an older mode of verification. If this is Lady Barrington's salve, it must be fine indeed. Why doubt it? This credentializing structure is most evident in instances where the recipe donor had recognizable expertise. When lay medical practitioner Lady Grace Mildmay titled her epilepsy remedy an "approved course . . . by Doctor Athill for children betwixt 3 and 10 years old," she prompted her reader to substitute Dr. Athill's specialized knowledge (confirmed in part by the specificity of information) for her own authentication.[53] Alternatively, compilers might heighten the recommending power of nonexpert practitioners by marking the recipe's multiple transmissions. Lady's Cotton's remedy for the dropsy (swelling) was given to Elizabeth Okeover, she noted, by someone named Dalton (245). Elizabeth Hirst's "yellow sanders" recipe, which involves having the patient drink her own urine baked in burnt ash tree, was given to her by Mr. Elton, but its ultimate source, the recipe documents, was Dr. Willis (80). By detailing a recipe's collective acceptance and resilience, compilers structured an accreted system of approval.[54] The names that populate recipe collections may thus at first glance appear to qualify information more by its "proven" quality in the past than its imagined testing in the future.

Yet past approval was not necessarily opposed to contingent future proving in recipe citational systems. To take as one example, consider the formation of authority in Rose Kendall and Ann Cater's recipe book, a compilation that cited, among others, the Countess of Warwick, Mr. Pigeon, Lady Barrington, Lady Maynard, Mrs. Mason, Lady Sillyard, Dr. Stephens, Lady Morley, Lady Howett, and Mrs. Herman. When the collection circulated to seventeenth-century readers Anne Wentworth and Elizabeth Clarke, how, we might wonder, did they interpret "To Make Clear Cakes of Gooseberry Lady Barrington's Way," which was signed "Approved by me" (4v)? While they would likely have assumed that the compiler(s) received the recipe from Lady Barrington (or copied it from someone else's collection with this attribution intact), the name "Lady Barrington" did not automatically guarantee the dish's value. Instead readers were called to test the testimony, which involved assessing multiple modes of *approval* against their own incarnation of gooseberry cakes. The name certainly served, as Foucault writes of the author-function, as a classifying device wavering between the poles of designation and description, distinguishing Lady's Barrington's delicious treats from other confectioners' versions.[55] Yet the compilers were hardly claiming Lady Barrington as the text's "author" (in a modern sense of the term), because she might readily have copied the recipe from a printed source or begged it from a friend. It was strikingly unusual for Elizabeth Freke to insist that "the Palsy Water Lady Freke" was falsely known as "the Lady of St. John Dropes" because "the original is my grandmothers' of Dorsettshire" (444). Attributing a recipe did not usually constitute a claim to ultimate origins but instead a means of differentiating it from other similar formulas.

The fact that Lady Barrington was said to have recommended, if not created, a formula for clear cakes, however, was not completely insignificant to its value. She served as a crucial corroborating witness in a collaborative experiment; that is, her name marked the relational quality that David Goldstein has seen as central to identification in the recipe genre.[56] Attributions thus functioned as a component within a credentializing system based on mobility.[57] We've seen that when women and men circulated, copied, and excerpted recipes they subjected their own truth claims to review by a community of knowers whose individual experiments then underwent similar reverification (even when the recipe was attributed to an "expert"). Recipe systems of naming thus marked the recipe's travels within a community of potential knowledge conferrers. Citations that seem strictly commemorative were not, as we might have first imagined, *outside* the production of knowledge, but one of its less obvious constituent elements. The "knowledge-effect," so to speak, emerged out of the circulation of independently insufficient confirming voices. It took a village, or at least textually connected set of kitchens, to qualify pudding making as knowledge.

It might also seem that the recipe's reliance on testimony made it an *impure* form of the genuine empirical practice carried out by learned men elsewhere in the culture. The Royal Society theoretically entrenched an idealized distinction between *approving* and *proving* through their motto—"*Nullius in verba*" (on no man's word)—a sentiment echoed by numerous reformers who preached that nothing should be credited except by direct personal observation. Yet, as sociologists of early modern science have so clearly demonstrated, witnessing was an explicit feature of all seventeenth-century sites of knowledge formation. According to Steven Shapin, the Royal Society fundamentally depended on the textual proliferation of firsthand observations by trustworthy reporters. In attending to the practical and rhetorical contours of truth making in early modern England, Shapin shows that the newly confirmed ideal of direct experience had limited practical value: reformers could not be skeptical of all knowledge derived from testimony and still allow knowledge to be communicated. Seventeenth-century experimental science was predicated on an understanding of knowledge as, by definition, social and sharable (as opposed to prior alchemical or esoteric formulations). After members of the Royal Society conducted experiments at Gresham Hall, or some other semipublic place, they made it their mission to circulate an account of the event in the form of an historical report detailing the location, date, and witnesses. "The thrust of Boyle's, and the Royal Society's, early program was to build a solid factual foundation for a reformed natural philosophy by soliciting more and more testimony and extending the networks of justified trust further and further," Shapin writes.[58] He argues that reformers grafted modes of verification onto preexisting networks of trust and credit in the culture. Only gentlemen, argues Shapin, were afforded "perceptual competence" in reporting on natural phenomena, centrally because they were economically independent and therefore positioned to be objective. Experimenters thus piggybacked their criteria for the reliability of witnessing on established social models.

To the dismay of feminist critics, Shapin dismisses the idea that early modern women could have played the role of scientific witness, in part because Shapin adheres to a narrow definition of genteel credibility.[59] Shapin's top-down model fails to acknowledge the legitimacy of early modern challenges to male elite authority or to the importance of competing civic and religious authorities as rival power centers. His understanding of gentlemanly competence thus rests on a view of early modern social structures that overestimate the currency of popular devaluations of women and nonelite men. Certainly people loudly and repeatedly proclaimed that only certain portions of the population could act as accurate reporters, but these viewpoints did not go unchallenged—in theory or in practice. In fact, the recipe archive precisely points us to one site where players other than elite men constructed alternate modes of authority.

If the scope of trust in Shapin's account is widened rather than rejected, however, his model provides an important analytical tool for understanding recipe knowledge formation, particularly in allowing us to see the way that collections created a community of knowers as the context for transforming eyewitness testimony into "knowledge." *Probatum est* in recipe writing performed in the kitchen what Shapin has identified as the "virtual witnessing" crucial to scientific protocols of the Royal Society. The intrusive voices of recipe compilers who chimed in with firsthand observations of the natural world as well as the sources they cited confirmed the techniques by which features of the natural world could be revealed. As Pennell has so astutely argued, the recipe's citational structure thus forms both a social and epistemological process; it etched lines of affiliation while lodging truth claims as utterances interpreted (and interpretable) within a community. Attributions and addresses to readers, in Pennell's reading, did more than signal networks and alliances; they generated an economy of knowledge.[60] Given that there was no Gresham College laboratory in which a community of ladies and housewives could gather to watch live demonstrations of the processes they undertook, the *textual* circulation of their materials became all the more critical in generating a site in which knowledge could be validated.

We have to remember as well that few people witnessed the experiments performed at Gresham College and thus the Royal Society also had to devise reliable textual and rhetorical means for proliferating and substantiating knowledge. Only five years after the founding of the Royal Society, Henry Oldenberg, in 1665, founded the *Philosophical Transactions* to serve this aim; it soon became the Society's central public face. As Peter Dear has shown, the *Philosophical Transactions* regulated the particular format and syntax that writers could use in encoding observations into recognizable knowledge.[61] Dear argues that the journal established rhetorics deemed appropriate to the epistemological basis for reformers' knowledge, a discourse designed to mark the reformers' distance from scholastic methods. Rather than start with a premise found in a textual source as part of a deductive argument, articles in the *Philosophical Transactions* were required to narrate a concrete event or moment of observing experienced by an identified author who remained highly present throughout the narrative.[62] Unlike modern experiments, which highlight the objective nature of knowledge, early reports were personally and socially saturated. Written in the first-person voice, lodged in the past tense, and peppered with concrete descriptive details, they thicken the immediacy of the encounter and endow the representation with an air of verisimilitude. "Scientific" writers followed what are now seen as techniques in creative writing. Henry Powers's report of his microscopic examinations of the sycamore locust in the *Philosophical Transactions*, for instance, hardly reads like a modern scientific account: "I could not only see its eyes," he declared, "which are red, goggled and prominent but also I could see them perfectly latticed."[63] According to the journal's protocols, an experiment had to emerge as a discrete historical occurrence fixed in time and space rather than a singular event anchoring a general statement. The mesmerizing detail of the locus's perfectly latticed red eyes made the experiment-event intensely present.

What form did articles in the *Philosophical Transactions* take? In addition to structured experiments seen by particular witnesses, the journal included entries solely devoted to recounting observations. Most reports were written as epistolary letters in a polite discursive style; some answered queries from previous writers. Authors felt free to register their disappointment, frustration, or surprise with results; that is, they did not attempt to detach the human actor from the scene of knowledge production. Occasionally first-person narratives flowed into a second-person recipe-like directive, but writers always re-anchored the form in a broader descriptive mode. Indeed, as Dear argues, an empirical commitment to the experience of the individual reporter was the only point of commonalty that diverse Royal Society members shared. The syntactical and rhetorical formal conventions of the *Transactions* generated the lingua franca that consolidated a group that otherwise might have splintered. Knowledge was entertained as an explicitly mediated product that had to be fabricated within a conventionalized literary and linguistic form. It becomes clear that the protocols of writing were not secondary to practice but implicated within it.

Household recipe writers developed their own vocabularies and systems of credit in ways that analogously sorted through the rhetoricity of knowledge and competing conceptions of experience. "The appending of a name to a recipe," Pennell writes, "is not merely a mark of donation, but also a register of witness and circulation; the recipe lives up to its title in being worthy of transmission" ("Perfecting Practice," 250). We have seen how truth making evolved in relation to practice and mobility, but there is more to say about how *witnessing* functioned as a rhetorical and syntactical operation in recipe collections. How was knowledge *qualified* in the framing devices and modes of address in these texts? What lexicons of proof did recipe communities employ?

Royalist supporter Philip Stanhope, Earl of Chesterfield, directly addressed the issue of evidentiary standards and methods in his medical recipe compilations, only the first two volumes of which have survived. Stanhope's collection is organized alphabetically, with red-letter capitals heading each neatly ruled page. The title page to the large folio (which extends over a thousand pages) reads: "A Booke of Severall Receipts for Severall Infirmities Both in Man and Woman, and most of them eyther tried by my selfe or my wife, or my Mother or approved by such persons as I dare give Creditt unto, that have Knowne the experiment of it themselves."[64] Labeling his book in such a way, Stanhope attempted to persuade readers of the veracity of his information by intermixing his own genteel standing (marked by his name, title, and sumptuous textual artifact), his role as practitioner, and his ability to vouch for the credibility of kin, friends, and experts. Declaring "most" information to be tested by intimates or recommended by people with firsthand experience, Stanhope fused testimony and practice.[65] His opening statement forced the reader to take seriously the conventional adjectival word "approved" attached to individual recipes in the text. In fact, Stanhope set up a sliding scale whereby he moved from hands-on trial, to the reliability of people he "dares" to consider most intimate, to credited sources. In addition to sources marked by their exotic or foreign status (e.g., "a German," "a Spanish physitian," "a Jew, physician to a Turk"), Stanhope tracked information as it circulated among—and was produced from the experience of—ladies, non-elite women, doctors, and family members, including his first wife (Katherine Chesterfield, daughter of Lord Hastings), mother, daughter-in-law, son (Arthur), brother-in-law (George Hastings), and sister. Stanhope also credited mobile information, from the "Syrup of Clove Gilleflowers" that Dr. Butler gave to Mrs. Moore, to a remedy derived from Dr. Frank, who bestowed it on Lady Gerrard of Dornely. His wife's recipe for fever reads: "I myself have proved, K. Chesterfield." Local doctors, ladies, and countrywomen joined in a network managed by Lord Chesterfield. In this textual community, unmediated experience collapsed into a virtual witnessing open to a wider array of reporters than the Royal Society typically sanctioned. While Stanhope's gentlemanly reputation served as the initial social anchor validating the collection, the fact that he could extend credit to female and nonnoble practitioners signaled elasticity of status in recipe modes of "truth telling."[66]

Elizabeth Freke, who, as a propertied gentlewoman living in Norfolk, did not occupy as elevated a social station as Lord Chesterfield, also grounded her knowledge in a mixture of personal practice and credited sources. Her indices include these headers: "A Table of the Receits: of Cakes, boiled meats & Physick: Collected by mee for my own use & most of them proved by Eliz. Freke" and "A Table of Physical Receits for my own use and Most of them Experyenced by mee Eliza. Freke with the Authors from whence I had some of them collected," found when the book is inverted (Figure 51).[67] Through these framing devices, Freke inscribed herself as collector, reader, primary user, person of experience, and prover. In choosing to speak directly to her reader about her proprietary knowledge, she placed herself on her reader's radar as a writing subject. Rather than accentuating her informants, as did Stanhope, Freke emphasized that the socially stratified sources that she convened were subject to her own reading and judgment. She indexed and footnoted sources with yet two additional tables, "An Alphabetical Table of all the Herbs plants, roots, trees I have taken out of Gerards herbal for my own use & convenience E Frek March 23, 1700," and "Of Flowres and Fruits, out of Cullpeper for my Memory" (290). By claiming "my" use and "my" memory, Freke nominated herself as the text's primary reader, despite the fact that she addressed an imagined audience throughout

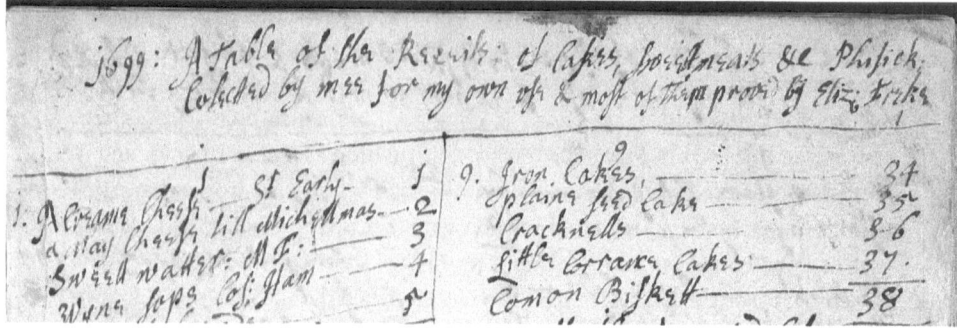

FIGURE 51. Header to the index in Elizabeth Freke's *Commonplace Book*, British Library, Add MS 45718, 1684–1714. By permission of the British Library.

the collection. When she declared that she had *partially* tested prescriptions (proven "most" recipes), Freke enjoined her future self or her implied reader to get to work and finish a task in process; that is, she enjoined later readers to filter textual sources with personal experimentation.

In the absence of direct statements about evidentiary standards (such as those seen in Stanhope's and Freke's collections), we can identify compilers' economies of trust by looking to inscriptions they made to individual recipes. Let's return to the Cater/Kendall collection, where, as we have seen, the compiler generated a mutually authorizing circuit of knowledge by marking Lady Barrington's clear cake recipe as "approved by me." How, we might ask, does the model of witnessing, which reformers drew from legal precedents and which guides Shapin's account of knowledge formation for experimentalists, work in this instance? In the realm of modern science, we typically distinguish "proving" (verifying by a set standard) from the "approval" of the witness, which confirms a preexisting truth. If this distinction were operative, however, what witness, in this recipe, is called to trial to substantiate what claim? The phrase "approved by me" leads one to believe that the compiler testifies to the truth of Lady Barrington's prior practice. Yet in Pennell's account of the recipe's structure of authorization, the *donor* is assumed to be the corroborating witness, the personified footnote substantiating the text's truth-value. The confusion of witness and actor muddies the clarity of a stable proven truth that *can* be distinguished from its later approval. Are these operations temporally or spatially distinct? Or conceptually inseparable?

Grace Mildmay's note about a recipe for cinnamon oil sent to her by Mr. Harris highlights the lexical ambiguity that contributed to this evidentiary uncertainty. When Mildmay writes in a letter, "I have proved and made oil of cinnamon only with water and by no means with sack," she plays on two modalities of the semantically capacious word "prove" that are differentiated in modern parlance: "to test" or "to authenticate."[68] Through this duality, Mildmay fuses authentication into labor of the *test*. She further complicates the matter by impeaching her chief witness because she *improves*, or perhaps *reproves*, in both senses of this term, Mr. Harris's recommendations; for Mildmay pointedly uses water rather than his recommended sack. The temporally unstable triad of donor, annotator, and future reader endows the recipe form with the degree of complexity that scholars are more apt to recognize when they grapple with linguistically and conceptually difficult texts. Shakespeare's poetic evocation of the pleasure-torment of sexual consummation in Sonnet 129 is a case in point, because scholars have thought long and hard about what "A bliss in proof and proved a very woe" might mean (1798). "Proving" as a test and a stated category of knowledge (that of being "proven") merged lexically in recipe discourse to create a productive intellectual quandary.

The diacritical model complicating when and by whom knowledge was conferred in recipe writing is further compounded when we take into consideration the English penchant for using the second-person imperative in recipes. Early modern Spanish, by comparison, customarily used the third-person voice. The English structure's implied reader—"you"—complicates the issue of witnessing. If "you" are enjoined to make the clear cakes according to Lady Barrington's instructions, do "you" add contingent additional approval to the truth of Barrington's knowledge? Is the implied reader, that is, a new potential witness whose presence is registered linguistically in the recipe's linguistic structure? Or has Lady Barrington now become a chief witness for the reader's expanded culinary repertoire? Grammatically, the genre interjects an unactualized future prover into the already complex matrix of the form. Even as they undertook the seemingly simple task of recording the best ways to make eye ointments and quince pastes, recipe writers navigated the question of conditional and processual truth making.

There is more to say about the use of the second-person imperative as the signature format for English recipe writing. In addition to creating a contractual form with an implied active reader, this linguistic structure split the writing subject into authoritative speaker and potentially skeptical receiver. If a compiler copied a yet untried recipe from a friend, she acted, at that moment, as the receiving "you" who might later make the dish and then, by virtue of now being the writing subject, convert into the approving prover of information for a future reader. In recording Lady Barrington's clear cakes, Rose Kendall and Anne Cater, for instance, heard her commanding voice urging them to take a quart of gooseberries and begin this process of making. After testing the information, Kendall and/or Cater assumed the mantle of that commanding voice, which was exhibited each time the collection was consulted. As both recipe producer and consumer, that is, the speaker linguistically inhabited temporary and shifting subject positions in relation to her text. She had to recognize that only the envisaged "you" could endow the donor or herself with the role of knowledge maker in a process that potentially proliferated collaborators and witnesses, some of which would then assume her place in the process. In this way, the recipe reader was trained—through the act of reading—to understand the operations of declaring, testing, doubting, and approving as distributed across ever-shifting positions.

While this may seem an overly ingenious reading of a fairly simple genre, we need only consider the gains made by literary criticism in exposing the complexities of the enunciating "I" as a speech act. Understanding the structures through which women could take up particular modes of address in poetic, philosophical, and religious writing has been important to scholars investigating early modern ideologies of gender. The "self" or "subject" that comes to life in poetry, for instance, has been seen as a template through which a reader might imagine a being in time and in relationship to persons and institutions. Despite the fact that they are reputedly simple formulas, recipes involved linguistic structures with similarly freighted meanings. Given abundant historical evidence of recipe circulation, we are in a position to see that their rhetorical operations fashioned and theorized epistemologies. Necessarily positioning a speaking subject in relation to past source, practice, witnesses, and the implied receiving "you," recipes *distributed* verification—as a recurrent process—across persons, speech acts, and labors.

When collectors appraised recipes for ink or lemon cream, they were swept up into scrutinizing lexicons for establishing truths. Elizabeth Digby, wife of Robert the first Baron of Digby, chose a vocabulary, for instance, that made transparent the status claim underwriting her knowledge. Her 1650 collection is introduced as "Receipts Approved by Persons of Qualitie and Judgment, collected by Elizabeth Digby, 1650" (Figure 52). The worthy persons who vouch for Digby's credibility (and allow her to nominate them as worthy)

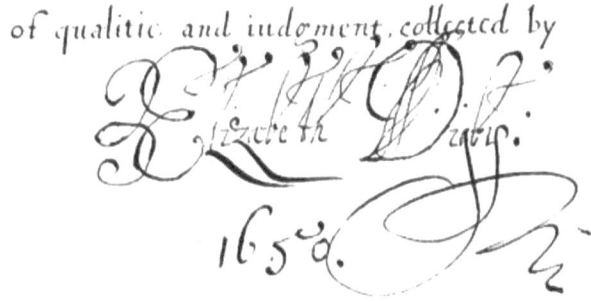

FIGURE 52. Title page to Elizabeth Digby's *Receipts*, British Library Egerton MS 2197. By permission of the British Library.

include Lady Grace Cavendish, Lady Stafford, Sir Fulke Greville, Queen Mary, and various doctors. Digby thus wielded the genteel standing that Shapin sees as critical to authenticating scientific disinterestedness, even as she extended her status-based ("quality") to non-elite informants.

Other recipe compilers concentrated their energies on selecting among linguistic options for guaranteeing and constituting knowledge. They deployed the word "prove" and its cognates to construct various claims to veracity—from the weakest forms of verification (the use of the word "approved" in a recipe title, with no supplementary support), to the strongest ("pro. myself"), with other formulations existing ambiguously on the spectrum.[69] When writers marked a formula with "probatum est," for instance, they employed a learned Latin phrase that tended to mystify agency (it "has been tested" by whom? the reader might wonder). To make matters more complicated, this phrase was associated with the *textual* tradition of books of secrets and medical treatises; the moment of proving thus inscribed the experimenter in the inherited traditions that empiricists typically found inadequate. Using this erudite phrase might or might not have legitimized collection as a learned tradition; for by the mid-seventeenth century, books of secrets had increasingly been identified as forms of entertainment trading in fantastical prescriptions that drifted far from the realm of practicality. Household recipe compilers adopted this authorizing tagline, ironically, just as it was being discredited in the reading public. The use of *probatum est* certainly made a claim to prior trial in practice, but the term introduced vexed problems. For some readers, it might have insinuated the writer in a reliable knowledge community predicated on learned medical authority. Yet given that it was the object of parody in some contexts, it might have exposed, for other readers, the compiler's distance from elite intellectual networks. The recipe collection *Natura Exenterata*, as we have seen, mocks the esoteric and theoretical world of medicine to which *probatums* were conventionally attached, calling attention to the limited value of the professional "Beard and Gowne" as signs of expertise. Yet the author tellingly recuperated the word "probatum" as signaling an empirical recipe practice opposed to empty learned discourse. It can thus be argued that recipes reclaimed and recoded a conventional medical "efficacy tag" for a different knowledge-culture.

Recipe writers had at their disposal a plethora of rhetorical options for positioning truth in relationship to a human proving subject. In what I call "signature probatums," writers preserved the passive construction of the Latin tagline but eschewed its disembodied tone. Ann Glyd, whom I discussed earlier, assiduously tested and recorded various truth claims. Her most common notion—"probatum Ann Glyd"—appropriated the prestige of learnedness, but also gave specificity to its otherwise seemingly universal quality. "Probatum," in the third person, singular, and passive form presented an air of certitude removed from a particular trial (it has been proved, sometime in the past). As in many of her other guarantors of truth, "probatum Ann Glyd" emphasized particularized human agency. Glyd also marked some recipes with personal testimony: "Pro my self" (21); "proved by myself" (23); "I myself have several times for horses feet proved it Ann Glyd" (66); proved by me Ann Glyd" (51); and "approved by me Ann Glyd" (60). In others, she opted to name others as provers: "probatum my Aunt Eavens" (53) or "proved by my cousin Grail" (52). Her statement, "I have proved with good effect Ann Glyd," emphasized "proving" as testing rather than "authentication," but she collapsed this distinction in other usages (62). She wrote "Approved by my selfe" beside an "Excellent Receipt of the cramp," for instance, but then crossed this note out and replaced it with "*Probatum* Ann Glyd" (80).[70] As Glyd's multiply purposed rhetorical forays indicate, the personalized *probatum* allowed the writer to have it all ways: to insert a writing subject who controlled the scene of proving into an established idiom that rested authority on depersonalized knowledge-making.

When recipe proving rested on particularized experience, it offered exactly the type of claim favored by the *Philosophical Transactions*.[71] When Glyd marked her currant jelly "July 9, 1700," she rendered her experimental making as a discrete moment in time (33). When Packe declared of her green plum jelly, "I have expearnced it Eleaven yeare," however, she vested her truth claim in replicability over time and thus severed its value from any singular discrete instance of proving (257). Along the same lines, Elizabeth Hirst bragged that her cure for a mad dog bite had been "often & effectually experimented" (6). And Glyd proclaimed of a fever remedy, "this I have given several times when infectious distempers have bine in my hous and the distemper hath spread no further Ann Glyd" (51). Okeover, Glyd, and Fanshawe customized their collections by obsessively marking their initials or names beside recipes; through proprietary, custodial, and agentive gestures, compilers, we see, developed numerous ways to personalize the otherwise disembodied second-person voice of the recipe. When Okeover inscribed "This I make" next to several recipes, she did more than mark a favorite recipe; her choice of the present tense signaled the recipe's ongoing use value as well as the knowledge value of making. We begin to see that recipe writing was not an ancillary legitimizing of what was already "known," but a fundamental defining of knowledge itself. In this respect, Spiller's work goes far to complicate Dear's conception of the Royal Society's broadcasting of practice as a secondary legitimizing act. "Once science is understood as a practice for creating knowledge," Spiller writes,

> the textual qualities to scientific texts cannot simply be understood as secondary to the scientific work that is at stake. Everything that comprises the physical existence of the text—its literary and rhetorical strategies; its illustrative and textual practices; the authors and the readers who created knowledge by making sense in and through texts—are expressions of the same practices for creating knowledge that define science itself. . . . It is not that science must necessarily . . . be mediated through the books, letters, illustrations and other textual forms in which it ends up being expressed. (*Science, Reading*, 5)

The difficulty in separating practice from medium comes across in one reader's note scribbled beside deleted medical recipes: "All theas receiptes ar verye falsly written. but being corrected heer they ar trew."[72] Claims that representations were wrongly written may have reflected concerns about accurate transcription or handwriting, but they also "made "trew" instructions a matter of content and form.[73]

The epistemological problems manifest in recipe claims to proof come to the fore in Shakespeare's *All's Well That Ends Well*, which, as I discussed in Chapter 4, reveals how domestic work was implicated in philosophical investigation of temporality. I return briefly to this play because it enables us to see another critical element of the recipe genre—its engagement with the nature of authorization, particularly its interest in the relations carried within lexicons of approval, proving, experience, reading, and empirical practice. It is, in fact, the "proven" status of the recipe that becomes its salient and signature feature for the play's heroine. When Helena seeks to gain the right to determine her own choice of husband by healing the king, she uses an immensely powerful recipe that she inherited from her physician father. But those around her do not immediately recognize the power of this recipe. Helena's argument for the legitimacy of her knowledge not only sheds light on debates in medical culture but also illuminates the epistemological dilemmas surrounding recipe practice.

In Shakespeare's immediate source, William Painter's *Palace of Pleasure*, the heroine learned her craft by watching her father work.[74] Shakespeare pointedly altered his source so that it is a treasured *written* recipe that is at the center of Helena's power. As well, when Helena seeks permission to treat the king at court, she does not argue simply for her father's expertise in classical or contemporary medicine. Instead she emphasizes that the remedy's tried-and-true information has been validated through a combination of experience, textual sourcing, accurate transmission, and corroboration:

> You know my father left me some prescriptions
> Of rare and prov'd effects, such as his reading
> And manifest experience had collected
> For general sovereignty, and that he will'd me
> In heedfull'st reservation to bestow them,
> As notes, whose faculties inclusive were,
> More than they were in note: Among the rest
> There is a remedy, approv'd, set down,
> To cure the desperate languishings whereof
> The king is render'd lost. (1.3.216–24)

In heralding the "approved" cure as having "prov'd effects," Helena interchanges claims to empirical proof with witnessing, a combination that, as we have seen, was typical in both recipe cultures in the early seventeenth century and in experimental reformers' writings later in the century. It is precisely the movement between *approval* and *proving* that is at stake in Helena's conceptualization of "experience." Who "approv'd" her father's remedies and by what means? And was the recipe's status as "set down" in writing, which she emphasizes, a marker of the cure's effectiveness? When her father collated his experience and reading to produce a written recipe, was he demanding an empirical re-proving of its "effects" by the future reader of his text?

Helena may also have recognized the limits of written knowledge by acknowledging the "secrecy" tradition from which the recipe genre emerged. Although technical "secrets" originally referred to esoteric knowledge whose causes remain occulted, recipe writers often recast the language of "secrecy" to refer to the private or protected nature of their information. Helena's father's instructions reveal a degree of guardedness, as he asks her to use "heedfull'st reservation" to bestow the prescriptions (1.3.211). Helena reemphasizes this point when she later tells the king that the recipe was

> . . . the dearest issue of [her father's] practice;
> And of his old experience th'only darling,
> He bade me store up, as a triple eye,
> Safer than mine own two, more dear. I have so. . . .
> I come to tender it and my appliance
> With all bound humbleness. (2.1.104–7; 111–12)

Treasured as a vital body part, the recipe can be revealed only through Helena's performance of the text, what she terms her "appliance." The cryptic phrase that Helena used earlier to validate her recipe requires further glossing in this light. Editors read her description of her father's recipes—"As notes, whose faculties inclusive were, / More than they were in notes"—as meaning that the recipes possessed more virtues than their writing indicated. But the phrase might additionally point to a surplus of knowledge that exceeds written instructions. Helena hints that the recipe is incomplete information dependent on a supplemental "appliance."[75] Practice may not just be the sign of legitimacy but the required *completion* of a partial textual instruction.

In recipe collections, we do find evidence of the value of withheld information. *Select Receipts*, signed by Ann Egerton and marked as "Taken out of Lady Barrett's Book case, Oct. the 24th 1711," included one recipe directly requesting that readers keep the information confidential: "A most excellent receipt for the Eyes, which I pray keep secret" (150). Was Elizabeth Fowler being coy when she broke off a recipe for orange biscuits with these words—"what more you must do next I cannot tell" (99)? Or was this simply an admission of the insufficiency of her knowledge? Mary Granville's failure to supply a promised recipe might have constituted a simple oversight, but it also might have indicated her decision to keep a particular formula out of circulation (27). The writer who most famously capitalized on this strategy was Hugh Plat, who hinted that his disclosure of information was deliberately transgressive. Plat claimed that he betrayed his wife's secrets by divulging her cherished cheese recipe (which she had refused to circulate); he elsewhere teasingly declined to disclose mysteries to his audience. Hannah Woolley had entrepreneurial interests in mind when she left some of her information incomplete. In *The Supplement to the Queen-Like Closet*, she informed readers that they could learn practices that could not be communicated in writing by coming directly to her shop and hiring her services (60–61). We return, then, to Helena's suggestion in *All's Well* that her inherited recipe might include *more* than is presented in its written incarnation; for her hint about the limits of textual knowledge now seems freighted with additional meanings. Her "notes" from her father champion a formula to which she has special proprietary oversight, one that must be proved in its "appliance" or use.

Helena also presents recipe experience as conflating past and present approval with practice and with textual sourcing. Skeptically labeled an "empiric" by the king, Helena is later praised by him as a "sweet practiser," both code words for those using empiricist methods (2.1.120, 186). Bequeathed to Helena in recipe form, the medical curatives exhibit the characteristics we've identified in manuscript collections of the day: they are marked, in the text, as mobile, contingent, and vested in readerly use. Placing the recipe at the intersection of reading, collection, experience, and "appliance"—and marking it as simultaneously "approved" and "prov'd"—*All's Well* hints at the vexed issues surrounding the *probatum ests* of the kitchen. Let's remember that when Helena beseeches the king for permission to treat him, she says that it will test the divine: "of heaven, not me, make an experiment," she begs (2.1.153). But this test modulates, in her next sentence, into a certainty emanating out of her "art": "But know I think, and think I know most sure, / My art is not past power, nor you past cure" (2.1.156–57). Her claim to "know most sure" can truly only materialize in Helena's iteration and actualization of the recipe script, in an action where her conditional knowledge will necessarily be reapproved: "proven" this time on a sovereign's body. In the early 1600s, when recipes were newly popular in print in England, Shakespeare positioned his heroine to grapple with a newly visible, yet unofficial, locale of knowledge production.

Although the recipe disappears from the plot of *All's Well* after the healing of the king, it persists as an overarching trope, manifest in the title's teleological "wellness" under which other plots coalesce. After Helena manipulates a form widely known to balance truth making and practice, she chooses to "prove" another text: the nasty letter in which the reluctant groom Bertram confesses that he has abandoned his wife and sets out "impossible terms" for a reunion. In Shakespeare's source, Helena receives a verbal report of her husband's disavowal of her. Yet Shakespeare again alters his source so that Bertram's bitter farewell, the equivalent of "when hell freezes over," comes in the form of a written note. In this letter, Bertram states that he will accept Helena as his wife only if she is able to extract a ring from his finger that he promises never to remove, and to have his child *before* he sexually consummates the marriage. Framed in the conditional, this letter becomes the catalyst for Helena's decision to create a "lawful deceit" and sexually substitute herself for Bertram's paramour in the dark. Grappling with how to make Bertram's instructions materialize, Helena moves from the epistemological conundrums of the recipe to another mode of "proving" with equally significant interpretative and bodily stakes.

In the play's notoriously jarring ending, characters struggle to reach consensus about what has truly happened; proof is the issue quintessentially at stake. Indeed the word "proof" and its cognates appear six times within fifteen lines in the final scene, and the issue of "proving" (meaning "substantiating") events is the lingering problem in the concluding lines. Helena produces as evidence Bertram's letter, which she has cleverly emended to suit her purposes; it requires only her pregnancy rather than an actual child. Her proof is accepted—though conditionally. Bertram offers a guarded—perhaps, coerced—emotional pledge: "If she, my liege, can make me know this clearly," he tells the king of Helena's claim to be pregnant with his child, "I'll love her dearly, ever ever dearly" (5.3.312–13) Helena's response repeats this conditionality: "If it appear not plain and prove untrue, / Deadly divorce step between me and you" (5.3.314–15). While epistemological cliffhangers are conventional in drama, its twist in *All's Well* is that it reincarnates (and exposes) the knotty conundrums of knowing explicitly attached to the recipe milieu. It is perhaps unexpected, or ironic, that Shakespeare's deliberately folklorish and unrealistic play registers timely meditations on early modern epistemologies. Shakespeare taps into the social and economic power of wielding a household knowledge that was nevertheless riddled with uncertainties and slippages. While we do not know whether all is indeed well at the end of this play, we do see ways that recipes alienated practice into literate forms that proliferated self-critical modes of knowing. These issues were, so to speak, on the table, in recipe culture.

Siting, Reading, Reflecting

Recipe writers not only traced their labors in curing epilepsy and conserving quinces but also contemplated the standards by which everyday truth claims might be judged. The transactional nature of recipe exchange, in fact, enabled the virtual witnessing that was a signature of knowledge production in scientific circles. "Practice," as we've seen, was not compromised by its mediation but converted into recognizable *knowledge* in part through its dissemination. The sociology of knowledge that has been undertaken with regard to the work of Royal Society reformers can thus be instrumental in preventing scholars from falsely identifying women's recipe exchange as an inexact version of a more "pure" form of knowledge making occurring in some other domain.[76] Through the recipe archive we are able to see the presence of otherwise unrecognized communities of reader-practitioners, *other* economies of knowledge enmeshed in the intertwined acts of making, writing, and reading.

Although household experiments might seem a far cry from those conducted by the Royal Society, both domestic and scientific experiments, as we have seen, flunk when graded according to modern standards of empirical verification; both were invested in interjecting a writing "I" and reading "you" into the transfer of information in ways that affirmed testimony and social relations. When I have laid out this argument in scholarly conversations, I've received diametrically opposite responses: the connection between domestic and scientific experiments either seems obvious or outlandish on the face of it. The fact that Robert Boyle and John Evelyn exchanged recipes with housewives and ladies either seems manifest evidence of a shared epistemological quest or is dismissed as incidental to the genuine innovations of science. Shapin, who takes a somewhat skeptical view of women's role in the rise of science, writes, "there is little reason to think that women were involved on anything but a casual basis in Boyle's program of technical labor: I know of no female laborant, operator, or chemical servant in Boyle's employ, nor is there even indirect evidence to suggest that women might have worked for him in these capacities" (*Social History*, 369). Shapin certainly *critiques* the sexism of a period that created social barriers for women who might otherwise have claimed scientific authority, noting in particular ways that Boyle staked his scientific credibility on a rejection of sexual alliances with women. Although Boyle learned handy tips from women (such as the nature of static electricity) and although he profited from the intellectual, emotional, and financial support of his sisters (Katherine Jones and Mary Rich), these women, Shapin concludes, simply were physically "not there" in Boyle's laboratory. He writes of Jones:

> There is no evidence that Lady Ranelagh was a physical presence in Boyle's laboratory, or indeed that she was at all concerned with the quotidian processes of chemical and pneumatic work that went on there. Nor is there any substantial evidence that she took a view of matters belonging to the practice of experimental natural philosophy: the cause of porosity, the correct mechanical explanation of colors or cold, or the specific gravity of talc. . . . Like many seventeenth-century gentlewomen, Lady Ranelagh thought it right that the woman of the house be able to practice elementary medicine, and she kept a collection of medical "receipts" which her brother intermittently acknowledged in his publication and which, indeed may have been an important source of his own work on medicinal "specifics." Lady Ranelagh's invisibility in experimental natural philosophy therefore stems substantially from her apparent lack of interest in the details of what was going on in her brother's laboratory at the back of her house and in the particular knowledge claims which flowed out of it. (*Social History*, 371–72)

Shapin's criteria for what counts as "experimental science" rests on the defined location of the laboratory and a firm distinction between pharmaceutical knowledge and "genuine" experimental inquiry. For women to be included in experimental work, they would have needed to construct an air pump, devise theories of causation, created nonutilitarian experiments, or, at least, have loitered in physical proximity to virtuosi at work.

Shapin has a point. If household recipes had laid out systematic processes or theorized causality in their experiments, historians of science might have credited their scientific contributions at this watershed moment. Recipe collections were instead miscellaneous in their topics and erratic in their truth claims. Some recipes emphasized community building and fantasy over and above a concern for standards of verification. And yet, when scholars assess the role of receipts in the history of science, they do not actually *read* household recipes or think about their affinities with the written transactions of the

Royal Society. Shapin pointedly makes his findings about women's lack of credibility as scientific reporters by rehearsing the culture's devaluation of Eve's daughters. Feminist scholarship, however, has richly shown that women's interactions in social life in the period often flew in the face of widespread claims to their disempowerment and that women exploited the fissures and contradictions in discourses of misogyny. Shapin's subsequent point, about the lack of evidence that women were physically "there" in the laboratory, oddly imposes an anachronistic modern division of specialized space on the early modern world, a division that Shapin elsewhere critiques in an astute discussion of "siting" knowledge production. Historical evidence suggests a more elasticized view of the domestic space as simultaneously kitchen, brew house, stillroom, garden, and laboratory.

Laboratories and other household spaces shared structural features, implements, and material goods. Inventorying Sir Kenelm Digby's laboratory at Gresham College and the 1707 Golden Phoenix laboratory (modeled on Boyle's laboratory at Jones's house), Lynette Hunter maintains that "virtually everything that [the laboratory worker] might have needed was readily available in the kitchen or still room of any substantial estate" (182). Knives, long-handled forks, trivets, straining ladles, jelly bags, pestles and mortars, furnaces, fires, braziers, tripod heating pots, ovens, distillation tubes, alembics, glass basins, gongs, earthen vessels, chopping plank, grinding stones, plate ware: these were precisely the implements required in recipe work. In the late seventeenth century, stillrooms increasingly became the provenance of women, and the phrase "still room" began to refer specifically to a space distinguished from the "laboratory," a site exclusively for experimentation that was still nonetheless lodged in the home.

Why would Lady Ranelagh need to be physically present in her brother's laboratory to experiment with natural substances when most everything required to do so was available elsewhere in her home? Looking for written testimony that women frequented the few sites where exceptional men conducted particular brands of experiments misses the larger point: the home *was itself* a locale of knowledge production, out of which scientific work was emerging, spatially and conceptually.[77] Long before the reformers erected spaces dedicated to scientific work, women and artisans engaged, as Smith argues, in the "work of making direct access to original nature count, both socially and intellectually" (20). Housewives and ladies had long delighted in "chemical practices," as Plat commented in his *Jewel House of Art and Nature*, published half a century before the Royal Society formed.[78] Recognizing broader participation in the rise of science requires recognition that modern divisions of public/private space as well as conceptual divisions between theory and practice had not emerged fully.[79] Experimentation, in the most capacious sense of the term, included a wide range of cultural activities and practices.

While recipes increasingly became interested in the lexicon of truth claims in the seventeenth century, it is more accurate to say that the scientific world moved closer to—and begin to systematize and theorize—the praxis that had been going on for quite some time piecemeal throughout England: in shops, mills, gardens, tradesmen's shops, and homes.[80] Reformers of the 1660s arrogated to themselves empirical features of craft knowledge that had previously been distributed broadly across artisans, gardeners, and housewives. Recovering the archive of seventeenth-century manuscript recipes thus helps us to rewrite a history that has obscured a full account of the multiplicity of cultures of experimentation.

From the late seventeenth century and through the eighteenth centuries, home recipe work was disaggregated from reformers' experimental writing because of several key cultural and discursive changes. By the end of the century, rural knowledge and artisanal lore, mocked by some as mere "ladies chemistry," began to be increasingly accepted as less creditable forms of knowing; vocational specialization had much to do with this devaluation.[81] Separately, the formal characteristics of published recipe writing and of scientific exchange diverged more sharply. As Sandra Sherman has comprehensively analyzed, eighteenth-century printed recipes evolved to take on characteristics of the modern cookbook, as writers staked their commercial appeal on the creation of a personalized, chatty writing persona; recipes drifted far from the world of *probatum est*.[82] At the same time, the rhetorical mode of presentation for the *Philosophical Transactions* gradually began to move toward the less subjective style of narration that now features in modern scientific reports.[83] These changes occurred against the backdrop of alterations of domestic labors that I have discussed in previous chapters: women of means began to delegate hands-on "experimental" work to servants; specialists took over the manufacture of household goods in a more developed market economy; and the locations of experimentation moved into specialized and less gender-inclusive sites. The result was that both the lexicons and conceptual domains of the laboratory and the kitchen diverged, just at the time that modern disciplinary divisions emerged. In the next centuries, recipes would sometimes loop into the vocabularies and standards shared by prestige knowledge systems (as seen in the movement toward home "economics" or the standardization of measurements); the case of seventeenth-century England provides an unusual alignment of household arts and experimental cultures.

The recipe archive helps us keep firmly in view the representational, textual, and linguistic character of knowledge production. Truth making took the form, in the broadest sense, of "writing practices," exchanges through which communities debated norms and standards of authentication. Features that appear innocuous and too familiar for analysis—casual citations, editorial glosses, ownership marks—turn out to be instrumental in converting tasks such as making lamb stews and brewing glossy ink into something knowable. How could one write recipes without being self-conscious about the epistemological stakes of the venture, about the *probatum ests* of the kitchen?

The punch line to a popular joke in the period hints that it was not merely members of an esoteric elite who grasped the conundrums inhering in recipe proof. In this joke, a learned man reading a "secret" undergoes a painful mode of ocular proving: "A Grave physicke Doctor reading by candle-light the secrets of Nature, and finding . . . that a large and a broad beard betokens a foole: He straight took the candle in one hand, and a looking glasse in th'other, and began to view what maner of beard his owne was. Now, holding the candle over neer: the flame set [the beard] on fire, and burnt it half off. Then all in a chafe, throwing downe the glasse, he took pen and ink, and wrot in the margin of this secret, *Probatum est.*" The reflexive nature of verification is, in this popular tale, vested precisely in a vexed scene of practice, one that involves physical testing and a self-scrutinizing scene of reading. While making the *probatum est* the butt of a joke, this anecdote brings to the fore the knotty operations of proving in seventeenth-century popular cultures of knowledge.

I close with a recipe that seems startlingly aware of the reflexive nature of knowledge production that the joke indicates. This recipe is housed in a collection where hands blur and textuality is at a premium, a compilation that includes an inventory of Lady Sleigh's library as well as Felicia Whitfield's citations of her published sources. A writer identified as R.S. has scribbled, at the bottom of a recipe for ink, "this receipt was writ with ink made by this receipt."[84] This notation makes the reflexive circuit of reading, material making, and verification strikingly visible. In this self-referential economy, one can test the veracity of information *through* the acts of reading and writing. The recipe offers instruction for how to produce the very substance that will allow the reader to reproduce the information of its making as well as its empirical mode of verification; the recipe's *probatum*, that is, rests explicitly in its legibility on the page. A recipe for ink, a recipe for thought.

CODA

The recipe world that I have presented emerges out of a particular time and place: early modern England. In identifying the vectors of taste, pleasure, knowledge, literacy, and memory as they saturated the early modern kitchen, I have tried to demonstrate how inadequate it is for scholars to regard recipes solely as *documenting* the domestic world of the past (although recipes certainly do have significant and recognizable documentary functions). As densely encoded textual and material forms, recipes also acted as relay points through which people learned, meditated, argued, networked, remembered, showed off, thought through problems, imagined, fantasized, played, and emoted. While dramatic shifts in cuisine, the rise of empirical methods, and a widening public dissemination of printed information make the early modern period a particularly rich site for recipe analysis, a similarly granulated and tailored account of these forms can be told for almost any time period and region. Recipes, since their emergence in the eighth century B.C. to the present, have acted, to different degrees, as mediating lens through which people have addressed social issues and materialized intellectual quandaries, often in passionate and personal ways.[1]

While some critics have characterized recipes as fundamentally conservative and regulatory in their impulse to shrink variation and monitor social behaviors, my case studies from the early modern English world point to the limits of such sweeping generalizations. If pressured to think in these terms, I would say that my archive prompts us instead to see the recipe's unusual expressive and intellectual potential. But, in fact, stating the issue as a matter of liberation *or* restriction narrows our understanding of the cognitive and cultural effects of recipe use. It is the form's *catalyzing* of reflection that is of chief importance to me, because this "readerly" operation has no inherent (and certainly no singular) ideological stake. The recipe's function as an incitement and framework for intellection is what current investigations, so taken with the antiquarian details of cordial waters and egg pastes, can all too easily miss.

The precise mechanism for how a recipe incites thought, reflection, and feeling is a matter of debate. The recipe can, as some commentators observe, guide even those readers determined to master the perfect pie pastry to become strikingly aware of the unexpectedly powerful psychic effects of seemingly straightforward technical instructions. In the *New Yorker*, Adam Gopnik vividly describes the failed promise of mastery—as well as the identificatory investments—prompted by the modern recipe, a form that, he writes,

> always contains two things: news of how something is made, and assurance that there's a way to make it, with the implicit belief that if I know how it is done I can show you how to do it. The premise of the recipe book is that these two things are naturally balanced; the secret of the recipe book is that they're not.
>
> The recipe is a blueprint but also a red herring, a way to do something and a false summing up of a living process that can be handed on only by experience, a knack posing as a knowledge. We say "What's the recipe?" when we mean "How do you do it?" And though we want the answer to be "Like this!" the honest answer is "Be me!"[2]

For Gopnik, the experience of consuming recipe books turns centrally on a false optimism and allure, as they incite belief that cooking is a knowledge that can be translated into and communicated through writing. Its "secret," as he explains, is the gap between ideal and realization, a gap exposed in intimately felt ways, I would argue, in the process of consuming recipes, both in reading and in practice. Gopnik puts his finger on the desire activated by this "promise" as well as the "honest" recognition of what the recipe user seeks. While recipe acts of making expose the inadequacy of textual instruction, according to Gopnik, they also uncover the complex desires for self-transformation driving recipe use.

Recipes, Gopnik contends, can act as an incitement for readers to acknowledge the sheer act of wanting that underpins hopes of mastery and identification:

> The desire to go on desiring, the wanting to want, is what makes you turn the pages—all the while aware that the next Boston cream

pie, the sweet-salty-fatty-starchy thing you will turn out tomorrow, will be neither more nor less unsatisfying than last night's was. When you start to cook, as when you begin to live, you think that the point is to improve the technique until you end up with something perfect, and that the reason you haven't been able to break the cycle of desire and disillusion is that you haven't yet mastered the rules. Then you grow up, and you learn that that's the game.

We need not agree that this process leads to an inevitable disillusionment, as Gopnik suggests, to recognize the vexed aspirations around recipe use that he so tellingly pinpoints: a fervent belief in structured rules that might guarantee material and personal transformation, a basic longing to be something other than oneself. *When you start to cook, as when you begin to live . . .* Perhaps I court charges of sentimentality (and indulge in my own sweeping generalizations) in believing that recipes fundamentally rest on fantasies that the world can be other than it is. You mix two substances together, and a miraculous new thing is born. You convert the entities of the raw natural world into ingredients that reconfigure its contours. You puzzle out a problem as you undertake an expressive and creating act of making. Rather than seeing recipes as indicating a supposedly mature recognition of the futility of text-based metamorphoses, as does Gopnik, I read them as prompting us to reveal our desires as a preliminary step toward other possible outcomes. (Who's to say, that is, that the Boston cream pie Gopnik criticizes can *never* match expectations?) As people lovingly turn the pages of recipe books (in Gopnik's description, in the intimate space of the bed), they indulge in imaginative identifications and fantasies that exceed a quest for improved technical skill. Recipe use thus makes legible the fantastical nature of fantasy—the pleasure of "wanting to want" and, perhaps, the intangible aims of desires circulating around culinary making (for example, the dream of personal comfort, communal identity, and, dare I say it, *love*, the thing that we are told *is* food). Recipes mobilize the psychic desire to go on desiring, a force tethered to the dream of effecting a transformative *otherness*; in the process, social kinds, structures, and identities take shape.

My account of early modern English recipes, one story within many intersecting cultural tales, remains woefully lacking unless accompanied by other stories that stretch to embrace the geographical and temporal character of recipe worlds. One might augment the story I've told, for instance, by moving forward in time in England to explain how Enlightenment thinking and

Victorian domesticity retailored the psychic and social investments of earlier manuscript and print recipe cultures. Or, one might map the recipe's transatlantic journeys, where it prompted strikingly new epistemological and social quandaries based on the collision of "new" and "old" worlds. My story remains incomplete in that it does not integrate additional archives and sources that might allow us to situate recipes in their global, imperial, and colonial contexts, networks that recipes themselves often occlude. Transglobal and transoceanic trade, which generated complex fantasies of familiarity and difference, silently underpin the acts of making and thinking undertaken in local kitchens. My book's investigation of recipes as sites of intellectual inquiry and social performance thus intends to supplement investigations of the recipe's saturation in commercial foodways as well as its mobilization on behalf of minoritarian identities and culture.

And there are darker stories to be told. The twentieth century bore witness to one instance in which recipes figured in an almost unspeakable story of individual and collective suffering and trauma. How could it be possible that Jews forcibly transported from parts of Poland, Germany, and the Czech Republic to the concentration transit "camp" Theresienstadt (or Terezin) would have the energy and drive to produce music, plays, courses in theology, art workshops, and—of all things—recipe collections? How could people who were battling horrific conditions of hunger, disease, fear, and imprisonment engage in something as frivolous as exchanging recipes? In 1969, a fragile hand-sewn manuscript found its way from Europe to Israel and finally to Manhattan. It landed, after a difficult geographical and temporal journey, in the hands of the daughter of Mina Pachter, whose writings are housed in the collection. In 1996, this document—which includes over seventy recipes for liver dumplings with ginger, coffee cake, fried noodles, stuffed eggs, and other foods—was translated, edited, and published as *In Memory's Kitchen: A Legacy from the Women of Terezin*.[3] That such a text existed is itself remarkable. At Terezin, only 19,000 of 144,000 people survived; 80,000 of the inhabitants were deported to death camps while others died of disease or starvation. Yet within this community, undernourished and captive women compared and collected food recipes that were clearly therapeutic rather than functional. Other memoirs that have survived from Terezin evidence that hungry internees discussed cooking at great length and debated competing ways to make particular dishes. Recording instructions for concocting cakes for which they longed created a second literate layer to their reminiscences. *In Memory's Kitchen* bespeaks the spiritual, social, and commemorative power of the recipe form; it exists as an assertion of the will to survive, as a source of comforting memory, and as a testament to the imagination. It's hard *not* to register the full import of words harbored within a recipe for stuffed eggs (*Gefullte Eier*): "Let fantasy run free."

Recipe stories—stylized in academic, elegiac, nostalgic, and celebratory modes—saturate twentieth- and twenty-first-century culture. In the present world, we fully recognize the community-building value of cheaply printed neighborhood, church, and school recipe collections, those compilations often unevenly stuffed into punch-hole or double-wire binders. Yet today people have also tapped into new media to create virtual global communities of crowd-sourced recipe websites (for instance, at epicurious.com or allrecipes.com). People join from geographically remote areas to witness hands-on demonstrations of cooking on popular television shows. Social media allows us to remark on our imitated versions of these preparations and to create anonymous large-scale conversations about techniques and ingredients. While the social and economic issues in these interactions are distinctly modern, today's digital, print, television, Internet, and scrapbook recipes produce variants of the basic promises we have seen in their early modern predecessors: that one *can* know how to be an authentic Indian within the United States; that one *can* go "back" to a pure, less commercialized agrarian farm world; that one *can* be mindful enough to access spirituality in quotidian actions; that one *can* peek into the intimate space of celebrity chefs; that one *can* be magically transported to exotic climes; that one *can* imagine sharing a lifestyle with legendary figures like William Shakespeare or Maya Angelou; or that one *can* hold onto the past by tracing a family lineage.

The handwritten pages and published books from long ago that I analyze draw our attention to the first moment when printed recipes appeared in England and joined a dialogue with people participating in a newly robust recipe scribal culture. These old collections, stored away in dusty special libraries but now newly entering the digital world, allow us to capture an earlier era's drive to metamorphose their social, natural, and intellectual landscapes, and even, somewhat whimsically, to contemplate performing superhuman feats in the kitchen: raising the dead, stilling time, altering natural elements, perpetuating the basic desire to desire that motors the promise of transformation.

NOTES

Preface

Note to epigraph: Disraeli, *Curiosities of Literature*, 1:129.
1. See Freedman, "Spices"; Albala, *Eating Right in the Renaissance*; and Morton, *The Poetics of Spice*.
2. Wheaton, *Savoring the Past*, 53. On emergent distinctions between French and English cuisine, see Mennell, *All Manners of Food*, 69–70; Pinkard, *A Revolution in Taste*; and Appelbaum, *Aguecheek's Beef*.
3. Bonnefons, *Les Délices de la Table*, 213–14; cited in Mennell, *All Manners*, 73.
4. L.S.R., *L'Art de bien Traiter*, 7; 1–2; cited in Mennell, *All Manners*, 73–74.
5. Flandrin, "Seasoning." Pinkard argues against a clear cause-and-effect model for medical and dietary changes (64–71). In registering the increased availability and decrease in prices for imported spices in England in the early seventeenth century, Braudel suggests a phenomena that Elias has mapped, whereby the diffusion of styles or goods (here spices) precedes their devaluation (*Structures of Everyday Life*, 1:22).
6. Thacker, preface, *The Art of Cookery*, first page, unpaginated front matter.
7. Addison, *Tattler*, no. 148 (Tuesday, March 21, 1709), 121.

Introduction

Note to epigraph: John Beale, letter to Hartlib, November 16, 1659, *A Complete Text and Image Database of the Papers of Samuel Hartlib*.
1. See Kim F. Hall, "Culinary Spaces, Colonial Spaces"; Wall, *Staging Domesticity*; and Snook, *Women, Beauty and Power*, esp. 21–37; 38–52.
2. Martino, *The Art of Cookery*, 130.
3. Pennell and DiMeo, introduction, *Reading and Writing Recipe Books, 1550–1800*, 15.
4. My textual-based investigation of recipes complements Julia Lupton's Heideggerian analysis of the contemplative and intellectual encounters that early modern dining provided for participants. Although Lupton uses a vocabulary that emphasizes the theatrical dimensions of banqueting, she is similarly concerned with the "digestive reflection" on personhood, knowledge, and relations that early modern food acts enabled ("Room for Dessert").

5. The important exception is Dimeo and Pennell, *Reading and Writing Recipe Books*.
6. DiMeo and Pennell, introduction, *Reading and Writing Recipe Books*, 10.
7. I intend "world making" in the sense used by Spiller in *Science, Reading, and Renaissance Literature*, 16–18.
8. See Eamon, *Science and the Secrets of Nature*. One of the key scholars to consider recipes as a cohesive object of study, Eamon examines modern science as rooted in popular printed "books of secrets" of the late Middle Ages and Renaissance. My purview is both narrower and more expansive than Eamon's, because I investigate recipes available to women (and therefore a subset of printed recipes) but also extend that domain to include manuscripts.
9. The most comprehensive studies of seventeenth-century recipes consist of dissertations and theses. In an invaluable investigation of early English recipe compilation and use, Elaine Leong explores lay medical practice. Her choice of topic leads her to exclude collections emphasizing culinary material, however, which influences her claims for a greater percentage of male involvement in recipe production than scholars have acknowledged. Her evidence might well look different if collections with fewer medical recipes were considered ("Medical Recipe Collections"). In "Opening Closets," Stine offers crucial research on the exchange of manuscript texts in the period as part of her study of vernacular medicine. Her decision to work with recipes that can be attributed does, as she acknowledges, tilt her sample toward elite women. While unearthing and analyzing recipes as important textual records, these studies offer limited generalizations about the class or gender dimensions of manuscript culture.
10. On the rise of the medical profession and its effect on women, see Nagy, *Popular Medicine*; Beier, *Sufferers and Healers*; and Pelling, *Medical Conflicts*. On the shift from production to consumption, see scholarship that follows and critiques Alice Clark's pathbreaking *Working Life of Women*, including Cahn, *Industry of Devotion*, and Korda, *Shakespeare's Domestic Economies*. On the civilizing process, see the classic work by Elias, *The Civilizing Process*.
11. See DiMeo, "Authorship and Medical Networks."
12. Dolan, *True Relations*.
13. The most analytical and generative work on early recipes is Pennell's "Perfecting Practice?" Spiller also sets an important agenda for recipe study in the introduction to her editions of facsimile collections, *Seventeenth-Century English Recipe Books*. See also DiMeo and Pennell, *Reading and Writing Recipe Books*.
14. *Susanna Packe Her Book*, 21. While modern cookbooks exhibit concern with nutrition and health, they are based on a fundamentally different understanding of the body: healthy foods are good for all people not just particular individuals, and seasoning is almost always primarily geared to taste with health considerations cropping up secondarily.
15. Markham, *The English Housewife*, 81–82. Throughout this book, I centrally cite Markham's 1623, 2nd and expanded edition. Named *The English Hus-wife*, this text was originally printed as a semi-separate book appended to *Countrey Contentments* in 1615. In 1623, an expanded version emerged as a stand-alone edition titled *Countrey Contentments, Or, The English Hus-wife*. In 1631 and in subsequent editions, it was called *The English House-wife*, but with variant spellings. In order to reduce confusion, I refer to all editions as *The English Housewife*, the name used by Markham's contemporaries and subsequent recipe writers; *Countrey Contentments* evolved into the name for Markham's husbandry manual. Editions of *The English Housewife* were published under slightly varying titles, in

1615, 1623, 1631, 1637, 1649, 1653, 1660, 1664, and 1683. The text was simultaneously collated into a collected works of Markham and published as part of *The Way to Get Wealth* in 1625, 1631, 1633, 1638, 1648, 1653, 1657, 1660, 1668, 1683, and 1695.

16. Pérez-Ramos, *Francis Bacon's Idea of Science*.

17. Wheaton, *Savoring the Past*, 28.

18. On the evolution of expertise, voice, and form in early modern recipes, see Sandra Sherman, *Invention of the Modern Cookbook*.

19. Perdita, because of its mission of disseminating writing by women, makes available a pool of recipes that excludes anonymous and male-compiled texts. For this reason, generalizing about recipes based on materials solely from this archive can skew the results.

20. For an example of a scholar grappling with problems of recipe attribution, see Aspin, "Who Was Elizabeth Okeover?"

21. While it is impossible to cite all significant recent scholarship devoted to recovering women's scribal communities, see, for a sample, Ezell, *Patriarch's Wife*; *Genre and Women's Life Writing in Early Modern England*, ed. Dowd and Eckerle; Frye, *Pens and Needles*; and *Early Modern Women's Manuscript Writing*, ed. Burke and Gibson.

22. On the recipe's conditional status, see Pennell, "Perfecting Practice." Goldstein provides an analysis of the structure and format of early modern recipes while making a larger argument about commensality and food (*Eating and Ethics*).

23. Partridge, *Treasurie*, 1573, B2.

24. Elizabeth Godfrey et al., *Collection of Medical and Cookery Receipts*, 11; Pudsey, *Lettice Pudsey Her Booke of Receipts*, F7v.

25. Dawson, *The Good Huswifes Jewell*, A4.

26. Doggett, *Recipe Book of Mary Doggett*, 190.

27. Newton, *A Booke of Usefull Receipts*, 152; Knight, *Mrs. Knight's Receipt Book*, 2; Murrell, *A Daily Exercise for Ladies and Gentlewomen* (1617), E4v.

28. Granville (Dewes), *Cookery and Medicinal Recipes*, 38–39.

29. Cruso, *Cookbook of Mary Cruso and Timothy Cruso*, fol. 11.

Chapter 1. Taste Acts

Note to epigraph: King, *The Art of Cookery*, 103–5.

1. Priscilla Ferguson, *Accounting for Taste*, 17.

2. Markham, *English Housewife* (1623), 59.

3. Haywood, *Female Spectator*, 3:154; Voltaire, *Philosophical Dictionary*.

4. In previous work exploring housework and English identity in plays, I mapped fantasies put forth by early English recipe books (*Staging Domesticity*, 18–58). Because my concern then was chiefly dramatic representations of housewifery, I did not investigate the complexity of the recipe world in and of itself. I repeat, refine, and elaborate some previous arguments as I extend my analysis chronologically. In doing so I heed the call made by Lehmann for additional research to be undertaken on the front matter of recipe books (*The British Housewife*, 13).

5. Bourdieu, *Distinction*, 6. When taste became Taste in the eighteenth century, Raymond Williams argues, it took on the meaning of a generalized polite quality, a faculty or power of the mind by which people accurately distinguish the good, bad, or indifferent (*Keywords*, 313–15).

6. Changes in food and changes in the marketing of recipe books appear to correlate as phenomena, because both move toward a culinary nationalism. But these stories do not predictably map onto each other: attention to the national contours of diet did not correspond exactly to when Englishness became a value endorsed by recipe reading. For this reason, we cannot make a causal historical argument about their relationship.

7. On the early modern closet as site of interpersonal male-male exchange and secrecy, see Stewart, "Early Modern Closet." On prayer closets and sexuality, see Rambuss, *Closet Devotions*. On the closet's relationship to public and private space, see McKeon, *Secret History of Domesticity*. On shifting and multiple meanings for closets, including their relation to gender, see Orlin, "Gertrude's Closet." On the closet as a space for female transgressive reading, see Roberts, "'Shakespeare Creepes into the Womens Closets.'" On Catholicism and closets, see Dolan, "Gender and the 'Lost' Spaces." Despite considerable analysis, there are still meanings to be mined in considering how the term signifies in recipes and how cabinets and closets filter meanings into the work of kitchens, stillrooms, reading rooms, and storage sites.

8. See Friedman, *House and Household in Elizabethan England*; Girouard, *Life in the English Country House*.

9. Orlin, "Gertrude's Closet." Only Kim Hall has commented on how the trope of the cabinet in recipe books might link it to cabinets used to display exotic, often New World, trifles ("Culinary Spaces, Colonial Spaces," 171–72).

10. See Kavey, *Books of Secrets*.

11. In *Chaste, Silent, and Obedient*, Hull argues that there were 163 books in five hundred editions written for women in this period, half of which were practical manuals (1–30). Though Hull's methods are self-confirming in one sense (she identifies any book having to do with cookery as "for women"), she makes a convincing case for an emergent female reading public in the 1570s.

12. Lehmann, *The British Housewife*, 30–33.

13. While we only have limited evidence about who actually bought these books, ownership marks suggest that non-elite women did read them. For examples, see the 1600 edition of Partridge's *Treasurie* in the Folger Library and the University of Toronto's copy of Plat's *Jewel House of Nature*.

14. Of the numerous how-to books printed in the late sixteenth century, recipes were unusual in targeting the class-hybrid and/or class-mobile woman. We cannot thus *fully* account for the trend toward recipe publishing by pointing to a general Protestant emphasis on industry.

15. Hackel, *Reading Material*, 101.

16. Recipe books that promised to open elite closets did *not* trade in the sexualized rhetoric of tantalizing disclosure that I have analyzed elsewhere as concerned with the stigma of print. See *The Imprint of Gender*, 169–226.

17. *Oxford English Dictionary (OED)*, v. 2; v. 1.

18. Hoby, *Private Life of an Elizabethan Lady*, 55.

19. Thomas Middleton and William Rowley, *The Changeling*, D1.

20. William Sherman, *Used Books*, esp. xiii–xv and chap. 1.

21. Brinsley, *Ludus Literarius*, 46–47; Hackel reads Brinsley's work when examining evidence of physical marks in books (*Reading Material*, 206).

22. See William Sherman, *Used Books*; and Helen Smith, *Grossly Material Things*, 185.

23. See Orgel, "Marginal Maternity," 275, 282.

24. Bayne, *Book of Recipes*, 46.
25. Okeover, *Collection of Medical Receipts*, fol. 125v.
26. Whitney, *A Choice of Emblems*, quoted in Cormack and Mazzio, *Book Use, Book Theory*, 3.
27. In the next ten editions of *The Treasurie*, signs of elaborate patronage relations and humanist trappings gradually fell away as its front matter emphasized instead the "commodity" of the book—both its anticipated use by readers as well as the writer's exchange of labor for money.
28. Murrell, *A New Booke of Cookerie*, title page.
29. The first two citations are to the 1608 *Closet for Ladies and Gentlewomen*, 44, 43; the next three are from Partridge's *Treasurie*, B4v. On early recipes as "alimentary symbols of class," see Albala, *Eating Right in the Renaissance*, 185.
30. Household accounts and descriptions of meals in other writings document aspiring culinary efforts and successes of gentry, yeomen, preachers, and merchants. See, for instance, William Harrison's denunciation of merchants' and householders' fare (*Description of England*, 128–30). For fictional references to the bawdy possibilities of social climbing through cookery, see Middleton, *Trick to Catch the Old-One*, F2v.
31. On Shakespeare's representation of foreign products and foods, see Fitzpatrick, *Food in Shakespeare*, 38–46; 83–106.
32. See Spiller, "Recipes for Knowledge."
33. In her insightful reading of *The Queens Closet Opened* and *The Court and Kitchen of Elizabeth Cromwel[l]*, Knoppers recovers these texts' reception history to show that they did not constrain consumers to read according to their overt political goals (*Politicizing Domesticity*, 94–139).
34. I rely extensively in my analysis, here and throughout, on Mennell's *All Manners of Food*.
35. Sandra Sherman, *Invention of the Modern Cookbook*, 122–27.
36. Rabisha, *Whole Body of Cookery*, A4v, A4.
37. Rabisha, *Whole Body of Cookery*. May's only mention of women is found in his allegory of Hospitality as a woman stripped of her title and "expos'd" while reposing on a bed awaiting rehabilitation by a noble patron (A3v).
38. Lamb, *Royal Cookery*, A3–A4.
39. Robert Smith, *Court Cookery*, A8.
40. Carter, "To The Reader," *Complete Practical Cook*.
41. On Woolley, see Hobby, *Virtue of Necessity*, 165–89; Theophano, *Eat My Words*, 197–202; and Goldstein, "Woolley's Mouse." Woolley denied authorship of *The Gentlewoman's Companion*, a text that made outspoken claims about female education.
42. On Woolley's social and economic commitment to recycling goods and discourses, see Goldstein, "Recipes for Authorship," 54–68.
43. In *Archimagirus . . . or Excellent and Approved Receipts and Experiments in Cookery*, Mayerne satirized recipe books. "I confesse, it may well be laid in my Dish, that I am no fit Cooke to dresse an Epistle, and to set it forth in the Kick-shaw Language, which these Chamaleon-Times love to feede on," he writes. "And, indeede, I am utterly unfit to write of Cookerie, who am not able to give an account of the very tearms of their Art" (A3–A3v).
44. Markham did not imagine the domestic closet to be a space for marking information but rather a place in which the housewife was to order marmalades, pastes, suckets, comfits, and other banqueting items (1623; 125).

45. Hall, "Culinary Spaces," esp. 168–77.
46. Goldstein, "Recipes for Authorship," 60.
47. See Ezell "Cooking the Books," 159–78.
48. On the use and affordability of eighteenth-century recipe books, see Lehmann, *British Housewife*, 61–127.
49. Bradley, *British Housewife*, 3:314. It was not just the French who were targeted in English recipe criticism. In a recipe for a roast pig, Bradley criticized Germans who "whip him to Death, but they deserve the same Fate for their Cruelty; there is no Occasion for such Barbarity to make a dainty Dish" (5:151). Eliza Smith's *The Compleat Housewife* identified the national components of the new cuisine as resting specifically on a geopolitical physiology.
50. See, for instance, Raffald, who advertised confections that one could buy in her store (*The Experienced English House-Keeper*), or Moxon, who saw her expertise as a vocation (*English Housewifery*).
51. Raffald, "To the Reader," in *The Experienced English House-Keeper*.
52. Glasse, *Art of Cookery*, 5th ed., frontispiece.
53. Annie Gray, "'A Practical Art,'" 50.
54. See also Raffald, dedicatory letter in *The Experienced English House-Keeper*.
55. Peckham, *Complete English Cook*, preface.
56. Ann Cook, *Professed Cookery*, iii.
57. Theophano, *Eat My Words*, 205.
58. See Lehmann's analysis of the price of books relative to wages in the eighteenth century (*British Housewife*, 62–66).
59. See Sandra Sherman, *Invention of the Modern Cookbook*, 30.
60. Bradley, *The British Housewife*, 1:9. Sandra Sherman reads this passage to show the relationship of printed recipe books to manuscript modes of authorization (*Invention of the Modern Cookbook*, 30)
61. Katharine Palmer, "A Collection of ye Best Receipts," 231.
62. Addison, *Spectator*, no. 10 (1711). On changes in practice and cultural attitudes toward housewifery, see Lehmann, *The British Housewife* , 68–79.
63. See Lehmann, *The British Housewife*, 67.
64. On women's domestic labor in relation to political and economic life, see Clark, *Working Life of Women*; and Erickson, *Women and Property*.
65. Voltaire, *Philosophical Dictionary*.
66. Carter, *The Complete Practical Cook*, "To the Reader," unpaginated. Flandrin notes that the physical ability to taste food began to be seen, within the new culinary regime, as an intrinsic quality rather than as an individual diner's manifestation of psycho-physiological humoral temperament. "From Dietetics to Gastronomy," 431.
67. While Raffald associated "beauty" with suspect ornamental aspects of cookery (*The Experienced English House-Keeper*, ii), she, at other points, caters to the pleasures of the eye and palate (iii). See Flandrin, "From Dietetics to Gastronomy," 418–32.
68. Nott's *Cook's and Confectioner's Dictionary* made the recipe book a connoisseur's object. In addition to showcasing the expertise of famed chef John Nott, this cookbook charted somewhat new territory through its inclusion of a copper-plate lined engraving frontispiece. While some recipe books, such as those by Smith and Carter, included copper plates of table settings as a graphic means of conveying information, Nott's book used a type of engraving associated with the prestigious print trade, the subject matter of which

signaled "refined" interest in philosophical questions and humanist iconographies. John Pine, a notable print shop operator, designer, engraver, and cartographer (later to become known for illustrated books of Horace, Virgil, *Robinson Crusoe*, and the Magna Carta), created the engraving for this recipe book. On Pine, see Hodnett, *Five Centuries of Book Illustration*, 85–86.

69. Gigante, *Taste: A Literary History*, 3. Gigante traces ways that taste as aesthetic discernment emerged from within its meaning as physical sensation (1–21).

70. Kant, *Anthropology from a Pragmatic Point of View*, 144.

71. Milton, *Paradise Lost*, ed. Hughes, bk. 5, lines 332–36.

72. Citing this scene in "Eating Songs" (1854), Leigh Hunt slyly observed: "the poet in our own country who has written with the greatest gusto on the subject of eating is Milton." Quoted in Gigante, *Taste*, 22.

73. Schoenfeldt, *Bodies and Selves in Early Modern England*, 136.

74. Goldstein, *Eating and Ethics*, 80.

75. See Moore, "Eve's Food Preparation"; Tigner, "Eating with Eve"; and Knoppers, *Politicizing Domesticity*, 140–64. Gigante surveys arguments about food in Eden, contextualized through reference to Milton's monism; Puritan communion rituals, divinity, and food; and the stomach's "transubstantiation" of material (*Taste: A Literary History*, 22–38). According to Gigante, Milton negotiated an embodied mode of taste while subsequent writers purged it of its physicality.

76. Gordon (Lord Byron), *Don Juan*, 13.99.8.

Chapter 2. Pleasure

Note to epigraphs: *A Gentlewomans Companion*, a conduct book and recipe text attributed, in the seventeenth century to Woolley, 37. Woolley, *Supplement*, 60. Jonson, *Neptune's Triumph*, 7:684. The first pages of the masque are not available on Early English Books Online, because there are pages missing in the edition used for digitalization.

1. Gascoigne, *The Steele Glas*, D1.
2. Sidney, *Apologie for Poetrie*, G2.
3. Greville, *Certaine Learned and Elegant Workes, Caelica*, Sonnet 24, 176. The sonnet concludes by overturning this valuation and arguing for a hidden ciphering of love within the body.
4. Plat, *Delightes*, C1v; Thomas Dawson, *Good Huswifes Jewell Wherein Is to Be Found Most Excellent and Rare Devises for Conceits in Cookerie*, title page; *A Good Huswifes Handmaide for the Kitchin . . . Hereunto Are Annexed, Sundrie Necessarie Conceits for the Preseruation of Health*, title page; and Murrell, *A Daily Exercise for Ladies and Gentlewomen Whereby They May Learne . . . Conceits in Sugar-Workes*, title page. Archer also comments on the shared terminology between recipe and poetic writing ("Quintessence," 120) as she astutely explores the interpenetration of literary and recipe cultures (114–34).
5. *Oxford English Dictionary*, "conceit," n.
6. Wheaton, *Savoring the Past*, 52–54.
7. In *Staging Domesticity* I explored "food wit" as a component of the uncanniness that helped to structure national ideology; I return here to contextualize this evidence differently.
8. Plato, *Dialogues of Plato, Gorgias*, Vol. 2:343–44.

9. "Of all the books produced since the most remote ages by human talents and industry those only that treat of cooking are, from a moral point of view, above suspicion. The intention of every other piece of prose may be discussed and even mistrusted; but the purpose of a cookery book is one and unmistakable. Its object can conceivably be no other than to increase the happiness of mankind," wrote Joseph Conrad in a preface to Jessie Conrad's *A Handbook of Cookery for a Small House*.

10. Masten, *Queer Philologies*.

11. With Rombauer's *The Joy of Cooking* as the noteworthy exception, modern cookbook titles typically do not celebrate the delights that *cooking* affords, instead opting to showcase a celebrity chef, famed restaurant, or particular cuisine, or the expertise that the book will bring.

12. Barthes, "Ornamental Cookery" in *Mythologies*, 78. On "food porn" (which originally meant cooking voyeurism), see McBride, "Food Porn"; and the Food Porn website (http://foodporndaily.com).

13. I disagree on this score with Ivan Day, who contrasts early modern recipe book graphics with the "artificial situation" of modern cookbooks that rely on high-resolution pictorial material ("From Murrell to Jarrin," 98).

14. M.B., *Ladies Cabinet Enlarged and Opened*, A2v.

15. Commendatory poem by A.B. to Bodenham, *Belvedere*, A3v.

16. While we have no firsthand accounts by recipe users to document their experience of reading (and indeed we might be skeptical about the validity of firsthand accounts), we know that recipe books catering specifically to female readerly pleasure sold well and were reprinted.

17. Although, as we have seen, May addressed his cookery books to chefs rather than to housewives, his works were bought and read by men and women across the social spectrum. Woolley and various female recipe manuscript collectors cite May.

18. May, *Accomplisht Cook*, A8.

19. Kim Hall, for instance, cites May to document the use of sugar at banquets, the decrease in popularity in conspicuous consumption after the civil war, and the positioning of women within the male-orchestrated banquet ("Culinary Spaces," 174–75).

20. Although Jonson designed *Neptune's Triumph* to be presented at court in 1623–24, James I cancelled the event. Two years later, Jonson imported some speeches verbatim into his play *The Staple of News*. On the overlap between poetry and recipes, see Archer, who offers a fascinating consideration of the affective and imaginative dimensions of recipe writing. She does come to a conclusion based on this analysis that differs from mine, because she argues that recipes facilitated the process by which housewifery was translated into female authorship ("Quintessence").

21. On medieval feasts, see Wilson, *Appetite and the Eye*; and Albala, *Banquet*.

22. Lévi-Strauss, *The Raw and the Cooked*.

23. On May's "Triumphs" and on the dessert course as a metaphysical operation tied to spatial arrangements, see Julia Lupton, "Room for Dessert." Lupton situates her analysis of the reflective rhythms of dessert and theater within the Heideggerian framework of "dwelling," routines of living associated especially with creaturely needs for shelter, sustenance, and sociability and organized around architectural concerns with setting, place, and locale.

24. Nashe, *Quaternio*, 157.

25. Wall, *Staging Domesticity*, 3.

26. Fumerton, *Cultural Aesthetics*, 111–67. On the banquet, see Stead, "Bowers of Bliss."
27. See Spencer, *British Food*, 116–22.
28. Heldke, "Foodmaking as Thoughtful Practice."
29. *Book of Ann Goodenough*, 40–41.
30. *Closet for Ladies* (1608), 17.
31. Wright, *The Female Vertuoso*, 23; cited by Archer, "The 'Quintessence of Wit,'" 114. Wright's play follows the plot of Shadwell's version, which was itself an adaptation of Moliere's work.
32. *Ladies Cabinet Enlarged*, 26–27.
33. Shakespeare, Sonnet 5, lines 9–14. All citations to Shakespeare will be to the Norton edition unless specified otherwise.
34. Side-by-side recipes in *The Ladies Cabinet Enlarged* present flowers with a naturalistic effect ("to Candy all kinds of flower as they grow with their stalkes on") and overtly artificial dimensions (covered in "rock candy") (14–15). Murrell contrasts three-dimensional fruit and flowers designed to seem real with those "covered with sparks of diamonds" (*Daily Exercise*, F2, E5). See Murrell's *A Daily Exercise* for an example of marzipan stamped with images of their ingredients (F2v). Manuscript recipe compilers experimenting with these options include Elizabeth Fowler (95), Granville (Dewes) (50), and Mrs. Knight (56).
35. Mueller also interprets culinary work as a domestic and gender-inclusive form of theater. While I am not persuaded by Mueller's argument that recipes addressed to women offered practitioners greater license than those written for men, I agree with her overarching conception of the theatrical opportunities that culinary work afforded ("Early Modern Banquet Receipts and Women's Theatre").
36. On the period's tendency to yoke the effects of natural magic, the illusions of machinery, and mysteries of courtly politics, see Jessica Wolfe, *Humanism*; and Butterworth, *Magic*.
37. *The Faerie Queene*, *Edmund Spenser's Poetry*, 2.12.55, ll. 1–2.
38. Donne, "That Women Ought to Paint," in *Juvenalia*, 7.
39. Yates, "Shakespeare's Messmates."
40. Stubbes, *Anatomie of Abuses*, 155.
41. Elizabeth Brunskill writes that medieval "sotelties usually expressed a religious or allegorical theme, with figures often bearing mottos that clarified their intent" ("Medieval Book of Herbs," 181–86).
42. Herbert, "The Banquet," in *The Temple*, 176. Gary Taylor mentions that communion was called "the banquet of most heavenly food" in *The Book of Common Prayer* ("Gender, Hunger, Horror," 33).
43. Jonson, *Bartholomew Fayre*, 48 (act 3, scene 6). I'm grateful to Linda McJannet, whose paper at the International Shakespeare Association, reminded me of this allusion ("'And Ginger Shall Be Hot I' Th' Mouth Too'").
44. De Acosta, *Naturall and Morall Historie*, 368.
45. Mayne, *The Citye Match*, 11 (scene 2).
46. See, for instance, Murrell, *Daily Exercise*, F3; Plat, *Delightes*, B9v. In *Bartholomew Fayre*, Cokes imagines serving gingerbread at his wedding in the shape of gloves that will enable the guests to eat their "fingers ends" (40) (act 3, scene 4).
47. See Orlin, *Private Matters and Public Culture*.
48. *Oxford English Dictionary*, "affection," n.1a.
49. Murrell, *A New Booke of Cookerie*, 44–45.

50. William Harrison, *Description of England*, esp. 123–32.

51. Because of my training as a literary scholar, I was surprised to find that early printed recipe books invited housewives to take pleasure in culinary artifice. So many literary texts echo sermons and conduct books that view housewifery as a moral *labor*. I note as well that recipes offer a rejoinder to feminist critics' tendency to dismiss domesticity as a site of gender restriction (frequently implicitly in their pejorative use of "domesticated" to mean politically neutralized).

52. On gender and cosmetics, see Dolan, "Taking the Pencil out of God's Hand." Moving beyond condemnations of face painting, Snook draws on recipes, among other materials, to argue that female practitioners viewed "beautifying physic" positively, as a "forum for the exercise of female authority in domestic medicine" (*Women, Beauty and Power*, 21–37; 47–52; quotation at 22).

53. As Archer suggests in her analysis of shifting meanings for the term "receipt," poems and recipes came to be defined in opposition to one another in the late seventeenth and eighteenth centuries ("Quintessence," 120).

54. Flandrin, "From Dietetics to Gastronomy," 363. Albala qualifies Flandrin's account by arguing that the late Renaissance was a distinct moment when cookery moved from a baroque to a mannerist style before giving way to neoclassicism (*Banquet*, 56–72).

55. Charles Carter, *Complete City and Country Cook*, vii.

56. A few playful confections survived in the eighteenth century, including "snow," a dish in which egg whites and sugar were whipped to form a stiff texture that then served as the basis for a winter scene decorated with sprigs of myrtle; "floating Island," in which fruit, chocolate, and cream were positioned by a sea of jelly to resemble an ocean scene; and the long-popular prickly confectionary hedgehog.

57. Glasse, *The Art of Cookery*, "To the Reader," i.

58. Shenstone, *Works in Verse and Prose*, 2:188.

59. Appelbaum traces the evolution of the myth of Cockaigne (*Aguecheek's Beef*, 118–54).

60. Jonson, "To Penshurst," in *Workes*, 820.

61. Nott, *Cook's and Confectioner's Dictionary*, preface, no pagination, irregular gatherings.

62. When Nott's book reprints the "Triumphs" pageant from May's text as part of its front matter, the spectacle is presented as an archaic practice no longer connected, in spirit or practice, with the foods presented in the recipe book.

63. Eliza Smith, *Compleat Housewife*, A2–2v.

64. See also Bradley, who argues against vegetarians who conscript Adam's diet as their natural and moral basis. As Bradley explicates the providential mandate given to Noah to eat meat, she argues for an evolving concept of a "natural" bodily constitution (*British Housewife*, 110).

65. Ovid, *Metamorphoses*, bk. 1, lines 117–21.

66. Kim Hall begins her analysis of the mystified foreign underpinnings of cookery in English books directed toward early modern women by tracing connections between the slavery-supported sugar trade and the recipe book industry ("Culinary Spaces, Colonial Spaces"). See also Sidney Mintz's classic work *Sweetness and Power*, which analyzes the global sugar system underwriting confectionery.

67. Peckham, *Complete English Cook*, preface, 5.

68. Addison, *Spectator* 10 (1711), cited by Lehmann, *British Housewife*, 69.
69. Herbert, *The Temple*, 41.

CHAPTER 3. LITERACIES

Note to epigraphs: Flyleaf of Fanshawe, *Memoirs*. Vives, *Instruction of a Christian Woman*, C3v. Goldberg, *Writing Matter*, 96.

1. The Wellcome Library online Manuscripts and Archives catalogue for Michel, *Her Book of Recepts*, an entry derived from Moorat, who, in the *Catalogue of Western Manuscripts*, designates over thirty manuscripts as illiterate.

2. In "Reading Graffiti," Scott-Warren explores ways that book graffiti was concerned with self-identification and place. He notes that the most common explanation for textual "graffiti" is that writers made "pen trials" to test whether ink was running properly from the quill (368).

3. *Oxford English Dictionary*, "illiterate," sense 1a.

4. Cressy, *Literacy and the Social Order*, 176–77. On ways that this mode of assessment underestimates female literacy, see Thomas, "Meaning of Literacy"; Spufford, "First Steps in Literacy," esp. 410–12; and Sanders, who offers a succinct review of literacy literature (*Gender and Literacy on Stage*, 197–98n3).

5. See Scott-Warren, "Reading Graffiti," 370.

6. Dolan, "Reading, Writing, and Other Crimes," 143. I am mindful of Dolan's caution about the bias in modern scholarship that leads us to overvalue literacy and to strive to *include* populations under this rubric without (1) understanding the ideologies carried by the term; and (2) appreciating that early modern people could achieve social standing precisely without deploying writing, this being a culture where "written and oral, literate and illiterate cultures interacted and overlapped" (150).

7. Pamela Smith, *The Body of the Artisan*, 8. While her interest is ultimately to distinguish text-based knowledge from that acquired by practice, Smith's work provides a framework for analyzing the material and technical dimensions of literacy in the early modern period, particularly in her attention to informal sites of knowledge production.

8. See Ferguson, *Dido's Daughters*, esp. 31–82; Dolan, "Reading, Writing, and Other Crimes"; Hackel, *Reading Material*; Thomas, "Meaning of Literacy"; Sanders, *Gender and Literacy*; Mazzola, *Learning and Literacy*, esp. 1–15; and Calabresi, "'You Sow,'" 85.

9. Ferguson, *Dido's Daughters*, 4. While Ferguson's ultimate concern is to press this definition of literacy as a site of social struggle within an analysis of imperial politics, her understanding of literacy as a social phenomenon attached in complex ways to class and gender ideologies has been crucial in rethinking literacy's parameters in other domains.

10. See Stallybrass, "Books and Scrolls" and "Library and Material Texts"; Chartier, *Order of Books*; Cormack and Mazzio, *Book Use, Book Theory*; Hackel, *Reading Material*; and William Sherman, *Used Books*. On the history of the book, see also Daybell and Hinds, *Material Readings of Early Modern Culture*; and Baron, *Reader Revealed*, 11–17.

11. Ezell, *Patriarch's Wife*; *Social Authorship*; "Domestic Papers"; and "Laughing Tortoise."

12. See Hackel, *Reading Material*; and Laroche, *Medical Authority*.

13. Goldstein and Leong have begun to unearth ways that recipe books can be of value for a history of early modern reading and writing practices. See Goldstein, *Eating and Ethics*, 135–70; and Leong, "Medical Recipe Collections." For an example of how my analysis might be extended to account for eighteenth-century American publics, see Catherine Kelly, who analyzes ways that domestic "accomplishments" were coterminous with, and part of, intellectual life ("Reading").

14. Vives, *Instruction of a Christian Woman*, K3r

15. Fleming, *Graffiti and the Writing Arts*, esp. 9–17.

16. Rainbowe, *Sermon Preached at the Funeral of the . . . Countess of Pembroke*, 39–40.

17. Crooke, *Microcosmographia*, 730. Cited by William Sherman, who notes that this definition points ahead to educational theories of bodily-kinetic intelligence and physical apprehension (*Used Books*, 41).

18. Heather Wolfe, "Women's Handwriting"; Spufford, "First Steps," 435.

19. Calabresi, "'You Sow, Ile Read,'" 83.

20. Coote, *English Schoole-Master*, A3.

21. Tutoft, Folger ms L.D.603; quoted in Wolfe, "Women's Handwriting," 23. According to Daybell, "basic reading and writing skills, along with other practical accomplishments, were increasingly deemed to be important for gentlewoman in their capacity as wives and mistresses of households" (*Women Letter-Writers*, 14).

22. *The Gentlewomans Companion* circulated under Woolley's name in four editions in the late seventeenth century, although she disavowed its authorship. On Woolley's concern that female readers spent too much time fussing about the mechanics of writing, see *Supplement*, 148.

23. On textiles and textile work, see Jones and Stallybrass, *Renaissance Clothing and the Materials of Memory*, esp. 134–71; and Frye, *Pens and Needles*, esp. 116–59.

24. *The Compleat Servant-Maid* (1683), A3v. For an overview of women's handwriting, see Daybell, *Women Letter-Writers*, esp. 61–90.

25. Barker, intro., *The Great Book of Thomas Trevillian*, 11.

26. *The Compleat Servant-Maid* (1685) insert between pp. 24 and 25 (the same copytext is found in the 1683 edition) On this particular *sententiae*, see Bull, *Laughing Philosopher*, 30. This adage later appeared in Quarles, *King Solomon's Recantations*, 13. On this saying in needleworks, see samplers compiled by the National Dames of the Colonial Society of America: http://www.nscda.org/samplers/samp_show_image.php?sampid=2441.

27. Elias, *The Civilizing Process*.

28. *The Compleat Servant-Maid*, 1683 edition in the British Library, following insert after p. 26.

29. Daybell comments, "Since most women were excluded from male centres of learning—the grammar schools, universities and Inns of Court—historians are deprived of institutional records which so well elucidate the education of boys and young men. By contrast, the majority of women were taught either within the household, a practice that has left comparatively few documentary sources beyond a small number of educational texts, occasional details of educational provision in household accounts, and passing references in autobiographical writings and correspondence, or in the Church, where they received religious education" (*Women Letter-Writers*, 11–12).

30. Theophano, *Eat My Words*, 157–64. Theophano examines cookbooks as part of her recovery of women's historical experience and lives.

31. *Maddison Family Recipe Book*, flyleaf, 211 (inverted).

32. *Oxford English Dictionary*, "madcap," sense B.

33. "An Exceding restorative for one yt is brought lowe" (Pudsey, *Receipts*, 3).

34. Hackel describes a provocative array of female ownership marks in books (*Reading Material in Early Modern England*, 214–21), including "Elizabeth Hunt her Book *not* his" in a printed midwifery manual (215). On ownership marks in herbals, see Laroche, *Medical Authority*, 67–101.

35. Buckhurst, *Jane Buckhurst Her Book*, flyleaf; and Price, *Compleat Cook*, which is signed: "This Booke was written by me: Rebecca Price in the Yare 1681" (2).

36. "Steal Not this Book for Fear of Shame for hear you see the owner's Name," Elizabeth Pearkes wrote in her copy of Nott's *Cook's and Confectioner's Dictionary* (edition in the Szathmary Collection, University of Iowa).

37. *Mrs Anne Brumwich Her Booke of Receipts*, opening pages. Dacres's compilation similarly includes two modes of address: "Mrs. Mary Dacres Her Booke 1666" followed by a less careful hand: "Mary Lady Dacres Her Booke 1686."

38. Amy Eyton and others, *Collection of Cookery Receipts*, 128 (inverted).

39. *Cookbook*, Folger Library MS V.b.13, 3.

40. Bent, *Receipts*, flyleaf; *Miss Caldwells Book*, 25a and 113a; Brown, *Medicinal and Cookery Recipes*, last page; and Lovelace, *Recipes Medical and Culinary*, fol. 3.

41. See Heather Wolfe, "Women's Handwriting."

42. See Pennell, "Perfecting Practice?" 241. Only five of the 120 extant manuscript recipe books that I have read attribute all or part of their writing to a scribe. Leong, whose work has been invaluable to this project, sees the use of professional scribes as more common in recipe collections; the fact that she limits her data to medical recipes might inflect her findings in this regard. Leong, "Medical Recipe Collections," chap. 2, 117–39.

43. Fanshawe, *Booke of Receipts*; Ladie Borlase, *Receiptes*; Ann Smith, *Cookbook*. Additionally Edward Birkhead declares himself the scripter for Mary Birkhead's recipes (*Recipe-Book of Mary Birkhead*, fol. 25).

44. Denbigh, *Receipts*, title page.

45. *Elizabeth Fowler Her Book*, 1684. See also Brockman's *Receipts and Exercises*, where the reader has practiced lacework capitals of the letter *E* and knots (flyleaf).

46. Elizabeth Hirst and others, *Medical and Cookery Receipts*, 6.

47. Lady Anne Percy, *Book of Receipts*.

48. On manicules, see William Sherman, *Used Books*, 25–52.

49. See Pennell's astute analysis of how the afterlife of recipe collections can stymie scholarship that seeks to understand the recipes' initial material contexts (the material forms that I recruit as the basis for understanding domestic literacies). Pennell offers four case studies showcasing ways that early recipes migrated from their original environments ("Making Livings").

50. Murrell, *Delightful Daily Exercise*, F3.

51. In *Writing Matter*, Goldberg argues that the violence enacted on subjects in the scriptive domain was displaced onto a student's control over tools of violence (60–107).

52. Shirley, *Accomplished Ladies Rich Cabinet of Rarities*, 191. The term "cutting" letters is common; see, for instance, *The Gentlewomans Companion*, 229.

53. Davies, *The Writing Schoolemaster*, A1v. Bruising was a cooking term as well, e.g., "bruise the nutmegs and Cynamon but not too small, and slice the ginger thin, and small." See Granville (Dewes), *Cookery and Medicinal Recipes*, 13.

54. Hall, *Receipt Book*, 27v. Hall's manuscript is also transcribed in Kowalchuk, "Recipes for Life."

55. See, for instance, *A Closet for Ladies and Gentlewomen* (1608), 34.

56. *The Boke of Carving* was excerpted in several of Murrell's books, including *Two Bookes of Cookerie and Carving*.

57. *The Genteel House-keeper's Pastime*, 4–5.

58. Rose, *A Perfect School of Instructions*, title page.

59. *Sermons of John Donne*, 7:222.

60. On recipes for "spread eagle," see Fowler, *Elizabeth Fowler Her Book*, 32v, #66; and Yate, *Receipt Book*, irregular gatherings. For an example of a collection that presents recipes calling for roasts to be wrapped in *writing* paper in order to prevent burning, see Shackleford's *Modern Art of Cookery Improved*, and Mrs. Johnson, *Receipts*.

61. Granville (Dewes), *Cookery and Medicinal Recipes*, 101.

62. W.M., *The Queens Delight*, 222, appended to *The Queens Closet Opened*.

63. On how particular styles of knots could be part of a family tradition or featured on family crests, see Frye, *Pens and Needles*, 122.

64. See, for example, an anonymous recipe for "cracknels" in Folger V.a.19, no pagination; *Cookery Book of Ann Goodenough*, 43; *Cookbook of Mary Puleston*, 55; and *Collection of Medical and Cookery Receipts*, Wellcome MS 7721, 21.

65. Hill, *Gardeners Labyrinth*, title page.

66. *Country Housewifes Garden*, 2–3.

67. Lawson addresses "the best way for planting . . . with the country housewifes garden for hearbes of common use, their vertues, seasons, profits, ornaments, variety of knots, models for trees, and plots for the best ordering of Grounds and Walkes" (title page). See Munroe on decoration and the kitchen garden (*Gender and the Garden*, 33–35). On how herbals and plant knowledge formed a basis for domestic design work, see Leah Knight, *Of Books and Botany*; Frye, *Pens and Needles*, 132, 192; and Laroche, *Medical Authority*.

68. But, for an exception, see Frye, *Pens and Needles*, and Munroe, *Gender and the Garden*.

69. Heather Wolfe, "Women's Handwriting," 21.

70. Comley, *A New Alphabet*, title page.

71. Kendall and Cater, *Cookery and Medicinal Recipes*, 17.

72. See the anonymous *Collection of Medical and Cookery Recipes*, New York Public Library, Whitney Cookery Collection no. 8, p. 11, recipe 72, where the "T" in "To make Syder" mutates into the standard calligraphical design of a woman's face. This same design face appears in Denbigh, *Cookery and Medical Receipts*, 25.

73. Plat, *Delightes for Ladies*, B9v.

74. Murrell, *Delightfull Daily Exercise* (1621), B3v.

75. See also Murrell, *Delightful Daily Exercise*, F9v.

76. Tusser, *Five Hundred Points of Good Husbandry*, A2.

77. Scott-Warren, "Reading Graffiti," 370.

78. See Fleming, *Graffiti*, esp. 9–27; Scott-Warren, "Reading Graffiti"; and Helen Smith, *Grossly Material Things*.

79. For an overview of the hornbook and the cultural meanings of alphabetization in the seventeenth century, see Crain, *The Story of A*, 15–52. On the crisscross as a feature of sewing literacy, see Calabresi, "'You Sow,'" 83.

80. Erasmus, *Declamation on the Subject of Early Liberal Education*, 339.

81. See Hammons, *Gender, Sexuality, and Material Objects*, 16.

82. Puttenham, *The Arte of English Poesie*, 146–47. On domestic posies, see Leah Knight, *Of Books and Botany*, 129–32.

83. Plat, *Jewel House of Art and Nature*, 34. Although *The Jewel House* was not addressed specifically to women, it was read by women. See, for evidence, the female signature in the copy housed in the University of Toronto Library.

84. Hammons, *Gender, Sexuality, and Material Objects*, 16.

85. Jonson, "Inviting a Friend to Supper" in *Complete Poems*, 1:23. Many thanks to Kasey Evans for encouraging me to think about this poem in the context of recipe work.

86. See Donaldson, "Destruction of the Book." Burton complains about recycled pages: "not only Libraries and shoppes, are full of our putid [sic] papers, but every close-stoole and jakes; they serve to put under pies, to lappe in Spice, and keepe rostemeat from burning" ("Democritus Junior to the Reader," *Anatomy of Melancholy*, 1621, 8).

87. Loewenstein, "The Jonsonian Corpulence."

88. Donne, "Upon Mr Thomas Coryat's Crudities," in *Complete English Poems* 11:27–35. Leah Knight notes that spices and plants might have rubbed off onto pages and enforced the "tendency in the period to imbue texts with pharmaceutical powers" (125).

89. Masten recasts Goldberg's "psychoanalytic graphology" as a "literosexuality" evidenced through the mechanism of printing as well as handwriting, one seen "not the flow of ink via phallic pens onto paper, but the linking of letters in the compositor's stick, the locking of letters into the printer's forme." *Queer Philologies*.

90. Calabresi, "'You Sow, Ile Read,'" 83. Calabresi's work on sewing as a form of literacy crucially enlarges our understanding of domestic artistic production. See also Jones and Stallybrass, *Renaissance Clothing*, 134–72.

91. Calabresi, "'You Sow, Ile Read,'" 86–89.

92. Scholars speculate that Treveylon may have been involved in textile trade and work. His "miscellanies" are housed in the British Library (1616) and the Folger Shakespeare Library (1608).

93. See *Oxford English Dictionary*, "cutwork," 2b.

94. Ciotti, *A Booke of Curious and Strange Inventions*, title page.

95. Burton, *The Anatomy of Melancholy*, ed. Shilletto, part 2, section 2, member 4; Vol. 2:112–13.

96. Woolley, *A Supplement to the Queen-Like Closet*, 1684; 131–32. Women, including someone identified only as "I.W.," limned pictures on glass, created cosmetics, produced intricate dyes, and fashioned wax fruits (*Her Book [of] Cookery*, University of Iowa Library, En6).

97. Parker, *Collection of Medical and Cookery Receipts*, fol. 2.

98. Archer, "Quintessence of Wit," 121.

99. Cotton, *Recipe Book*.

100. "To make a Jacobine" is inscribed on the flyleaf to M.W., *Cookery and Medicinal Recipes*, Folger V.b.316. On Elizabeth Cromwell's recipes, see Knoppers, *Politicizing Domesticity*, 114–39.

101. Mary Forster and others, *Collection of Cookery Receipts*.

102. Davies, *Writing Schoolemaster*, R1.

103. While Goldberg acknowledges contradictions that riddle the disciplinary process (including the strangely doubled and anatomized hand that appears visually in handwriting manuals), he deemphasizes the deconstructive and critical potential of this imagery (*Writing Matter*). For assessments that implicitly or explicitly critique Goldberg's claims, see Mazzola, *Learning and Literacy*; Stallybrass, "'Adorn'd with Variety of Loose, and Easy Fig-

ures and Flourishes': The Aesthetics and Politics of Calligraphic Virtuosity," unpublished paper; and Altman, review of *Writing Matter*.

104. Hyrde, preface to Erasmus, *Devout Treatise*. See also my *Staging Domesticity*, 12–17.

105. Sandra Sherman, "'The Whole Art and Mystery of Cooking,'" 123.

106. *Receipt Book of Penelope Jephson*, flyleaf. See also Eyton and others, *Collection of Cookery Receipts*, flyleaf; and Elizabeth Brockman, *Receipts and Exercises*, 12. Baumfylde's collection, as Catherine Field observes, unwittingly commented on the unregulated assembly of collaborative scripts that made up the compilation itself: "many hands hands" appears scrawled on the flyleaf. Field is largely concerned to establish recipe books as expressive life writing ("'Many Hands Hands'").

107. *Edmund Spenser's Poetry*, 518; Sidney, *Major Works*, 215.

108. Okeover, *Collection of Medical Receipts*, 225 and 229.

Chapter 4. Temporalities

Note to epigraphs: Mayerne, "Publisher to the Reader," *Archimagirus anglo-gallicus*, A2v–A3; Child, *American Frugal Housewife*, 3, quoted by Goldstein, "Recipes for Authorship," 239.

1. Although my citations to Shakespeare are from *The Norton Shakespeare*, I retain the name "Helena," which was used intermittently in early texts and is deployed in most modern editions.

2. Garrett Sullivan interprets Helena's tears within the framework of potentially productive acts of "forgetting" in this play and in early modern culture (*Memory and Forgetting*, 44–64, esp. 44–45).

3. *Cookery Book of Ann Goodenough*, 40–41.

4. Hilary Rose, "From Household to Public Knowledge," xii–xiii.

5. Lewis, *Receipts in Cookery*, verso of first page. An inscription notes that the text was written "out of a Booke which was the La: Marquis Dorsetts."

6. *Recipe Book of Mary Doggett*, 1.

7. *Oxford English Dictionary*, IV 19, 2a, 3, 1.

8. Seasoning's semantic range also extended to include the act of alleviating or moderating a substance (*Oxford English Dictionary*, "season, v.," 1d) and the act of bringing (people, things, houses) into health or a healthy condition (4e).

9. On dietaries, see Albala, *Eating Right in the Renaissance*. For the most influential work on humoral theory and early modern literature, see Paster, *Humoring the Body*, and Schoenfeldt, *Bodies and Selves*.

10. In exploring Woolley's thrifty recycling of materials and writings, Goldstein similarly notes that "preservation" embraced both a technical act and a philosophical category important for understanding Woolley's relationship to social and national communities ("Recipes for Authorship," 239–92).

11. Turner, *The Seconde Part of William Turners Herball*, 35v.

12. Doggett offered "An Excellent water for the preservacion of Man or Woman long to Live" (*Her Book of Receipts*, 3). Lady Sedley asserted of a cordial: "whosoever useth this water ever and anon, and not often, it preserveth him long in good liking, and shall make one seem young a long time." Cited in Guthrie, "Lady Sedley's Receipt Book," 152.

13. Granville (Dewes), *Cookery and Medicinal Recipes*, 38–39. This manuscript is not continuously paginated.

14. Battista Guarini, *Il pastor fido*, 27.

15. Crowne, *The Married Beau*, p. 51, sig. H2.

16. Whitney, *A Sweet Nosgay*, C5.

17. In *Staging Domesticity* I identified ways that early modern stage representations portrayed the specter of mortality haunting kitchen work. I leveraged this evidence to enlarge the meaning of "domesticity" as made manifest in domestic work (*Staging Domesticity*, 189–220). I return to consider the way that recipe presentations of domesticity and violence address the timely fleshliness of being a creature. On violence and mortality in aristocratic banqueting, see Fumerton, *Cultural Aesthetics*, chap. 4, esp. 128–36.

18. Partridge, *Widdowes Treasure*, A2v.

19. *Ladie Borlase's Receiptes*, 132.

20. *The Compleat Servant-Maid* (1683), 174.

21. Cavendish, "Natures Cook," in *Poems, and Fancies*, 127.

22. Yates, "Shakespeare's Messmates." Yates is interested in Shakespearean texts to the extent that they test Donna Harraway's conception of a shared ecological hospitality in which humans are one merely one constituent party. Yates uses Hamlet's joke about Polonius as being eaten at "dinner" as the jumping-off point for an ecological analysis of relations in which "cooking" signifies transformative operations generally.

23. On *mummia* and "corpse pharmacology" in early modern Europe, see Sugg, *Murder After Death*, 40; and Camporesi, *Bread of Dreams*, esp. 40–55.

24. Oates, "Food Mysteries," 25.

25. Yates's theorization of the verb "kitchening," read through Shakespearean works, derives out of a conceptual and discursive matrix compatible with "seasoning" ("Shakespeare's Messmates").

26. Fumerton, *Cultural Aesthetics*, 135.

27. See Painter, *The Palace of Pleasure*, vol. 1, novel 38, 172.

28. See Floyd-Wilson, *Occult Knowledge*; and Field, "'Sweet Practicer.'"

29. Parker, *Collection of Medical and Cookery Receipts*, fol. 13v; Okeover, *Collection of Medical Receipts*, fol. 132v; and *Queens Closet Opened*, 117–18. Field notes that fistula recipes appear in collections attributed to Baumfylde and Corlyon ("'Sweet Practicer'").

30. See, for example, Woolley, *An Accomplish'd Ladies Delight*, p. 285, #63.

31. *Recipe Book . . . of Archdale Palmer*, ed. Uden, 29 in facsimile, 168 in transcription pagination.

32. Barrett, *Select Receipts*, 26–27.

33. Corlyon, *A Booke of Divers Medecines*, fol. 145v.

34. *A Closet for Ladies and Gentlewomen* (1608), 176.

35. W.M., *The Queens Closet Opened*, 71.

36. The recipe archive could further contribute to critical debates about *All's Well* in two salient ways: (1) it might offer a rebuttal to critics who interpret Helena's medical skill as a transgressive intellectual transvestism or poaching of professional knowledge, and (2) it might help to make sense of the eroticized representation of the king's healing as an instance of "queer physic" (see my *Staging Domesticity*, 161–88). Analyses of recipes and *All's Well* by Field ("'Sweet Practicer'") and by Floyd-Wilson (*Occult Knowledge*) refine scholarly understanding early modern female agency.

37. *Oxford English Dictionary*, "preserve," v. 2 and 4a, 1b, 5c, 5b, respectively.

38. Helena, the person able to "quicken a rock," emerges as the agent *and* object of enlivening in the final scene, the resolution to the riddle: "one that's dead is quick" (2.1.72, 5.3.300–301). The animated king and Helena's materializing tears repeat in the play's final representation of Helena's resurrected and quickened (pregnant) body, which is used to evidence the truth of *past* actions rather than to celebrate the future reproduction of family and social world.

39. Schwarz, *What You Will: Gender, Contract, and Shakespearean Social Space*.

40. See my *Staging Domesticity*, 18–58. On early modern women's use of medicinal recipes as a means of "therapeutic determination," see Stobart, "'Lett Her Refrain from All Hot Spices.'" Representations flaunting female medical housewifery embrace the powerful cosmic implications of domesticity rather than revealing "kitchen avoidance," the rich term that Yates uses in identifying an early modern habit of turning away from human implication in an organic sphere of decay ("Shakespeare's Messmates").

41. On rue, see Laroche, *Medical Authority*, 1 and 67.

42. See *All's Well*, 4.2.36; 2.2.22; 5.3.164, 5.3.323.

43. For an overview of the segregation of medical and culinary practice/knowledge, see Fitzpatrick, *Renaissance Food*, 55–72.

44. Richard Halpern inadvertently alludes to how distillation's everyday context might dovetail with the sonnets' unusual representation of sexuality: "Somehow the sonneteers' rhetoric of seduction has gotten twisted in the direction of family values," Halpern writes. "Indeed, the sense of imminent demise that pervades the poem works less to whip up a desperate sexual longing than to mortify desire into something merely prudent. It makes sex seem as exciting as putting up preserves" ("Shakespeare's Perfume," 8). Halpern's point is a good one. Sex in Sonnets 5 and 6 might seem dryly functional and drained of erotic energy as it is made to serve a larger social and aesthetic duty. Yet literary representations that I examine elsewhere show that functional domestic work was often highly eroticized (Wall, *Staging Domesticity*, 51–53).

45. Although the most popularly recognized apparatus for distillation in modern times is the "still," which is popularly identified with making alcoholic beverages, distillation was earlier used for various industrial, pharmaceutical, and chemical processes. Persian experimenters created the alembic around 800 A.D. Writers spanning the thirteenth to sixteenth centuries—including friar Roger Bacon, friar John of Rupescissa, physician Petrus Bonus of Ferrara, and teacher Andreas Libavius—outlined procedures for transmuting substances into magical elixirs. Unlike alchemists, medicinal distillers in the craft tradition (such as Hieronymus Brunschwig) concentrated on the curative properties of herbs and plants as well as the purification of waters; distillation was a requisite skill of pharmacology.

46. This assumption is based, in part, on the fact that a later sonnet (54) specifically describes the products of distilled roses as "sweetest odors" (12). In the earlier two poems, however, distilled roses are not specified as sweet-smelling dematerialized aesthetic objects.

47. See *Medicinal and Cookery Recipes of Mary Baumfylde*, fol. 35; and *Lettice Pudsey Her Booke of Receipts*, fol. 13.

48. Brunschwig, *The Vertuose Boke of Distyllacyon*, Q3.

49. See, for one example, Ralph Knevet's 1631 play *Rhodon and Iris*, where a servant describes her mistress's potion making: "With limbecks, viols, pots, her Closet's fill'd / Full of strange liquors by rare art distill'd" (E3).

50. W.M., "To the Ingenious and Courteous Reader," *Queens Closet Opened*, A3v.

51. On the recipe as "memorandum" rather than instruction, see Woolley, *Queen-Like Closet*, 314.

52. The phrase is Theophano's in *Eat My Words*, 49. Goldstein sees the early modern manuscript collection as a "textually congealed act of commensality" that offered a "textual crystallization of the material act of food-sharing" (*Eating and Ethics*, 145).

53. Pennell and DiMeo, introduction, *Reading and Writing Recipe Books*, 14. See also Theophano, *Eat My Words*, 85–116. On commemorative practices in Dorothy Wake Pennyman's recipe book, see Pennell, "Making Livings, Lives and Archives," 234–36.

54. *Cookbook of Mary Puleston*, 92–93.

55. *Receipt Book of Mary Hookes*, 33, 41, 35.

56. Priscilla Ferguson, *Accounting for Taste*, 17 (emphasis added).

57. Jones and Stallybrass, *Renaissance Clothing and the Materials of Memory*.

58. Bromehead, *Collection of Medical and Cookery Recipes*, fol. 1.

59. *Mrs Fanshawes Booke of Receipts of Physickes*. See also Goldstein's compelling analysis of Fanshawe's recipe collection and memoirs (*Eating and Ethics*, 153–70).

60. Spurling, *Elinor Fettiplace's Receipt Book*, xi.

61. Spurling, *Elinor Fettiplace's Receipt Book*, 21; 35.

62. Catchmay, *A Booke of Medicens*, 2v.

63. On Westcombe's discharge and baronetcy, see *Calendar of Treasury Books*, 1480–89.

64. *Autobiography and Correspondence of Mary Granville, Mrs. Delany*, 1:300.

65. Laroche argues that an herbal owners' decision not to cancel the signatures of previous owners was an implicit memorialization (*Medical Authority*, 75–84).

66. Theophano, *Eat My Words*, 49–51. Theophano offers a sustained exploration of cookbooks as sites of memory.

67. See, for example, *Autobiography and Correspondence of Mary Granville, Mrs. Delany*, 1:337.

68. Augusta Hall (Lady Llanover), *Good Cookery Illustrated*. "Granville Fish Sauce" appears on p. 176 and as recipe 36 in the appendix, pp. 425–26.

69. Hall created this imaginative cookbook, *Good Cookery Illustrated*, by sandwiching a recipe book within a fictional tale in which a traveler unexpectedly discovers fine dining at a remote Welsh hermitage. His conversation with an elderly hermit residing in a Welsh cave becomes the occasion for Hall to satirize modernity. The Traveler's pretentious claims about advances of machinery and industry are proven wrong, and the Hermit emerges as a culinary expert. Their exchange becomes the framework for a cookbook made up of four hundred pages of discursive instructions and a one-hundred-page appendix filled with recipes. The *historical* nature of the cookery is indicated by the fact that Hall includes recipes from seventeenth-century sources such as May's *Accomplisht Cook*. On this text, see Freemon, who observes that the Granville fish sauce is "thought to be named after Lady Llanover's illustrious ancestor, sir Richard Granville" but could have been named for Mary Granville Delany (*First Catch Your Peacock*, 308).

70. Bayne, *Book of Recipes*.

71. Spurling similarly constructed a family history in editing Elinor Fettiplace's recipe book, which she inherited (*Elinor Fettiplace's Receipt Book*).

72. *Recipe Book of Hopestill Brett*, 16v.

73. A note inscribed in a recipe collection attributed to Martha Hodges reveals similar genealogical detective work: "Our Great Grandmother Hodges her receipt book. She was

mother to Mrs. Priaulx who was the Grandmother of Mrs. Sarah Tilley by Mrs. Howes marrying her daughter Mrs. Mary Priaulx. Her name is written by herself at the other end." *Collection of Cookery Receipts by Martha Hodges, Robert Foster and Others*, opening page.

74. On the scholarly problems of using recipes to construct medical and social networks, see DiMeo, "Authorship and Medical Networks."

75. The practice of recording family histories in medical recipe collections is documented by Leong ("Medical Recipe Collections," 34–36) and Stine ("Opening Closets," 198). On Bibles, books of hours, and childbirth books as storage sites for family histories, see William Sherman, *Used Books*, 59–60.

76. Springatt and others, *Collection of Cookery and Medical Receipts*, fol. 1v.

77. While the Folger W.a.283 conventionally provides family births and deaths for the Stevens family of Oxfordshire, other recipe users meditated broadly on death in their inscriptions. Witness the following lines that haunt recipe collections: "Doe not deare soule this sacrifice refuse, / That in thy grave I doe interre my muse" (adaptation of lines by John Donne in Bridget Parker, *Collection of Medical and Cookery Receipts*, fol. 76v); "For I know that thou will bring me to death and to the place appointed for all living" (Elizabeth Whiteaker, *Collection of Cookery Receipts*); "Margaret Oliver her Book and might God give her Grace in it to Look / And when her passing bell doth toll the Lord of heaven receive her Soul" (handwritten annotation in the University of Iowa copy of Sarah Harrison's *The House-keeper's Pocket-Book*); "The leaf is green the rose is red / [SUCH] is my Book when I am ded / When I am ded Tole much the Bell / Then take my Book and use it well" (John Hadley's inscription to his wife in the University of Iowa copy of Nott's *Cook's and Confectioner's Dictionary*).

78. Randolph (Blome), *Cookbook*, 1697, unclear pagination, image 104 on the Perdita Database.

79. Lynda Payne comments on Blome's recording of her father's autopsy, in *With Words and Knives*, 75–76.

80. The printed ode is traditionally dated 1735, although the date is contested by some scholars. The Yale Library catalogue states that Joanna Lipking attributes the poem to Mary Castillion Randolph on the basis of the marginal note that Lady Oxenden died on All Saints' Day (the date for the first Lady Oxenden's death in 1697, which would have the book written when Mary Castillion Randolph was alive). I do not need to settle the question of attribution, because the provenance is not significant to my analysis of the recipe text's reception as a commemorative form joining other types of memorials.

81. See McGovern, *Anne Finch and Her Poetry*, 121–23.

82. *Book of Cookery Recipes*, fol. 1.

83. Hudson, *Cookery Receipts*, opening page.

Chapter 5. Knowledge

Note to epigraph: "Philatros," preface, *Natura Exenterata*, unpaginated. This text is attributed to Aletheia Talbot based on the portrait of her included in contemporary editions and on external references.

1. Brumwich, *Booke of Receipts*, flyleaf. This folio is signed by Rhoda Fairfax, Ursula Fairfax, Rhoda Hussey, Hanna Garthnait, and Dorothy Cartwright. The Wellcome catalogue identifies the daughter of Edward Trotman, a lawyer in Gloucester, as its original compiler.

2. Baron Ferdinando Fairfax of Cameron II was an MP from York, of Scottish peerage, who married Rhoda, daughter of Thomas Chapman of Hertfordshire and widow of Thomas Hussey of Lincolnshire. Twenty years before she died, Hussey apparently gave the collection to her daughter Ursula Fairfax, who married William Cartwright in 1669.

3. See Leong, "Medical Recipe Collections," 129.

4. For an overview of debates about the "rise of science" paradigm, see Shapin, *Scientific Revolution*; Pérez-Ramos, *Francis Bacon's Idea of Science*; and Peter Harrison, "Was There a Scientific Revolution?"

5. Eamon, *Science and the Secrets of Nature*; Dear, *Revolutionizing the Sciences*; and Daston, "The Factual Sensibility."

6. Smith and Findlen state, "Artist-artisans . . . articulated a body of claims about nature and about the nature of authority that helped form the basis of the new science," introduction to *Merchants and Marvels*, 17. For foundational research in this area, see Pamela Smith, *Body of the Artisan*; Harkness, *Jewel House*; and Findlen, *Possessing Nature*. See also Santillana, "The Role of Art in the Scientific Renaissance"; *Science and the Arts in the Renaissance*, ed. Shirley and Hoeniger; *Picturing Science, Producing Art*, ed. Jones and Hoeniger.

7. See Hunter, "Sisters of the Royal Society"; Nagy, *Popular Medicine*; and Laroche, *Medical Authority*.

8. On the status of the recipe in cultures of experimentation, see Pennell, "Perfecting Practice?"; Spiller, introduction, *Seventeenth-Century English Recipe Books*; and Field, "'Sweet Practicer.'"

9. Susanna Packe, *Her Book*. The Folger catalogue guesses, "This Susanna Packe may be the third daughter of Sir Christopher Packe, Lord Mayer of London, who married Sir Thomas Bellot, bart., in 1675." Because the spelling is even more variable than those in comparable recipe books, it is likely that someone without extensive formal education wrote the text. The evidence is hardly conclusive.

10. Although Leong offers valuable evidence that recipe claims about experience become pointedly more serious over the course of the century, I do not agree with her claim that the word "proved" was a "trope rather than a reflection of actual practice" ("Medical Recipe Collections," 112). Stine states recipe claims to proof "did not necessarily mean that a remedy had been tried first hand, only that it was said to have been used to good effect by a reliable source" ("Opening Closets," 44). Rebecca Bushnell argues that "books of secrets," the genre from which recipes emerged, compromised their claims about proving when they acknowledged the imaginative and recreational value of their information (*Green Desire*, 176–81). See also Pennell's skepticism about conventional markers of proof ("Perfecting Practice?" 255n28). On *probatum* as an "efficacy tag" in medieval writings see C. Jones, "Formula and Formulation."

11. On the problem of distinguishing prescriptive and descriptive documents, see Dolan, *True Relations*, esp. 111–53.

12. Hirst, *Mrs. Elizabeth Hirst her book*, 6, 2, 38.

13. As I mention in the Preface, the varying hands in this collection, its circulation among family members, and the simple problem that the family included three persons named "Elizabeth Okeover" prevent proof positive identification of whose learning the book documents. Nevertheless recipes attributed to a singular hand, "Elizabeth Okeover," formed the bulk of a 250-page collection. See Aspin's quest to establish the provenance of this collection: "Who Was Elizabeth Okeover?"

14. Elizabeth Browne et al., *Collection of Cookery and Medical Recipes*, 65; Anstey and Fenwick, *Cookery Book*, 117.

15. As Pollock has demonstrated in her case study of Grace Mildmay, home treatments that look ridiculous to modern readers were not significantly different from those recommended by formally trained physicians of the day (*With Faith and Physic*).

16. Rebecca Laroche documented early modern women's recipe experimentation with pH balance in her 2011 curated exhibit at the Folger Shakespeare Library, "Beyond Home Remedy: Women, Medicine, Science."

17. *Second Part of the Good Hus-Wives Jewell*, 31 (numbered 25).

18. Over the course of the seventeenth century, writers begin to use more precise measurements, registering a nascent desire for standardization that would be fully effected only in the nineteenth century. See, for instance, collections attributed to Katherine Davies, *Medicinal and Cookery Receipts*; and the *Receipt Book of Penelope Jephson*.

19. Harkness points to Bacon's sleight-of-hand, since he embraced artisanal methods and information but was reluctant to count manual laborers as knowledge producers (*Jewel House*, 246–48).

20. Pamela Smith's work builds on scholarship by Edgar Zilsel and Paolo Rossi.

21. Pérez-Ramos, *Francis Bacon's Idea of Science*, 48. On maker's knowledge and books of secrets, see Kavey, *Books of Secrets*, 114–15; and Spiller, introduction, *Seventeenth-Century*, xii–xvi.

22. Bushnell, *Green Desire*, 161–68. Pamela Smith issues this challenge: "The story of local modes of cognition and the vernacular knowledge systems such as those of the 'old women' and 'herbalists' mentioned by almost early modern botanist as the basis of his specimens and local plant knowledge has yet to be written" (*Body of the Artisan*, 240–41). For scholars who have taken up this challenge, see Laroche, *Medical Authority and Englishwomen's Herbal Texts*; and Leah Knight, *Of Books and Botany*.

23. The Hartlib Scriptorium was a communication hub for transmitting scientific information between Britain and the Continent. On Jones's connection to chemistry and natural philosophy, see DiMeo, "Katherine Jones, Lady Ranelagh"; and Archer, "Women and Alchemy in Early Modern England," esp. chap. 7. See also Frances Harris, "Living in the Neighbourhood of Science: Mary Evelyn, Margaret Cavendish and the Greshamites."

24. In the Boyle family recipe collection, Jones or a female cousin cited "My brother Robert distilled roses." On the basis of this citation and others, this collection is commonly attributed to Katherine Jones, though DiMeo skeptically limits Jones's contributions ("Katherine Jones, Lady Ranelagh").

25. "Sarah Horsington Her Manuscript, 1666," cited by Hunter, "Sisters," 192–94. The manuscript is located in the William Andrews Clark Memorial Library.

26. The Lowdham collection cites Boyle's cure for kidney stones; his trick of boiling an egg in vinegar to create "strange forms"; his knowledge of the secret virtues of walnut tree liquor; his treatment for "nephritical distempers"; and his methods for making preservative spirits of wine. Lowdham, mss. 137 (inverted).

27. For a *poetic* recipe for making ink, see Beau Chesne and Baildon, *A Book Containing Divers Sorts of Hands*. On the commercial history of ink, see Johns ("Ink"), who also issues a call for scholars not to look through the ink on the page but to investigate its production history.

28. See also Dekker, *Satiro-Mastix* C3; and Jonson, *Workes*, 450.

29. Partridge, *The Widdowes Treasure*, 1588, B5v–B6.

30. On characteristics of recipes, see Goody, "The Recipe, the Prescription and the Experiment."

31. Lewis, *Receipts in Cookery* . . . *owned by the Lady Marquess Dorset*, 52.

32. *The Recipe Book . . . of Archdale Palmer*, 70 in facsimile, 188 in transcription pagination.

33. Vaughan, *Magia Adamica; or, The Antiquitie of Magic*, 118. Cited by Picciotto, *Labors of Innocence*, 144.

34. On problems in recipe attribution, see DiMeo, "Authorship and Medical Networks."

35. See Aspin's account of the intersection and transmission of two recipe collections connected to the Okeover family ("Who Was Elizabeth Okeover?"). Leong traces lines of transmission for collections moving within the Johnson-Phillip family in Lincolnshire and the Fairfax family.

36. Bacon, *Novum Organvm*, aphorism 25. In *The History of the Royal Society*, Sprat also gendered inductive methods in ways that would make it unlikely to be identified in women's domestic work: "the *Wit* that is founded on the *Arts* of Men's Hands, is masculine and durable" (415).

37. See Merchant, *Death of Nature*; Schiebinger, *The Mind Has No Sex?*

38. See Findlen, *Possessing Nature*; Marchitello, *Machine in the Text*.

39. Spiller argues that early printed books of secrets, which illustrated the Aristotelian idea of experiment as visual demonstration of truth, absorbed Baconian models in the seventeenth century so as to emphasize the role of human *techne* in understanding the workings of nature (Introduction, *Seventeenth-Century English Recipe Books*, xvi). Eamon argues that popular traditions tested knowledge by reproducing natural effects (*Science and the Secrets of Nature*, 10).

40. See Findlen and Smith, *Merchants and Marvels*; Smith, *Business of Alchemy*, 7.

41. See also Bono, *The Word of God and the Languages of Man*. As Kavey explains, sixteenth-century books of secrets "presented readers with models of the natural world that were susceptible to human manipulation, pointed to the agents of natural change that were vulnerable to such efforts, and issued instructions for producing particular changes that would suit or satisfy human desires. . . . The effect of all these books was to authorize readers' perceptions of the natural world and recognize their position, and sometimes even centralize their position, in it" (*Books of Secrets*, 3).

42. *Sor Juana Anthology*, 225–26.

43. Goldstein warns about the risks of using recipes as proof of practice (*Eating*, 159–60). Sandra Sherman argues that the eighteenth-century printed cookbook creates a pedagogic intimacy that emerged out of previous manuscript writing ("'The Whole Art and Mystery of Cooking,'" 12).

44. See Eamon, *Science and the Secrets of Nature*, 131–33; Pennell, "Perfecting Practice?" 250–53.

45. Dear, "Miracles," 666.

46. For differing accounts of the social history of the fact, see Poovey, *History of the Modern Fact*; Shapiro, *Culture of Fact*.

47. On Bacon's articulation of ways that "learned experience" must create artificial situations to observe nature (including acts of variation, production, translation, inversion, compulsion, application, or conjunction, and changes of experiment), see Eamon, *Science and the Secrets of Nature*, 286.

48. Spiller, introduction, *Seventeenth-Century English Recipe Books*, x.

49. Eamon, by contrast, sees early modern recipes as reinforcing distinctions between application and reflection (*Science and the Secrets of Nature*, 281). Eamon's rigorous account of the hermeneutics of knowledge, found in the revivified "venatic" paradigm (or the "hunt" for knowledge) in the seventeenth century, points to the importance of experientially-rooted explanation. See also Dear, *Revolutionizing the Sciences*; Pamela Smith, *The Body of the Artisan*; and Daston, "The Factual Sensibility."

50. We might remember that Plat was an inveterate entrepreneur of knowledge. As he supervised the family's brewery and dispensed medicine in the city, Plat interviewed servants, millers, grocers, flax wives, lace makers, purse makers, victuallers, vintners, brewers, herb wives, apothecaries, cooks, bakers, painters, scriveners, goldsmiths, merchants, mariners, coal makers, tailors, and drapers (*Jewel House*, 142–80). For an example of a manuscript recipe writer who exhorted future readers to "make careful practice," see Katherine Packer, *A Boocke*, title page.

51. Spiller, introduction, *Seventeenth-Century English Recipe Books*, xxxvii, xxxvi. Leong sees printed recipe collections' emphasis on practice as part of a call for medical reform ("Medical Recipe Collections," 51).

52. See Pennell on the intersection of social and epistemological features of the recipe ("Perfecting Practice?" 247–53). On recipe citation in manuscript and in print, see Goldstein, *Eating*, 145–53.

53. Pollock, *With Faith and Physic*, 113. Philip Stanhope was unusual in including details about the religious and national identities of informants when tracking recipe sources; he mentions an ague remedy given by a Jew (who was a Turk's physician) to a friend (*A Booke of Severall Receipts*, 2) and an Italian doctor's remedy for the gout acquired from Mrs. June Perrot of Lumbersford, friend of Lady Herbert (293).

54. Although published recipe books of the later seventeenth century were interested in validating the expertise of a singular compiling "author," some adapted the citational structure common in the manuscript world to the format of print. See *The Queens Closet Opened* (which lists esteemed noble persons who *approved* the recommended practices) and Kenelm Digby's citation-filled *Closet*, based on a manuscript.

55. Foucault, "What Is an Author?"

56. Goldstein, *Eating*, 155–61. For Goldstein, recipe relationality creates "surrogate spaces of commensality" (170).

57. Pennell, "Perfecting Practice?" 250–51.

58. Shapin, *The Scientific Revolution*, 205.

59. Kavey argues that recipe compilers could qualify as scientific witnesses (*Books of Secrets*, 34). See also Pennell, "Perfecting Practice?" 247–51; Leong, "Medical Recipe Collections," 56; Stine, "Opening Closets," 13; DiMeo, "Katherine Jones, Lady Ranelagh," 162–66.

60. Seeing the recipe as a "transmission" rather than a "prescription" enables Pennell to "fit it in alongside other readings in the histories of women, notably of social networks, knowledge formation and communication and domestic technology" ("Perfecting Practice?" 252–53).

61. Dear, "Totius in Verba." Dear sees the construction of facts as dependent on rhetorical, literary, and generic features of scientific writing ("Miracles," 663).

62. Atkinson, "Philosophical Transactions." Dear notes that Newton falsified his methods so that they "fit" the narrative requirements of the Society ("Totius in Verba," 154–55).

63. Henry Powers, *Experimental Philosophy*, 32; cited by Dear, "Totius in Verba."

64. Stanhope, *A Booke of Severall Receipts*.

65. *Natura Exenterata* similarly promotes first-person practice but includes a hefty list of actual "approvers." On the relation of legal and scientific vocabularies, see Stine, "Opening Closets," and Shapin, *A Social History of Truth*.

66. Stanhope's tome circulated this model of authorization extensively. Leong has identified at least four manuscript collectors who copied sections of Stanhope's works, including Sarah Hughes, Katherine Browne, and Lady Borlase (Leong, "Medical Recipe Collections," 137n76). See *Pharmaceutical Recipes*, Folger V.b.286; *Select and Very Choice and Rare Receipts*, Folger V.a.365; Brown, *Medicinal and Cookery Recipes*; and Hughes, *Her Receipts of Her Whole Booke*. Stanhope's daughter-in-law, Lady Anne Percy, became an "after-the-fact" corroborating witness when she produced her own collection, some of which modified recipes in her father-in-law's compilations. See Percy, *Book of Receipts*.

67. *Commonplace Book of Elizabeth Freke*. See also Dorothy Stone's collection, *Cookery book*, which ends with this assurance: "Note that those Receipts which have this Mark Opposite them in the Margent are known Aprove'd to be good as any now Extant" (130).

68. Pollock, *With Faith and Physic*, 142.

69. For examples showing the spectrum on which approval and proving were conferred, see Jephson, *Receipt Book*, 97; and Glyd, *Recipe-Book*, 21, 23, 44, 51, 52, 53, 60, 63. Glyd marks her kidney stone cure, "this to my knowledge hath been proved, and hath brought away gravel Ann Glyd" (48); she writes of her treatment for a wound made by a rusty nail, "I myself have several times for horses feet proved it Ann Glyd" (66).

70. See also Okeover, who marks "I pro:" beside a burn recipe. While this could mean "I proved," she also routinely abbreviates "probatum" to "pro," suggesting the fascinating possibility that the note means "I probatum," or "I has been proved" (*Collection of Medical Receipts*). Stanhope claims that his remedy for a severed artery was "approved *in* Lord Brooke" (emph. mine; *A Booke of Severall Receipts,* B, 178 B6).

71. Sandra Sherman emphasizes that chatty references to personal practice in seventeenth-century recipe books paved the way for the development of the modern cookery book in the eighteenth century (*Invention*, 12).

72. William Sherman, 18 (citing Huntington Library mss. HEH RB 432871). When recipe writers worried about textual accuracy, they registered proper editorial care as part of the construction of valid testimony. The compiler of Okeover's collection, for instance, attended to errata, repeating three times that a particular remedy had been mistakenly cancelled (*Collection of Medical Receipts*).

73. See, for instance, Mrs. Maddison, who declares of her dropsy cure: "I cannot write it right" (*Maddison Family Recipe Book*, 40), and Sarah Hughes who, throughout recipes that she translates from Spanish, comments on the intellectual problems of cultural, linguistic, and culinary translation (*Her Receipts*).

74. See Painter, *Palace of Pleasure*, novel 38, 1:172.

75. My thanks to Peter Stallybrass for calling to my attention the commercial aspects of the recipe's suppression of knowledge. He has unearthed eighteenth-century published recipes that deliberately omit crucial details that may then be purchased at a vendor.

76. In their account of the emergence of the public sphere, Andrew Barnaby and Lisa Schnell write that "the question of the human-as-knower in the seventeenth century was more properly a social issue than a purely philosophical one. To seventeenth-century thinkers, solutions to the problem of 'right knowing' were intimately connected to a

broader series of issues involving communities of knowledge and of knowers" (*Literate Experience*, 2).

77. Shapin, "The House of Experiment"; Archer, "Women and Alchemy."

78. While Plat appealed to "every gentlewoman that delights in chemical practices" (*The Jewel House*, 1594, 20), he declined to publish experiments "more fit for a philosopher's laboratory than a gentlewoman's closet" (34).

79. Aspin writes, "Much work has been done by historians of medicine to show that, far from being merely an underdeveloped version of modern medicine, the medical culture of early modern England was a rich matrix of overlapping spheres of competence and activity, populated by a range of claimants to medical expertise" ("Who was Elizabeth Okeover?" 531). On the professionalization of medicine and its effects on women, see Beier, *Sufferers and Healers*; Pelling, *Medical Conflicts in Early Modern London*; Nagy, *Popular Medicine*; Stine, "Opening Closets"; and Hunter, "Women and Domestic Medicine."

80. Bushnell argues that debates about nature that took place in universities, gentleman's societies, and literary salons had a counterpart with those in the "nursery, market garden, and in the pages of common gardening manuals" (*Green Desire*, 5–6).

81. See Thomas, *Man and the Natural World*, 74; Bushnell, *Green Desire*, 171–72.

82. Sandra Sherman, *Invention*.

83. See Dear, "Totius in Verba"; Atkinson, "Philosophical Transactions."

84. Sleigh and Whitfield, *Collection of Medical Receipts*, inverted 144.

Coda

1. On the recipe as embedded discourse, see Leonardi's path-breaking essay, "Recipes for Reading." On the perils of the recipe, see British cookery writer Nigel Slater, *Appetite*, 9.

2. Gopnik, "What's the Recipe? Our Hunger for Cookbooks."

3. De Silva, ed., *In Memory's Kitchen: A Legacy from the Women of Terezin*.

WORKS CITED

Works Before 1800

Manuscripts

Anon. *Book of Cookery Recipes*, seventeenth century. Whitney Cookery Collection. Manuscripts and Archives Division. New York Public Library, MssCol 3318, vol. 6.
Anon. *Collection of Medical and Cookery Receipts in Various Hands*, later seventeenth century. Wellcome Library, MS 7721.
Anon. *Collection of Medical and Cookery Recipes*. Whitney Cookery Collection. Manuscripts and Archives Division. New York Public Library, MssCol 3318, vol. 8.
Anon. *Cookbook*, 1678–ca. 1689. Folger Shakespeare Library, MS V.b.13.
Anon. *Cookbook*, ca. seventeenth century. Folger Shakespeare Library, MS V.a.19.
Anon. *Cookery and Medicinal Recipes*, 1675–ca. 1750. Folger Shakespeare Library, MS V.a.429.
Anon. *Her Book [of] Cookery*, 1700–1799. Szathmary Culinary Manuscripts Collection, MsC0533, University of Iowa Library, series 4, En6.
Anon. *Pharmaceutical Recipes*, ca. 1690, ca. 1750–ca. 1870. Folger Shakespeare Library, MS V.b.286.
Anon. *Receipt Book*, ca. 1704–1787. Folger Shakespeare Library, MS W.a.283.
Anon. *Select and Very Choice and Rare Receipts*, ca. 1675. Folger Shakespeare Library, MS V.a.365.
Anstey, Mary Ann, and Diana Matilda Fenwick. *Cookery Book, with Some Medical and Household Receipts*, 1798–1828. Wellcome Library, MS 960.
Ayscough, Lady. *Receits of Phisick and Chirurgery*, 1692. Wellcome Library, MS 1026.
Barrett, Lady. *Select Receipts*, ca. 1700. Wellcome Library, MS 1071.
Baumfylde, Mary. *Medicinal and Cookery Recipes of Mary Baumfylde*, 1626, ca. 1702–1758. Folger Shakespeare Library, MS V.a.456.
Bayne, Anne. *Book of Recipes*, ca. 1700. Szathmary Culinary Manuscripts Collection, MsC0533, University of Iowa Library, series 4, En13.
Bent, Mary. *Receipts*, 1664–1729. Wellcome Library, MS 1127.
Birkhead, Mary. *Recipe-Book of Mary Birkhead Containing Culinary and Medicinal Recipes*, begun March 25, 1681. British Library, Egerton MS 2415.
Borlase, Ladie. *Receiptes*, 1655. Szathmary Culinary Manuscripts Collection, MsC0533, University of Iowa Library, series 4, En12. Reprinted in *Ladie Borlase's Receiptes Booke*, ed. David Schoonover. Iowa City: Iowa University Press, 1998.

Boyle Family, perhaps Lady Ranelagh. *Collection of Receipts*, ca. 1675–ca. 1710. Wellcome Library, MS 1340.

Brett, Hopestill. *Recipe Book of Hopestill Brett*, 1678–1700. Esther Aresty Collection, Kislak Center for Special Collections, University of Pennsylvania Library, MS codex 626.

Brockman, Elizabeth. *Receipts and Exercises*, ca. 1674–87. British Library, MS 45199.

Bromehead, Mary. *Collection of Medical and Cookery Recipes*, 1761. Whitney Cookery Collection. Manuscripts and Archives Division. New York Public Library, MssCol 3318, vol. 13.

Brown, Katherine. *Medicinal and Cookery Recipes*, 1650–62. Folger Shakespeare Library, MS V.a.397.

Browne, Elizabeth, Penelope Humphreys, Sarah Studman, and Mary Dawes. *Collection of Cookery and Medical Recipes*, 1697–1791. Wellcome Library, MS 7851.

Brumwich, Anne, and others. *Mrs Anne Brumwich Her Booke of Receipts or Medicines for Severall Sores and Other Infermities*, ca. 1625–1700. Wellcome Library MS 160.

Buckhurst, Jane. *Jane Buckhurst Her Book*, 1653. Folger Shakespeare Library, MS V.a.7.

Caldwell, Miss. *Miss Caldwells Book. Manuscript Recipe Book*, 1757–90. Szathmary Culinary Manuscripts Collection, MsC0533. University of Iowa Library, series 4, En14.

Catchmay, Lady Frances. *A Booke of Medicens*, ca. 1625. Wellcome Library, MS 184a.

Clifford, Ann. *The Diary of Anne Clifford, 1616–1619*, ed. Katherine O. Acheson. New York: Garland, 1995.

Corlyon. Mrs. *A Booke of Divers Medecines, Broothes, Salves, Waters, Syroppes, and Oyntementes of Which Many or the Most Part Have Been Experienced and Tryed by the Speciall Practize of Mrs Corlyon*, ca. 1606. Wellcome Library, MS 213.

Cotton, Catharine. *Recipe Book*, 1698. Esther Aresty Collection, Kislak Center for Special Collections, University of Pennsylvania Library, MS codex 214.

Cruso, Mary. *Cookbook of Mary Cruso and Timothy Cruso*, 1689. Folger Shakespeare Library, MS X.d.24.

Dacres, Mary. *Recipe Collection of Mary, Lady Dacres, for Cookery and Domestic Medicine*, 1666–1696. British Library, MS 56248.

Davies, Katherine. *Medicinal and Cookery Receipts*, seventeenth century. British Library, Egerton MS 2214.

Dawson, Jane. *Cookbook of Jane Dawson*, 1675. Folger Shakespeare Library, MS V.b.14.

Denbigh, Hester. *Cookery and Medical Receipts*, 1700. Whitney Cookery Collection. Manuscripts and Archives Division. New York Public Library, MssCol 3318, vol. 11.

Digby, Elizabeth. *Receipts Approved by Persons of Qualitie and Judgment*, 1650. British Library, Egerton MS 2197.

Doggett, Mary. *Recipe Book of Mary Doggett*, 1682. British Library, Add MS 27466.

Eyton, Amy, and others. *Collection of Cookery Receipts, with a Few Medical and Household Receipts*, 1691–1738. Wellcome Library, MS 2323.

Fanshawe, Ann. *Memoirs*, 1676. British Library, MS 41161.

———. *Mrs Fanshawes Booke of Receipts of Physickes*, 1651–1707. Wellcome Library, MS 7113.

Forster, Mary, and others. *Collection of Cookery Receipts, with Some Medical and a Few Household Receipts*, 1758. Wellcome Library, MS 2410.

Fowler, Elizabeth. *Elizabeth Fowler Her Book*, 1684. Folger Shakespeare Library, MS V.a.468.

Freke, Elizabeth. *Commonplace Book of Elizabeth Freke*, 1684–1714. British Library, Add MS 45718.

Fuller, Elizabeth. *Collection of Cookery and Medical Receipts*, 1712–1822. Wellcome Library, MS 2450.

Glyd, Ann. *Recipe-Book of Anne, Wife of Richard Glydd*. Brockman Papers vol. 129, British Library, Add MS 45196.
Godfrey, Elizabeth, and others. *Collection of Medical and Cookery Receipts*, 1686. Wellcome Library, MS 2535.
Goodenough, Ann. *Cookery Book of Ann Goodenough*, ca. 1700–ca. 1775. Folger Shakespeare Library, MS W.a.332.
Granville, Anne (Dewes). *Cookery and Medicinal Recipes of the Granville Family*, ca. 1640–ca. 1750. Folger Shakespeare Library, MS V.a.430.
Hadley, John. Owner, John Nott, *The Cook's and Confectioner's Dictionary*, London, 1733. Edition at the University of Iowa Library. TX705 .N68 1733.
Hall, Constance. *Receipt Book*, 1672. Folger Shakespeare Library, MS V.a.20.
Hartlib, Samuel. *A Complete Text and Image Database of the Papers of Samuel Hartlib*, ca. 1600–1662. Sheffield University Library. 2nd ed. Shelfmark Sheffield HRIOnline, Humanities Research Institute, 2002. Ref. 62/25/1A–4B.
Hirst, Elizabeth, and others. *Mrs. Elizabeth Hirst her book, A Collection of Medical and Cookery Receipts*, 1684–1725. Wellcome Library, MS 2840.
Hodges, Martha, and others. *Collection of Cookery Receipts by Martha Hodges, Robert Foster and Others*, 1675–1725. Wellcome Library, MS 2954.
Hookes, Mary. *Receipt Book of Mary Hookes*, ca. 1675–1725. Folger Shakespeare Library, MS V.b.342.
Hudson, Sarah. *"Her Book": A Collection of Cookery Receipts, with a Few Medical Receipts*, 1678. Wellcome Library, MS 2954.
Hughes, Sarah. *Mrs Hughes Her Receipts of Her Whole Booke*, 1637. Wellcome Library, MS 363.
Jackson, Jane. *A Very Shorte and Compendious Methode of Phisicke and Chirurgery*, 1642. Wellcome Library, MS 373.
Jephson, Penelope Patrick. *Receipt Book of Penelope Jephson*, 1671; 1674–75. Folger Shakespeare Library, MS V.a.396.
Juana, Sor. *A Sor Juana Anthology*, trans. Alan S. Trueblood. Cambridge, Mass.: Harvard University Press, 1988.
Johnson, Mrs. *Receipts for Cookery and Pastry Work*, 1700. Folger Shakespeare Library, MS W.a.311.
Kendall, Rose, and Anne Cater. *Cookery and Medicinal Recipes*, 1675–ca. 1750. Folger Shakespeare Library, MS V.a.429.
Knight, Mrs. *Mrs. Knight's Receipt Book*, 1740. Folger Shakespeare Library, MS W.b.79.
Lewis, Anthony. *Receipts in Cookery, Confectionery. Gardening, Medicine*, owned by the Lady Marquess Dorset, ca. 1606/7. British Library, Sloane MS 556.
Longe, Sarah. *Mrs. Sarah Longe Her Receipt Booke*, 1610. Folger Shakespeare Library, MS V.a.425.
Lovelace, Anne. *Recipes Medical and Culinary*. British Library, Add MS 34722.
Lowdham, Caleb, and Jane Lowdham, late seventeenth century to early eighteenth century. Wellcome Library, MS 7073.
Maddison Family Recipe Book, ca. 1600–1710. Esther Aresty Collection, Kislak Center for Special Collections, University of Pennsylvania Library, MS codex 252.
Michel, Elizabeth. *Her Book of Recepts*, mid-eighteenth century to 1801. Wellcome Library, MS 3539.
Miller, Mary. *Her Booke of Receipts*, 1660. Wellcome Library, MS 3547.
Morton, Lady. *The Lady Mortons Boke of Receipts*, . . . 1693. Whitney Cookery Collection. Manuscripts and Archives Division. New York Public Library, MssCol 3318, vol. 4.

Newton, Jane. *A Booke of Usefull Receipts for Cookery* . . . , ca. 1675–ca. 1700. Wellcome Library, MS 1325.
Okeover, Elizabeth. *Collection of Medical Receipts, with a Few Cookery Receipts*, ca. 1675–ca. 1725. Wellcome Library, MS 3712.
Oliver, Margaret. Owner of Sarah Harrison, *The House-keeper's Pocket-Book*, London, 1733. Inscribed edition in University of Iowa Library. TX705.H37 1748.
Packe, Susanna. *Her Book 1674*. Folger Shakespeare Library, MS V.a.215.
Packer, Katherine. *A Boocke of Very Good Medicines for Several Deseases, Wounds, and Sores Both New and Olde*, 1639. Folger Shakespeare Library, MS V.a.387.
Palmer, Archdale. *The Recipe Book, 1659–1672, of Archdale Palmer, Lord of the Manor of Wanlip*. Leicestershire: Sycamore Press, 1985.
Palmer, Katharine. *A Collection of ye Best Receipts*, 1700–1739. Wellcome Library, MS 7976.
Parker, Bridget. *Collection of Medical and Cookery Receipts*, ca. 1663. Wellcome Library, MS 3768.
Pearkes, Elizabeth. Owner, John Nott's recipe book, *The Cook's and Confectioner's Dictionary*, London, 1733. Inscribed edition in the University of Iowa Library. TX705.N68 1733.
Percy, Lady Anne. *Manuscript Cookery Book*, 1650. Whitney Cookery Collection. Manuscripts and Archives Division. New York Public Library, MssCol 3318, vol. 2.
Price, Rebecca. *The Compleat Cook; or, The Secrets of a Seventeenth-Century Housewife*, ed. and intro. Madeleine Masson. London: Routledge and Kegan Paul, 1974.
Pudsey, Lettice. *Lettice Pudsey Her Booke of Receipts*, ca. 1675. Folger Shakespeare Library, MS V.a.450.
Puleston, Mary. *Cookbook of Mary Puleston*, before 1764. Folger Shakespeare Library, MS W.b.102.
Randolph, Grace (Blome). *Cookbook*, 1697. Folger Shakespeare Library, MS V.b.301.
Sleigh, Elizabeth, and Felicia Whitfield. *Collection of Medical Receipts, with Some Cookery Receipts*, 1647–1722. Wellcome Library, MS 751.
Smith, Ann. *Cookbook of Ann Smith*, 1690. Folger Shakespeare Library, MS V.a.434.
Springatt, Frances, and others. *Collection of Cookery and Medical Receipts*, 1686–1824. Wellcome Library, MS 4683.
Stanhope, Philip. *A Booke of Severall Receipts for Severall Infirmities Both in Man and Woman*. Wellcome Library, MS 761.
Staveley, Jane. *Receipt Book*, 1693–94. Folger Shakespeare Library, MS V.a.401.
Stone, Dorothy. *Cookery book*, ca. 1725. Folger Shakespeare Library, MS W.a.315.
W., M. *Cookery and Medicinal Recipes*, ca. 1700–ca. 1850. Folger Shakespeare Library, MS V.b.316.
Whiteaker, Elizabeth. *Collection of Cookery Receipts*, ca. 1725. Wellcome Library, MS 4997.
Yate, Joane. *Receipt Book*, 1682. Whitney Cookery Collection. Manuscripts and Archives Division. New York Public Library, MssCol 3318, vol. 3.

Printed Works

Addison, Joseph. *Spectator*, no. 10 (1711).
———. *Tattler* 148 (Tuesday, March 21, 1709).
Anon. *A Closet for Ladies and Gentlewomen, or the Art of Preserving, Conserving, and Candying with the Manner Howe to Make Divers Kinds of Syrups: And All Kind of Banqueting Stuffes. Also Divers Soveraigne Medicines and Salues, for Sundry Diseases*. London, 1608.
Anon. [Attributed to Hannah Woolley.] *The Compleat Servant-Maid; or, The Young Maidens Tutor Directing Them How They May Fit, and Qualifie Themselves for Any of These Employ-*

ments . . . Composed for the Great Benefit and Advantage of All Young Maidens, 1677. Reprinted 1683.

Anon. *The Court & Kitchin of Elizabeth, Commonly Called Joan Cromwel[l] the Wife of the Late Usurper.* London, 1664.

Anon. *The Genteel House-keepers Pastime, or, The Mode of Carving at the Table Represented in a Pack of Playing Cards.* London, 1693.

Anon. [Attributed to Hannah Woolley.] *The Gentlewomans Companion; or, A Guide to the Female Sex Containing Directions of Behaviour, in All Places, Companies, Relations, and Conditions, from Their Childhood Down to Old Age: Viz. as, Children to Parents. Scholars to Governours . . . Whereunto Is Added, a Guide for Cook-maids, Dairy-maids, Chamber-maids, and All Others That Go to Service.* London, 1673.

Anon. *A Good Huswifes Handmaide for the Kitchin Containing Manie Principall Pointes of Cookerie, Aswell How to Dresse Meates, After Sundrie the Best Fashions Used in England and Other Countries. . . . Hereunto Are Annexed, Sundrie Necessarie Conceits for the Preservation of Health. Verie Meete to Be Adjoned to the Good Huswifes Closet of Provision for Her Houshold.* London, 1594.

Anon. [Attributed to M.B.] *The Ladies Cabinet Enlarged and Opened Wherein Is Found Hidden Severall Experiments in Preserving and Conserving, Physicke, and Surgery, Cookery and Huswifery.* London, 1654.

Anon. *The Ladies Companion, or, A Table Furnished with Sundry Sorts of Pies and Tarts, Gracefull at a Feast, with Many Excellent Receipts for Preserving, Conserving, and Candying of All Manner of Fruits. . . . By Persons of Quality Whose Names Are Mentioned.* London, 1653.

Anon. *A Propre New Booke of Cokery.* London, 1545.

Anon. *The Rare Triumphes of Love and Fortune Plaide Before the Queenes Most Excellent Maiestie: Wherin are manye fine conceites with great delight.* London, 1589.

Anon. *Town and Country Cook; or Young Woman's Best Guide.* London, 1780).

Bacon, Francis. *The Novum Organum.* London, 1676.

Beau Chesne, John de, and M. John Baildon. *A Book Containing Divers Sorts of Hands.* London, 1571.

Blague, Thomas. *A Schole of Wise Conceytes Wherein as Every Conceyte Hath Wit, So the Most Have Much Mirth . . . translated out of divers Greeke and Latine wryters.* London, 1572.

Bodenham, John. *Belvedere, or, the Garden of the Muses.* London, 1600.

Bradley, Martha. *The British Housewife: or, the Cook, Housekeeper's, and Gardiner's Companion.* London, 1760.

Brinsley, John. *Ludus Literarius, or the Grammar School.* London, 1627.

Brooks, Catharine. *The Complete English Cook.* London, 1767.

Brunschwig, Hieronymus. *The Vertuose Boke of Distyllacyon of the Waters of All Maner of Herbes.* London, 1527.

Burton, Robert. *The Anatomy of Melancholy.* Oxford, 1621.

———. *The Anatomy of Melancholy*, ed. A. R. Shilletto. 3 vols. London, 1893.

Carter, Charles. *The Compleat City and Country Cook: Or, Accomplish'd Housewife.* London, 1736.

———. *The Complete Practical Cook: or, A New System of the Whole Art and Mystery of Cookery.* London, 1730.

Carter, Susannah. *The Frugal Housewife, or Complete Woman Cook. Wherein the Art of Dressing All Sorts of Viands, with Cleanliness, Decency, and Elegance, Is Explained in Five Hundred Approved Receipts.* London, 1772.

Cartwright, Charlotte. *The Lady's Best Companion; or, Complete Treasure for the Fair Sex. Containing the Whole Arts of Cookery, Pastry, Confectionary, Potting, Pickling, Preserving, Candying, Collaring, Brewing, &c.* . . . Blackburn, 1799.

Cavendish, Margaret. *Poems, and Fancies Written by the Right Honourable, the Lady Margaret Newcastle.* London, 1653.

Ciotti, Giovanni. *A Booke of Curious and Strange Inventions.* London, 1596.

Comley, William. *A New Alphabet of the Capitall Romane Knotted Letters.* London, 1622.

Cook, Ann. *Professed Cookery: Containing Boiling, Roasting, Pastry, Preserving, Potting, Pickling, Made-Wines, Gellies, and Part of Confectionaries.* Newcastle, 1735.

Cooper, Joseph. *The Art of Cookery Refin'd and Augmented Containing an Abstract of Some Rare and Rich Unpublished Receipts of Cookery Collected from the Practise of That Incomparable Master of These Arts, Mr. Jos. Cooper, Chiefe Cook to the Late King.* London, 1654.

Coote, Edmund. *The English Schoole-Master.* London, 1627.

Crooke, Helkiah. *Microcosmographia.* London, 1615.

Crowley, Robert. *A Setting Open of the Subtyle Sophistrie of Thomas Watson Doctor of Divinitie.* London, 1569.

Crowne, John. *The Married Beau, or, The curious impertinent, a comedy, acted at the Theatre-Royal, by Their Majesties servants.* London, 1694.

Davies, John. *The Writing Schoolemaster.* London, 1631.

Dawson, Thomas. *A Booke of Cookerie and the Order of Meates to Bee Served to the Table, Both for Flesh and Fish Dayes, with Divers Approved Medicines for Grievous Diseases. With Certaine Points of Husbandry.* London, 1620.

———. *The Good Huswifes Jewell Wherein Is to Be Found Most Excellent and Rare Devises for Conceits in Cookerie . . . Whereunto Is Adjoyned Sundry Approved Reseits for Many Soveraine Oyles, and the Way to Distill Many Precious Waters, with Divers Approved Medicines for Many Diseases. Also Certaine Approved Points of Husbandry.* London, 1587.

———. *The Second Part of the Good Huswives Jewell Where Is to Be Found Most Apt and Readiest Wayes to Distill Many Wholsome and Sweet Waters. In Which Likewise Is Shewed the Best Maner in Preserving of Divers Sorts of Fruits, & Making of Sirrops with Divers Conceits in Cookerie with the Booke of Carving.* London, 1597.

de Acosta, José. *The Naturall and Morall Historie of the East and West Indies.* London, 1604.

de Bonnefons, Nicolas. *Les Délices de la Table.* Paris, 1662.

Dekker, Thomas. *Satiro-Mastix, Or, The untrussing.* London, 1602.

Des Périers, Bonaventure. *The Mirrour of Mirth and Pleasant Conceits Containing Many Proper and Pleasaunt Inventions, for the Recreation and Delight of Many.* London, 1583.

Digby, Kenelm. *The Closet of the Eminently Learned Sir Kenelme Digbie Kt. Opened . . . Published by His Son's Consent.* London, 1669.

Donne, John. *Juvenalia, or Certain Paradoxes and Problems.* London, 1633.

———. *The Sermons of John Donne*, ed. Evelyn M. Simpson and George R. Porter. 10 vols. Berkeley: University of California Press, 1954–1962.

———. "Upon Mr Thomas Coryat's Crudities." In *The Complete English Poems*, ed. A. J. Smith. London: Penguin, 1971.

Erasmus, *A Declamation on the Subject of Early Liberal Education for Children*, trans. Beert C. Verstraete, vol. 26, *The Collected Works of Erasmus*, ed. J. K. Soward. Literary and Educational Writings 4. Toronto: University of Toronto Press, 1985.

Farley, John. *The London Art of Cookery.* London, 1783.

Gascoigne, George. *The Steele Glas.* London, 1576.

Glasse, Hannah. *The Art of Cookery, Made Plain and Easy; Which Far Exceeds Any Thing of the Kind Ever Yet Published*. London, 1747. Initially attributed to "A Lady."
——. *The Art of Cookery, Made Plain and Easy*. London, 1775.
Greville, Fulke. *Certaine Learned and Elegant Workes of the Right Honorable Fulke Lord Brooke Written in His Youth*. London, 1633.
Grey, Elizabeth (Countess of Kent). *A Choice Manuall, or Rare and Select Secrets in Physick and Chyrurgery*. London, 1653. Reprinted London, 1661.
Guarini, Battista. *Il pastor fido, or The faithfull shepherd*. London, 1647.
Harrison, Sarah. *The House-Keeper's Pocket-Book, and Compleat Family Cook. Containing Above Three Hundred Curious and Uncommon Receipts in Cookery, Pastry, Preserving, Pickling, Candying, Collaring, &c. with Plain and Easy Instructions for Preparing and Dressing Every Thing Suitable for an Elegant Entertainment*. . . . London, 1733.
Harrison, William. *The Description of England: The Classic Contemporary Account of Tudor Social Life*, ed. Georges Edelen. New York: Dover, with the Folger Shakespeare Library, 1994.
Haywood, Eliza. *The Female Spectator*. London, 1748.
——. *A New Present for a Servant Maid*. London, 1771.
Henderson, William. *The Housekeeper's Instructor*. London, 1790.
Herbert, George. *The Temple*. London, 1633.
Hill, Thomas. *The Gardeners Labyrinth*. London, 1594.
Hitchcock, Robert. *The Quintesence of Wit Being a Corrant Comfort of Conceites, Maximes, and Poleticke Devises*. London, 1590.
Holland, Mary. *The Complete British Cook*. London, 1800.
Hyrde, Richard. Preface to *A Devout Treatise upon the Pater Noster* by Desiderius Erasmus. Trans. Margaret Roper. London, 1526.
Jonson, Benjamin. *Barthol[o]mew Fayre*. London, 1631.
——. *The Complete Poems*, ed. George Parfitt. London: Penguin, 1996.
——. *Neptune's Triumph for the Returne of Albion*. 1623. Reproduced in *Ben Jonson*, ed. C. H. Herford Percy and Evelyn Simpson. Oxford: Clarendon, 1941.
——. *The Workes of Benjamin Jonson*. London, 1616.
Kant, Immanuel. *Anthropology from a Pragmatic Point of View*, trans. Victor Lyle Dowd. Carbondale: Southern Illinois University Press, 1996.
King, William. *The Art of Cookery*. London, 1708.
Knevet, Ralph. *Rhodon and Iris*. London, 1631.
Lamb, Patrick. *Royal Cookery, or the Complete Court Cook*. London, 1710.
Lawson, Williams. *The Country Housewifes Garden for Hearbes of Common Vse, Their Vertues, Seasons, Profits, Ornaments, Varietie of Knots*. . . . London, 1618.
M., W. *The Queens Closet Opened: Incomparable Secrets in Physick, Chirurgery, Preserving, Candying, and Cookery; as They Were Presented to the Queen by the Most Experienced Persons of Our Times, Many Whereof They Were Honoured with Her Own Practice, When She Pleased to Descend to These More Private Recreations . . .* , by W.M. One of Her Late Servants. London, 1655.
——. *The Queens Closet Opened*. London, 1671.
——. *The Queens Delight, or the Art of Preserving, Conserving, and Candying*. Cornhill, 1654. Appended to *The Queens Closet Opened*. London, 1655.
Markham, Gervase. *Countrey Contentments, or The English Huswife: Containing the Inward and Outward Vertues Which Ought to Be in a Compleate Woman: As Her Skill in Physicke, Surgerie, Extraction of Oyles . . . Brewing, Baking, and all Other Things Belonging to an Houshold. Cookery*. London, 1623. First published 1615. Reprinted as *The English House-Wife*, with

variously spelled titles in 1631, 1637, 1649, 1653, 1660, 1664, and 1683. Reprinted as part of *The Way to Get Wealth* in 1625, 1631, 1633, 1638, 1648, 1653, 1657, 1660, 1668, 1683 and 1695.

Martino, Maestro. *The Art of Cookery: The First Modern Cookery Book*, ed. Luigi Ballerini. Berkeley: University of California Press, 2005.

May, Robert. *The Accomplisht Cook, or, The Art and Mystery of Cookery*. London, 1660.

Mayerne, Theodore. *Archimagirus anglo-gallicus; or, Excellent & Approved Receipts and Experiments in cookery*. London, 1658.

Mayne, Jasper. *The Citye Match*. London, 1639.

Middleton, Thomas. *A Trick to Catch the Old-One*. London, 1608.

Middleton, Thomas, and William Rowley. *The Changeling*. London, 1653.

Milton, John. *Paradise Lost*, in *John Milton: Complete Poems and Major Prose*, ed. Merritt Y. Hughes. Indianapolis: Odyssey Press, 1957.

Moxon, Elizabeth. *English Housewifery. Exemplified in Above Four Hundred and Fifty Receipts*. Leeds, 1749.

Munday, Anthony. *A Banquet of Daintie Conceits Furnished with Verie Delicate and Choyse Inventions, to Delight Their Mindes, Who Take Pleasure in Musique, and There-Withall to Sing Sweete Ditties*. London, 1588.

Murrell, John. *A Daily Exercise for Ladies and Gentlewomen Whereby They May Learne and Practice the Whole Art of Making Pastes, Preserves, Marmalades, Conserves, Tartstuffes, Gellies, Breads, Sucket Candies, Cordiall Waters, Conceits in Sugar-Workes of Severall Kindes... Used Both by Honourable and Worshipfull Personages. By John Murrell, Professour Thereof*. London, 1617.

———. *A Delightful Daily Exercise*. London, 1617.

———. *A Delightfull Daily Exercise for Ladies and Gentlewomen*. London, 1621.

———. *Murrels Two Bookes of Cookerie and Carving*. London, 1631.

———. *A New Booke of Cookerie Wherein Is Set Forth the Newest and Most Commendable Fashion for Dressing or Sowcing, Eyther Flesh, Fish, or Fowle. Together with Making of All Forts of Jellyes, and Other Made-dishes for Service; Both to Beautifie and Adorne Eyther Nobleman or Gentlemans Table*. London, 1615.

Nashe, Thomas. *Quaternio, or A fourefold way to a happie life set forth in a dialogue betweene a countryman and a citizen*. London, 1633.

Nott, John. *The Cook's and Confectioner's Dictionary: or the Accomplish'd Housewife's Companion... Revised and Recommended by John Nott, Cook to His Grace the Duke of Bolton*. London, 1723.

Ovid. *Metamorphoses*, trans. Arthur Golding, ed. John Frederick Nims. Philadelphia: P. Dry, 2000.

Painter, William. *The Palace of Pleasure*, ed. Joseph Jacobs. London, 1890.

Palmer, Archdale. *The Recipe Book, 1659–1672, of Archdale Palmer, Gent.*, ed. Grant Uden. Wymondham: Sycamore, 1985.

Partridge, John. *The Treasurie of Commodious Conceits & Hidden Secrets and May Be Called, the Huswives Closet, of Healthfull Provision*. London, 1573.

———. *The Treasurie of Commodious Conceites, and Hidden Secrets: Commonly called, The good huswives closet of provision, for the health of her houshold*. London, 1584.

———. *The Widdowes Treasure Plentifully Furnished with Sundry Precious and Approved Secrets in Phisicke and Chirurgery, for the Health and Pleasure of Mankinde*. London, 1588.

Peckham, Ann. *The Complete English Cook, or Prudent Housewife*. London, 1771.

Phiston, William. *The Welspring of Wittie Conceites Containing, a Methode, Aswell to Speake, as to Endight (Aptly and Eloquently of Sundrie Matters: as (also) . . . great varietie of pithy sentences, vertuous sayings, and right morall instructions.* London, 1584.

Plat, Hugh. *Delightes for Ladies.* London, 1602.

———. *The Jewel House of Art and Nature.* London, 1594; reprinted 1653.

Plato. *The Dialogues of Plato*, ed. and trans. Benjamin Jowett. 5 vols. Oxford: Clarendon, 1892.

Puttenham, George. *The Arte of English Poesie*, ed. Frank Whigham and Wayne A. Rebhorn. Ithaca, N.Y.: Cornell University Press, 2007.

Quarles, Francis. *King Solomon's Recantations.* London, 1688.

Rabisha, William. *The Whole Body of Cookery Dissected, Taught and Fully Manifested, Methodically, Artificially and According to the Best Tradition o[f] the English, French, Italian, Dutch, &c.* London, 1661.

Raffald, Elizabeth. *The Experienced English House-Keeper, for the Use and Ease of Ladies, House-Keepers, Cooks, &c. Wrote Purely from Practice.* Manchester, 1769. Reprinted 1784.

Rainbowe, Edward. *A Sermon Preached at the Funeral of the Right Honorable Anne Countess of Pembroke.* London, 1677.

Rose, Giles. *A Perfect School of Instructions for the Officers of the Mouth Shewing the Whole Art of a Master of the Household . . . by Giles Rose, One of the Master Cooks in His Majesties Kitchen.* London, 1682.

Shackleford, Ann. *The Modern Art of Cookery Improved; or, Elegant, Cheap, and Easy Methods, of Preparing Most of the Dishes Now in Vogue.* London, 1767.

Shakespeare, William. *The Norton Shakespeare*, ed. Stephen Greenblatt et al. New York: W. W. Norton, 1997.

———. *The Riverside Shakespeare.* Boston: Houghton Mifflin, 1974.

Shenstone, William. *The Works in Verse and Prose, of William Shenstone.* Dublin, 1764.

Shirley, John. *The Accomplished Ladies Rich Closet of Rarities: Or, The Ingenious Gentlewoman and Servant-maids Delightfull Companion.* London, 1687.

Sidney, Philip. *An Apologie for Poetrie.* London, 1595.

———. *Sir Philip Sidney: The Major Works*, ed. Katherine Duncan-Jones. Oxford: Oxford University Press, 2002.

Smith, E[liza]. *The Compleat Housewife: Or, Accomplished Gentlewoman's Companion: Being a Collection of Upwards of Five Hundred of the Most Approved Receipts in Cookery, Pastry, Confectionary, Preserving, Pickles, Cakes, Creams, Jellies, Made Wines, Cordials.* London, 1736.

Smith, Robert. *Court Cookery, or the Complete English Cook.* London, 1723.

Spenser, Edmund. *Edmund Spenser's Poetry*, ed. Hugh Maclean and Anne Lake Prescott. 3rd ed. New York: W. W. Norton, 1993.

Sprat, Thomas. *History of the Royal Society.* 4th ed. London, 1734.

Stubbes, Philip. *The Anatomie of Abuses*, ed. Margaret Jane Kidnie. Tempe: Arizona Center for Medieval and Renaissance Studies, in conjunction with Renaissance English Text Society, 2002.

Talbot, Aletheia. *Natura Exenterata . . . Where are contained, Her choicest Secrets digested into Receipts.* London, 1655.

Thacker, John. *The Art of Cookery.* London, 1758.

Turner, William. *The Seconde Part of William Turners Herball.* London, 1562.

Tusser, Thomas. *Five Hundred Points of Good Husbandry.* London, 1638.

Vaughan, Thomas. *Magia Adamica; or the Antiquitie of Magic, and the Descent thereof from Adam downwards, proved.* London, 1650.

Vives, Juan. *The Instruction of a Christian Woman*, trans. Richard Hyrde. London, 1529.
Voltaire, *The Philosophical Dictionary*, trans. Tobias Smollett. In *The Works of Voltaire*, 13:44–58. Paris: E. R. Du Mont, 1901.
W., A. *A Book of Cookrye; Very Necessary for All Such as Delight Therein*. London, 1587.
White, John. *A Rich Cabinet, with Variety of Inventions; unlock'd and opened, for the recreation of ingenious spirits at their vacant houres Being receits and conceits of severall natures, and fit for those who are lovers of naturall and artificiall conclusions*. London, 1651.
W[hitney], Is[abella]. *A Sweet Nosgay or Pleasant Posye*. London, 1573.
Woolley, Hannah. *An Accomplish'd Ladies Delight in Preserving, Physick, Beautifying, and Cookery, Containing I. the art of preserving and candying fruits & flowers . . . , II. the physical cabinet, or, excellent receipts in physick and chirurgery . . . 3. the compleat cooks guide*. London, 1675.
———. *The Ladies Delight: Or, A Rich Closet of Choice Experiments & Curiosities*. London, 1672.
———. *The Ladies Directory in Choice Experiments & Curiosities of Preserving in Jellies, and Candying Both Fruits & Flowers*. London, 1662.
———. *The Queen-Like Closet; or, Rich Cabinet Stored with All Manner of Rare Receipts for Preserving, Candying & Cookery. Very Pleasant and Beneficial to All Ingenious Persons of the Female Sex*. London, 1675.
———. *A Supplement to the Queen-Like Closet, or, a Little of Every Thing Presented to All Ingenious Ladies, and Gentlewomen*. London, 1674.

Works After 1800

Albala, Ken. *The Banquet: Dining in the Great Courts of Late Renaissance Europe*. Champaign: University of Illinois Press, 2007.
———. *Eating Right in the Renaissance*. Berkeley: University of California Press, 2002.
Altman, Joel B. Review of *Writing Matter*. *Shakespeare Quarterly* 43:1 (1992): 92–97.
Appelbaum, Robert. *Aguecheek's Beef, Belch's Hiccup, and Other Gastronomic Interjections*. Chicago: University of Chicago Press, 2006.
Archer, Jayne Elisabeth. "The 'Quintessence of Wit': Poems and Recipes in Early Modern Women's Writing." In *Reading and Writing Recipe Books, 1550–1800*, ed. Michelle DiMeo and Sara Pennell, 114–34. Manchester: Manchester University Press, 2013.
———. "Women and Alchemy in Early Modern England." Ph.D. diss., University of Cambridge, 2000.
Aspin, Richard. "Who Was Elizabeth Okeover?" *Medical History* 44 (2000): 531–40.
Atkinson, Dwight. "Philosophical Transactions of the Royal Society of London, 1675–1975: A Sociohistorical Discourse Analysis." *Language in Society* 25:3 (September 1996): 333–71.
Barker, Nicolas, intro. and ed. *The Great Book of Thomas Trevillian: A Facsimile of the Manuscript in the Wormsley Library*. London: Roxburghe Club, 2000.
Barnaby, Andrew, and Lisa Schnell. *Literate Experience: The Work of Knowing in Seventeenth-Century English Writing*. London: Palgrave, 2002.
Baron, Sabrina Alcorn, ed. *The Reader Revealed*. Seattle: University of Washington Press; Washington, D.C.: Folger Shakespeare Library, 2001.
Barthes, Roland. *Mythologies*, trans. Richard Howard. New York: Hill and Wang, 1972.
Beier, Lucinda McCray. *Sufferers and Healers: The Experience of Illness in Seventeenth-Century England*. London: Routledge and Kegan Paul, 1987.

Bono, James. *The Word of God and the Languages of Man: Interpreting Nature in Early Modern Science and Medicine*. Madison: University of Wisconsin Press, 1995.

Bourdieu, Pierre. *Distinction: A Social Critique of the Judgment of Taste*, trans. Richard Nice. Cambridge, Mass.: Harvard University Press, 1984.

Braudel, Fernand. *Structures of Everyday Life*, trans. Sian Reynolds, vol. 3 of *Civilization and Capitalism, 15th–18th Century*. 3 vols. New York: Harper and Row, 1981.

Brunskill, Elizabeth. "Medieval Book of Herbs and Medicines" *Northwestern Naturalist*, n.s., 1 (1953–54): 181–86.

Bull, John, trans. *The Laughing Philosopher*. London: Sherwood and Jones, 1825.

Burke, Victoria and Jonathan Gibson, eds. *Early Modern Women's Manuscript Writing: Selected Papers from the Trinity/Trent Colloquium*. Burlington, Vt.: Ashgate, 2004.

Bushnell, Rebecca. *Green Desire: Imagining Early Modern English Gardens*. Ithaca, N.Y.: Cornell University Press, 2003.

Butterworth, Phillip. *Magic on the Early English Stage*. Cambridge: Cambridge University Press, 2005.

Cahn, Susan. *Industry of Devotion: The Transformation of Women's Work in England, 1500–1650*. New York: Columbia University Press, 1987.

Calabresi, Bianca F. C. "'You Sow, Ile Read': Letters and Literacies in Early Modern Samplers." In *Reading Women: Literacy, Authorship and Culture in the Atlantic World, 1500–1800*, ed. Heidi Brayman Hackel and Catherine E. Kelly, 79–104. Philadelphia: University of Pennsylvania Press, 2008.

Calendar of Treasury Books, ed. William A. Shaw, vol. 7, 1681–1685 (1916), 1480–89. British History Online. http://www.british-history.ac.uk/report.aspx?compid=83942.

Camporesi, Pierre. *Bread of Dreams: Food and Fantasy in Early Modern Europe*, trans. David Gentilcore. Chicago: University of Chicago Press, 1989.

Chartier, Roger. *The Order of Books: Readers, Authors, and Libraries in Europe Between the Fourteenth and Eighteenth Centuries*, trans. Lydia G. Cochrane. Stanford, Calif.: Stanford University Press 1994.

Child, Lydia Maria. *The American Frugal Housewife*. 8th ed. Boston: Carter and Hendee, 1832.

Clark, Alice. *Working Life of Women in the Seventeenth Century*. 1919. London: Routledge and Kegan Paul, 1982.

Conrad, Joseph. Preface to *A Handbook of Cookery for a Small House*, by Jessie Conrad. New York: Doubleday, 1923.

Cormack, Bradin, and Carla Mazzio, eds. *Book Use, Book Theory: 1500–1700*. Chicago: University of Chicago Library, 2005.

Crain, Patricia. *The Story of A: The Alphabetization of America from "The New England Primer" to "The Scarlet Letter."* Stanford, Calif.: Stanford University Press, 2000.

Cressy, David. *Literacy and the Social Order: Reading and Writing in Tudor and Stuart England*. Cambridge: Cambridge University Press, 1980.

Daston, Lorraine. "The Factual Sensibility." *Isis* 79 (1988): 452–67.

Day, Ivan. "From Murrell to Jarrin: Illustrations in British Cookery Books 1621–1820." In *The English Cookery Book: Historical Essays*, ed. Ellen White, 98–150. Totnes: Prospect, 2004.

Daybell, James. *Women Letter-Writers in Tudor England*. Oxford: Oxford University Press, 2006.

Daybell, James, and Peter Hinds, eds. *Material Readings of Early Modern Culture: Texts and Social Practices, 1580–1730*. New York: Palgrave Macmillan, 2010.

Dear, Peter. "Miracles, Experiments and the Ordinary Course of Nature." *Isis* 81:4 (1990): 663–83.

———. *Revolutionizing the Sciences: European Knowledge and Its Ambitions, 1500–1700.* Princeton, N.J.: Princeton University Press, 2001.

———. "Totius in Verba: Rhetoric and Authority in the Early Royal Society." *Isis* 76:2 (1985): 154–61.

De Silva, Cara, ed. *In Memory's Kitchen: A Legacy from the Women of Terezin,* trans. Bianca Steiner Brown. Northvale, N.J.: Jason Aronson, 1996.

DiMeo, Michelle. "Authorship and Medical Networks: Reading Attributions in Early Modern Manuscript Recipes." In *Reading and Writing Recipes Books, 1550–1800,* ed. Michelle DiMeo and Sara Pennell, 25–46. Manchester: Manchester University Press, 2013.

———. "Katherine Jones, Lady Ranelagh (1615–91): Science and Medicine in a Seventeenth-Century Englishwoman's Writing." Ph.D. diss., University of Warwick, 2009.

DiMeo, Michelle, and Sara Pennell, ed. *Reading and Writing Recipe Books, 1550–1800.* Manchester: Manchester University Press, 2013.

Disraeli, Isaac. *Curiosities of Literature.* 4 vols. Boston: William Veazie, 1858.

Dolan, Frances. "Gender and the 'Lost' Spaces of Catholicism." *Journal of Interdisciplinary History* 32:4 (2002): 641–65.

———. "Reading, Writing, and Other Crimes." In *Feminist Readings of Early Modern Culture: Emerging Subjects,* ed. Valerie Traub, M. Lindsay Kaplan, and Dympna Callaghan, 142–67. Cambridge: Cambridge University Press, 1996.

———. "Taking the Pencil out of God's Hand: Art, Nature and the Face-Painting Debate in Early Modern England." *PMLA* 108:2 (1993): 224–39.

———. *True Relations Reading, Literature, and Evidence in Seventeenth-Century England.* Philadelphia: University of Pennsylvania Press, 2013.

Donaldson, Ian. "Destruction of the Book." *Book History* 1 (1998): 1–10.

Dowd, Michelle M. and and Julie A. Eckerle, eds. *Genre and Women's Life Writing in Early Modern England.* Aldershot, U.K.: Ashgate, 2007.

Eamon, William. *Science and the Secrets of Nature: Books of Secrets in Medieval and Early Modern Culture.* Princeton, N.J.: Princeton University Press, 1994.

Elias, Norbert. *The Civilizing Process,* trans. Edmund Jephcott. 2 vols. Oxford: B. Blackwell, 1978.

Erickson, Amy. *Women and Property in Early Modern England.* London: Routledge, 1993.

Ezell, Margaret J. M. "Cooking the Books; or, The Three Faces of Hannah Woolley." In *Reading and Writing Recipe Books, 1550–1800,* ed. Michelle DiMeo and Sara Pennell, 159–78. Manchester: Manchester University Press, 2013.

———. "Domestic Papers: Manuscript Culture and Early Modern Women's Life Writing." In *Genre and Women's Life Writing in Early Modern England,* ed. Michelle M. Dowd and Julie A. Eckerle, 33–48. Aldershot, U.K.: Ashgate, 2007.

———. "The Laughing Tortoise: Speculations on Manuscript Sources and Women's Book History." *English Literary Renaissance* 38:2 (2008): 331–55.

———. *The Patriarch's Wife: Literary Evidence and the History of the Family.* Chapel Hill: University of North Carolina Press, 1987.

———. *Social Authorship and the Advent of Print.* Baltimore: University of Maryland Press, 1999.

Ferguson, Margaret. *Dido's Daughters: Literacy, Gender, and Empire in Early Modern England and France.* Chicago: University of Chicago Press, 2003.

Ferguson, Priscilla. *Accounting for Taste: The Triumph of French Cuisine.* Chicago: University of Chicago Press, 2004.

Field, Catherine. "'Many Hands Hands': Writing the Self in Early Modern Women's Recipe Books." In *Genre and Women's Life Writing in Early Modern England,* ed. Michelle M. Dowd and Julie A. Eckerle, 49–63. Aldershot, U.K.: Ashgate, 2007.

———. "'Sweet Practicer, Thy Physic I Will Try': Helena and Her 'Good Receipt' in *All's Well, That Ends Well*." In *All's Well That Ends Well: New Critical Essays*, ed. Gary Waller, 194–208. New York: Routledge, 2007.
Findlen, Paula. *Possessing Nature: Museums, Collecting, and Scientific Culture in Early Modern Italy*. Berkeley: University of California Press, 1994.
Fitzpatrick, Joan, ed. *Food in Shakespeare: Early Modern Dietaries and the Plays*. Aldershot, U.K.: Ashgate, 2007.
———. *Renaissance Food from Rabelais to Shakespeare*. Aldershot, U.K.: Ashgate, 2010.
Flandrin, Jean-Louis. "From Dietetics to Gastronomy: The Liberation of the Gourmet." In *Food: A Cultural History from Antiquity to the Present*, ed. Jean-Louis Flandrin, Massimo Montanari, Albert Sonnenfeld, 418–32. New York: Columbia University Press, 1999.
———. "Seasoning, Cooking and Dietetics in the Late Middle Ages." In *Food: A Cultural History from Antiquity to the Present*, ed. Jean-Louis Flandrin, Massimo Montanari, Albert Sonnenfeld, 313–27. New York: Columbia University Press, 1999.
Fleming, Juliet. *Graffiti and the Writing Arts of Early Modern England*. Philadelphia: University of Pennsylvania Press, 2001.
Floyd-Wilson, Mary. *Occult Knowledge, Science, and Gender on the Shakespearean Stage*. Cambridge: Cambridge University Press, 2013.
Food Porn website. http://foodporndaily.com.
Foucault, Michel. "What Is an Author?" In *Language, Counter-Memory, Practice*, ed. Donald F. Bouchard, trans. Donald F. Bouchard and Sherry Simon, 113–38. Ithaca, N.Y.: Cornell University Press, 1977.
Freedman, Paul. "Spices in the Middle Ages." *History Compass* 2:1 (2004): 1–5.
Freemon, Bobby. *First Catch Your Peacock: The Classic Guide to Welsh Food*. 1980. Talybont, Ceredigion, Wales: Y Lofla Cyf, 1996.
Friedman, Alice. *House and Household in Elizabethan England*. Chicago: University of Chicago Press, 1989.
Frye, Susan. *Pens and Needles: Women's Textualities in Early Modern England*. Philadelphia: University of Pennsylvania Press, 2010.
Fumerton, Patricia. *Cultural Aesthetics: Renaissance Literature and the Practice of Social Ornament*. Chicago: University of Chicago Press, 1991.
Gigante, Denise. *Taste: A Literary History*. New Haven, Conn.: Yale University Press, 2005.
Girouard, Mark. *Life in the English Country House: A Social and Architectural History*. New Haven, Conn.: Yale University Press, 1978.
Goldberg, Jonathan. *Writing Matter: From the Hands of the English Renaissance*. Stanford, Calif.: Stanford University Press, 1990.
Goldstein, David. *Eating and Ethics in Shakespeare's England*. Cambridge: Cambridge University Press, 2013.
———. "Recipes for Authorship: Indigestion and the Making of Originality in Early Modern England." Ph.D. diss., Stanford University, 2004.
———. "Woolley's Mouse: Early Modern Recipe Books and the Uses of Nature." In *Ecofeminist Approaches to Early Modernity*, ed. Jennifer Munroe and Rebecca Laroche, 105–28. New York: Palgrave Macmillan, 2011.
Goody, Jack. "The Recipe, the Prescription and the Experiment." In *The Domestication of the Savage Mind*. 129–45. Cambridge: Cambridge University Press, 1977.
Gopnik, Adam. "What's the Recipe? Our Hunger for Cookbooks." *New Yorker*, November 23, 2009. http://www.newyorker.com/magazine/2009/11/23/whats-the-recipe.

Gordon, George, Lord Byron. *Don Juan*, ed. Leslie Marchand. Boston: Houghton Mifflin, 1958.
Granville, Mary. *The Autobiography and Correspondence of Mary Granville, Mrs. Delany*, 2nd ser., 3 vols., ed. the Right Honorable Lady Llanover. London, 1862.
Gray, Annie. "'A Practical Art': An Archeological Perspective on the Use of Recipe Books." In *Reading and Writing Recipe Books, 1550–1800*, ed. Michelle DiMeo and Sara Pennell, 47–67. Manchester: Manchester University Press, 2013.
Guthrie, Leonard. "The Lady Sedley's Receipt Book, 1686, and other Seventeenth Century Receipt Books." *Proceedings of the Royal Society of Medicine* 6 (1913): 150–70.
Hackel, Heidi Brayman. *Reading Material in Early Modern England: Print, Gender, Literacy*. Cambridge: Cambridge University Press, 2005.
Hall, Augusta Waddington (Lady Llanover), *Good Cookery Illustrated. And recipes communicated by the Welsh hermit of the cell of St. Gover, with various remarks on many things past and present*. London: R. Bentley, 1867.
Hall, Kim F. "Culinary Spaces, Colonial Spaces: The Gendering of Sugar in the Seventeenth Century." In *Feminist Readings of Early Modern Culture: Emerging Subjects*, ed. Valerie Traub, Lindsay Kaplan, and Dympna Callaghan, 168–90. Cambridge: Cambridge University Press, 1996.
Halpern, Richard. "Shakespeare's Perfume." *Early Modern Culture: An Electronic Seminar*, 2 (2001): 8. http://emc.eserver.org/1-2/halpern.html.
Hammons, Pamela. *Gender, Sexuality, and Material Objects in English Renaissance Verse*. Burlington, Vt.: Ashgate, 2010.
Harkness, Deborah. *The Jewel House: Elizabethan London and the Scientific Revolution*. New Haven, Conn.: Yale University Press, 2007.
Harris, Frances. "Living in the Neighbourhood of Science: Mary Evelyn, Margaret Cavendish and the Greshamites." In *Women, Science and Medicine*, ed. Lynette Hunter and Sarah Hutton, 198–217. Stroud, Gloucestershire: Sutton, 1997.
Harrison, Peter. "Was There a Scientific Revolution?" *European Review* 15:4 (2007), 445–57.
Heldke, Lisa. "Foodmaking as Thoughtful Practice." In *Cooking, Eating, Thinking*, ed. Deane Curtin and Lisa Heldke, 203–29. Indianapolis: Indiana University Press, 1992.
Hobby, Elaine. *Virtue of Necessity: English Women's Writing, 1649–1688*. Ann Arbor: University of Michigan Press, 1989.
Hoby, Margaret. *The Private Life of an Elizabethan Lady*, ed. Joanna Moody. Phoenix Mill: Sutton, 1998.
Hodnett, Edward. *Five Centuries of Book Illustration*. Aldershot, U.K.: Scolar, 1988.
Hull, Suzanne. *Chaste, Silent and Obedient: English Books for Women, 1475–1640*. San Marino, Calif.: Huntington Library, 1982.
Hunter, Lynette. "Sisters of the Royal Society: The Circle of Katherine Jones, Lady Ranelagh." In *Women, Science and Medicine 1500–1700: Mothers and Sisters of the Royal Society*, ed. Lynette Hunter and Sarah Hutton, 178–97. Thrupp, Stroud, Gloucestershire: Sutton, 1997.
———. "Women and Domestic Medicine: Lady Experimenters, 1570–1620." In *Women, Science and Medicine 1500–1700: Mothers and Sisters of the Royal Society*, ed. Lynette Hunter and Sarah Hutton, 89–107. Stroud, Gloucestershire: Sutton, 1997.
Johns, Adrian. "Ink." In *Materials and Expertise in Early Modern Europe*, ed. Ursula Klein and E. C. Spary, 101–124. Chicago: University of Chicago Press, 2010.
Jones, Ann Rosalind, and Peter Stallybrass. *Renaissance Clothing and the Materials of Memory*. Cambridge: Cambridge University Press, 2000.

Jones, Caroline, and F. David Hoeniger, eds. *Picturing Science, Producing Art*. New York: Routledge, 1998.
Jones, Claire. "Formula and Formulation: Efficacy Phrases in Medieval English Medical Manuscripts." *Neuphilologische Mitteilungen* 99:2 (1998): 199–209.
Kavey, Allison. *Books of Secrets: Natural Philosophy in England, 1550–1600*. Urbana: University of Illinois Press, 2007.
Keller, Evelyn Fox. *Reflections on Gender and Science*. New Haven, Conn.: Yale University Press, 1985.
Kelly, Catherine E. "Reading and the Problem of Accomplishment." In *Reading Women: Literacy, Authorship and Culture in the Atlantic World, 1500–1800*, ed. Heidi Brayman Hackel and Catherine E. Kelly, 124–43. Philadelphia: University of Pennsylvania Press, 2009.
Knight, Leah. *Of Books and Botany in Early Modern England: Sixteenth-Century Plants and Print Culture*. Burlington, Vt.: Ashgate, 2009.
Knoppers, Laura. *Politicizing Domesticity from Henrietta Maria to Milton's Eve*. Cambridge: Cambridge University Press, 2011.
Korda, Natasha. *Shakespeare's Domestic Economies: Gender and Property in Early Modern England*. Philadelphia: University of Pennsylvania Press, 2002.
Kowalchuk, Kristine. "Recipes for Life: Seventeenth-Century Englishwomen's Household Manuals." Ph.D. diss., University of Alberta, 2012.
Laroche, Rebecca. "Beyond Home Remedy: Women, Medicine, and Science." Exhibition at the Folger Shakespeare Library, January–May, 2011.
———. *Medical Authority and Englishwomen's Herbal Texts, 1550–1650*. Farnham, U.K.: Ashgate, 2009.
Lehmann, Gilly. *The British Housewife: Cookery Books, Cooking and Society in Eighteenth-Century Britain*. Blackawton, Totnes, Devon: Prospect, 2003.
Leonardi, Susan. "Recipes for Reading: Summer Pasta, Lobster la Riseholme, and Key Lime Pie." *PMLA* 104 (1989): 340–47.
Leong, Elaine. "Medical Recipe Collections in Seventeenth-Century England: Knowledge, Text, and Gender." Ph.D. diss., Oxford University, 2005.
Lévi-Strauss, Claude. *The Raw and the Cooked*, trans. John and Doreen Weightman. New York: Harper and Row, 1969.
Llanover, Lady. *Good Cookery Illustrated: And Recipes Communicated by the Welsh Hermit of the Cell of St. Gover*. London, 1867.
Loewenstein, Joseph. "The Jonsonian Corpulence, or The Poet as Mouthpiece." *ELH* 53 (1986): 491–518.
Lupton, Julia. "Room for Dessert: Sugared Shakespeare and the Dramaturgy of Dwelling." In *Culinary Shakespeare*, ed. David Goldstein and Amy Tigner. Pittsburgh: Duquesne University Press, forthcoming.
Marchitello, Howard. *Machine in the Text: Science and Literature in the Age of Shakespeare and Galileo*. New York: Oxford University Press, 2011.
Masten, Jeffrey. *Queer Philologies: Sex, Language and Affect in Shakespeare's Time*. Philadelphia: University of Pennsylvania Press, forthcoming.
Mazzola, Elizabeth. *Learning and Literacy in Female Hands, 1520–1698*. Farnham, U.K.: Ashgate, 2013.
McBride, Ann E. "Food Porn." Forum. *Gastronomica* 10:1 (2010): 38–46.
McGovern, Barbara. *Anne Finch and Her Poetry: A Critical Biography*. Athens: University of Georgia Press, 1992.

McJannet, Linda. "'And Ginger Shall Be Hot i' th' Mouth Too': Eastern Spices in London Comedies." Unpublished paper. Presented at the International Shakespeare Association. Prague, 2011.

McKeon, Michael. *The Secret History of Domesticity: Public, Private, and the Division of Knowledge*. Baltimore: Johns Hopkins University Press, 2006.

Mennell, Stephen. *All Manners of Food: Eating and Taste in England and France from the Middle Ages to the Present*. Urbana: University of Illinois Press, 1996.

Merchant, Carolyn. *The Death of Nature*. San Francisco: Harper and Row, 1980.

Mintz, Sidney. *Sweetness and Power: The Place of Sugar in Modern History*. New York: Penguin, 1986.

Moorat, S. A. J. *Catalogue of Western Manuscripts on Medicine and Science in the Wellcome Historical Medical Library*. London: Wellcome Institute for the History of Medicine, 1962–1973.

Moore, George. "Eve's Food Preparation: Art and Experience in Eden." http://www.southernct.edu/organizations/hcr/2004/nonfiction/eve.htm.

Morton, Timothy. *The Poetics of Spice: Romantic Consumerism and the Exotic*. Cambridge: Cambridge University Press, 2000.

Mueller, Sara. "Early Modern Banquet Receipts and Women's Theatre." *Medieval and Renaissance Drama in England* 24 (2011): 106–30.

Munroe, Jennifer. *Gender and the Garden in Early Modern English Literature*. Burlington, Vt.: Ashgate, 2008.

Nagy, Doreen. *Popular Medicine in Seventeenth-Century England*. Bowling Green, Ohio: Bowling Green State University Popular Press, 1988.

Oates, Joyce Carol. "Food Mysteries." 1993. In *Not for Bread Alone: Writers on Food, Wine, and the Art of Eating*, ed. Daniel Halpern, 25–37. New York: Harper Perennial, 2008.

Orgel, Stephen. "Marginal Maternity: Reading Lady Anne Clifford's *A Mirror for Magistrates*." In *Printing and Parenting in Early Modern England*, ed. Douglas Brooks, 267–89. Aldershot, U.K.: Ashgate, 2004.

Orlin, Lena Cowen. "Gertrude's Closet." *Shakespeare Jahrbuch* 134 (1998): 44–67.

———. *Private Matters and Public Culture in Post-Reformation England*. Ithaca, N.Y.: Cornell University Press, 1994.

Paster, Gail Kern. *Humoring the Body: Emotions and the Shakespearean Stage*. Chicago: University of Chicago Press, 2004.

Payne, Lynda. *With Words and Knives: Learning Medical Dispassion in Early Modern England*. Aldershot, U.K.: Ashgate, 2007.

Pelling, Margaret, with Frances White. *Medical Conflicts in Early Modern London: Patronage, Physicians, and Irregular Practitioners, 1550–1640*. Oxford: Clarendon, 2003.

Pennell, Sara. "Making Livings, Lives and Archives: Tales of Four Eighteenth-Century Recipe Books." In *Reading and Writing Recipe Books, 1550–1800*, ed. Michelle DiMeo and Sara Pennell, 225–46. Manchester: Manchester University Press, 2013.

———. "Perfecting Practice? Women, Manuscript Recipes and Knowledge in Early Modern England." In *Early Modern Women's Manuscript Writing: Selected Papers from the Trinity/Trent Colloquium*, ed. Victoria Burke and Jonathan Gibson, 237–58. Burlington, Vt.: Ashgate, 2004.

Pennell, Sara, and Michelle DiMeo. Introduction, *Reading and Writing Recipe Books, 1550–1800*, ed. Michelle DiMeo and Sara Pennell, 225–46. Manchester: Manchester University Press, 2013.

Pérez-Ramos, Antonio. *Francis Bacon's Idea of Science and the Maker's Knowledge Tradition*. Oxford: Oxford University Press, 1988.
Picciotto, Joanna. *Labors of Innocence in Early Modern England*. Cambridge, Mass.: Harvard University Press, 2010.
Pinkard, Susan. *A Revolution in Taste: The Rise of French Cuisine, 1650–1800*. Cambridge: Cambridge University Press, 2010.
Pollock, Linda. *With Faith and Physic: The Life of a Tudor Gentlewoman, Lady Grace Mildmay 1552–1620*. London: Collins and Brown, 1993.
Poovey, Mary. *A History of the Modern Fact: Problems of Knowledge in the Sciences of Wealth and Society*. Chicago: University of Chicago Press, 1998.
Rambuss, Richard. *Closet Devotions*. Durham, N.C.: Duke University Press, 1998.
Roberts, Sasha. "'Shakespeare Creepes into the Womens Closets about Bedtime': Women Reading in a Room of Their Own." In *Renaissance Configurations: Voices/Bodies/Spaces, 1580–1690*, ed. Gordan McMullan, 30–63. New York: St. Martins, 1998.
Rombauer, Irma. *The Joy of Cooking*. New York, Scribner, 2006.
Rose, Hilary. "From Household to Public Knowledge, to a New Production System of Knowledge." Foreword to *Women, Science and Medicine*, ed. Lynette Hunter and Sarah Hutton, xi–xx. Thrupp, Stroud, Gloucestershire: Sutton, 1997.
Sanders, Eve. *Gender and Literacy on Stage in Early Modern England*. Cambridge: Cambridge University Press, 1998.
Santillana, Giorgio. "The Role of Art in the Scientific Renaissance." *Critical Problems in the History of Science*, ed. Marshall Clagett, 33–65. Madison: University of Wisconsin Press, 1959.
Schiebinger, Londa. *The Mind Has No Sex? Women in the Origins of Modern Science*. Cambridge, Mass.: Harvard University Press, 1989.
Schoenfeldt, Michael. *Bodies and Selves in Early Modern England: Physiology and Inwardness in Spenser, Shakespeare, Herbert, and Milton*. Cambridge: Cambridge University Press, 1999.
Schwarz, Kathryn. *What You Will: Gender, Contract, and Shakespearean Social Space*. Philadelphia: University of Pennsylvania Press, 2011.
Scott-Warren, Jason. "Reading Graffiti in the Early Modern Book." *Huntington Library Quarterly* 73:3 (2010): 363–81.
Shapin, Steven. "The House of Experiment in Seventeenth-Century England." *Isis* 79:3 (1988): 373–404.
———. *The Scientific Revolution*. Chicago: University of Chicago Press, 1996.
———. *A Social History of Truth: Civility and Science in Seventeenth-Century England*. Chicago: University of Chicago Press, 1994.
Shapiro, Barbara. *A Culture of Fact: England, 1550–1720*. Ithaca, N.Y.: Cornell University Press, 2003.
Sherman, Sandra. *Invention of the Modern Cookbook*. Santa Barbara, Calif.: Greenwood, 2010.
———. "'The Whole Art and Mystery of Cooking': What Cookbooks Taught Readers in the Eighteenth Century." *Eighteenth Century Life* 28:1 (2004): 115–35.
Sherman, William. *Used Books: Marking Readers in Renaissance England*. Philadelphia: University of Pennsylvania Press, 2008.
Shirley, John W., and F. David Hoeniger, eds. *Science and the Arts in the Renaissance*. Washington, D.C.: Folger Shakespeare Library, 1985.
Slater, Nigel. *Appetite: So What Do We Want to Eat Today?* London: Fourth Estate, 2000.

Smith, Helen. *Grossly Material Things: Women and Book Production in Early Modern England.* Oxford: Oxford University Press, 2012.

Smith, Pamela. *The Body of the Artisan: Art and Experience in the Scientific Revolution.* Chicago: University of Chicago Press, 2004.

———. *The Business of Alchemy: Science and Culture in the Holy Roman Empire.* Princeton, N.J.: Princeton University Press, 1994.

Smith, Pamela, and Paula Findlen. Introduction to *Merchants and Marvels: Commerce, Science, and Art in Early Modern Europe,* ed. Smith and Findlen, 1–25. New York: Routledge, 2002.

Snook, Edith. *Women, Beauty and Power in Early Modern England.* New York: Palgrave Macmillan, 2011.

Sonnenfeld, Albert, Jean Louis Flandrin, and Massimo Montanari, eds. *Food: A Cultural History from Antiquity to the Present.* New York: Columbia University Press, 1999.

Spencer, Colin. *British Food: An Extraordinary Thousand Years of History.* London: Grub Street, 1933.

Spiller, Elizabeth. "Recipes for Knowledge: Maker's Knowledge Traditions, Paracelsian Recipes and the Invention of the Cookbook, 1600–1660." In *Renaissance Food from Rabelais to Shakespeare,* ed. Joan Fitzpatrick, 55–72. Aldershot, U.K.: Ashgate, 2009.

———. *Science, Reading, and Renaissance Literature: The Art of Making Knowledge, 1580–1670.* Cambridge: Cambridge University Press, 2004.

———. Introduction and ed. *Seventeenth-Century English Recipe Books: Cooking, Physic and Chirurgery in the Works of Elizabeth Grey and Aletheia Talbot.* The Early Modern Englishwoman: A Facsimile Library of Essential Works, ser. 3, vols. 3–4. Burlington, Vt.: Ashgate, 2008.

Spufford, Margaret. "First Steps in Literacy: The Reading and Writing Experiences of the Humblest Seventeenth-Century Spiritual Autobiographers." *Social History* 4:3 (1979): 407–35.

Spurling, Hilary, ed. *Elinor Fettiplace's Receipt Book.* London: Viking, 1986.

Stallybrass, Peter. "'Adorn'd with Variety of Loose, and Easy Figures and Flourishes': The Aesthetics and Politics of Calligraphic Virtuosity." Unpublished paper.

———. "Books and Scrolls: Navigating the Bible." In *Books and Readers in Early Modern England,* ed. Jennifer Andersen and Elizabeth Sauer, 42–79. Philadelphia: University of Pennsylvania Press, 2002.

———. "The Library and Material Texts." *PMLA* 119:5 (2004): 1347–52.

Stead, Jennifer. "Bowers of Bliss: The Banquet Setting." In *"Banquetting Stuffe": The Fare and Social Background of the Tudor and Stuart Banquet,* ed. C. Anne Wilson, 115–57. Edinburgh: Edinburgh University Press, 1986.

Stewart, Alan. "The Early Modern Closet Discovered." *Representations* 50 (1995): 76–100.

Stine, Jennifer. "Opening Closets: The Discovery of Household Medicine in Early Modern England." Ph.D. diss., Stanford University, 1996.

Stobart, Anne. "'Lett Her Refrain from All Hot Spices': Medicinal Recipes and Advice in the Treatment of the King's Evil in Seventeenth-Century South-West England." In *Reading and Writing Recipe Books, 1550–1800,* ed. Michelle DiMeo and Sara Pennell, 203–24. Manchester: Manchester University Press, 2013.

Sugg, Richard. *Murder After Death: Literature and Anatomy in Early Modern England.* Ithaca, N.Y.: Cornell University Press, 2007.

Sullivan, Garrett. *Memory and Forgetting in English Renaissance Drama.* Cambridge: Cambridge University Press, 2005.

Taylor, Gary. "Gender, Hunger, Horror: The History and Significance of the Bloody Banquet." *JEMCS (Journal of Early Modern Cultural Studies)* 1:1 (2001): 1–45.

Theophano, Janet. *Eat My Words: Reading Women's Lives Through the Cookbooks They Wrote*. New York: Palgrave, 2002.
Thomas, Keith. *Man and the Natural World: Changing Attitudes in England, 1500–1800*. Oxford: Oxford University Press, 1996.
———. "The Meaning of Literacy in Early Modern England." In *The Written Word: Literacy in Transition*, ed. Gerd Baumann, 97–131. Oxford: Oxford University Press, 1986.
Tigner, Amy. "Eating with Eve." *Milton Quarterly* 44:4 (2010): 239–53.
———. "Preserving Nature in Hannah Woolley's *The Queen-Like Closet, or Rich Cabinet*." In *Ecofeminist Approaches to Early Modernity*, ed. Jennifer Munroe and Rebecca Laroche, 105–28. New York: Palgrave Macmillan, 2011.
Wall, Wendy. *The Imprint of Gender: Authorship and Publication in the English Renaissance*. Ithaca, N.Y.: Cornell University Press, 1993.
———. *Staging Domesticity: Household Work and English Identity in Early Modern Drama*. Cambridge: Cambridge University Press, 2002.
Wheaton, Barbara. *Savoring the Past: The French Kitchen and Table from 1300 to 1789*. New York: Touchstone, 1983.
Williams, Raymond. *Keywords*. New York: Oxford University Press, 1985.
Wilson, C. Anne, ed. *The Appetite and the Eye*. Edinburgh: Edinburgh University Press, 1991.
Wolfe, Heather. "Women's Handwriting." In *The Cambridge Companion to Early Modern Women's Writing*, ed. Laura Lunger Knoppers, 21–39. Cambridge: Cambridge University Press, 2009.
Wolfe, Jessica. *Humanism, Machinery, and Renaissance Literature*. Cambridge: Cambridge University Press, 2004.
Yates, Julian. "Shakespeare's Messmates." In *Culinary Shakespeare*, ed. David Goldstein and Amy Tigner. Pittsburgh: Duquesne University Press, forthcoming.

INDEX

acrostics, 149–50
Addison, Joseph, xi, 57, 60, 110
aesthetics, 21, 47–50, 58–63, 71, 78–79, 98–101
ague recipe, 8, 194, 280 n.53
Ainsly, Robert, 195–97
Albala, Ken, 172–73, 261 n.29, 266.n.54
All's Well That Ends Well (Shakespeare), 18, 168–69, 177–83, 207, 242–46, 272 n.2, 273 n.36, 274 n.38
animals, 8, 59–60, 75–76, 79–80, 84, 89–90, 102, 104–5, 107, 139, 141, 162, 175–76
annotations, 5, 14, 30–31, 113, 123, 126, 131–37, 160, 163–65, 192–93, 195, 198–210, 214–18, 225, 230–31, 235, 239–41, 250, 269 n.35, 269 n.36, 272 n.106, 275–76 n.73, 276 n.77, 281 n.69, 281 n.70
Appelbaum, Robert, 102
appetite, ix, 20, 45, 58–61, 94, 95, 107, 108, 161–62, 214
approval, 213–18, 229–40, 242–44, 281 n.69
Archer, Jayne Elisabeth, 85, 159, 263 n.4, 264 n.20, 266 n.53, 280 n.54, 281 n.65, 281 n.70
Aristotelianism, 228, 229
Aristotle, 226
art: and cookery, 3, 36, 38, 39, 58–64, 65–101, 170–71 (*see also* conceits); relationship to nature, 86–92, 101–9
artisanal knowledge/literacy, 115, 220–21, 249–50
Ash, Rebekah, 141
Aspin, Richard, 282 n.79
attribution of recipes, 11–13, 18, 113, 125–26, 225, 229–35
Averie, Joseph, 131

Bacon, Francis, 210, 220–21, 225–26, 228, 278 n.19, 279 n.47
Bales, Peter, 161
banqueting, 29, 74–75, 81–82, 88, 90, 91, 93–97, 149, 152, 257 n.4, 264 n.19
Barker, Nicolas, 120
Barrett, Lady, 178, 223, 224, 243
Barrington, Lady, 229–31, 236–38
Barthes, Roland, 71
Baumfylde, Mary, 130, 159, 169, 272 n.106
Bayne, Anne, 30, 195–97
Beale, John, 1
beef, xi, 96
Bent, Mary, 130
Best, Arabella, 123
Bett, Edmund, 192
Bible, 16, 39, 50–51, 107–8, 198–99, 201
Binoit, Peter, 149–50
blast salve recipe (for infected wounds), 214–15
Blome, Grace. *See* Randolph, Grace Blome
Bonnefons, Nicholas, x
books of secrets, 4, 24, 67, 211, 239, 277 n.10, 279 n.39, 279 n.41
Borlase, Lady (Alice Bankes), 131, 139, 156–57, 175–76
Bourdieu, Pierre, 21
Boyle, Robert, 210, 221–22, 228, 232, 246–48
Boyle family recipe book, 223, 224, 278 n.24
Bradley, Martha, 47, 49, 50, 56, 99, 100, 262 n.49, 266 n.64
Brayman Hackel, Heidi, 30, 115, 116
Brett, Hopestill, 197–99
Breughel, Pieter (*Land of Cockaigne*), 102, 104
Brinsley, John, 30

Brockman, Elizabeth, 164, 165
Bromehead, Mary, 191
Brooks, Catharine, 49–51
Broughton, Dorothy, 190
Brown, Katherine, 130
Brumwich, Anne, 209–10
Buckhurst, Jane, 126
Burton, Robert, 157, 271 n.86
Bushnell, Rebecca, 221, 277 n.10, 282 n.80
Byron, Lord (George Gordon), 63, 153

cabinets, 29, 34, 41, 88, 260 n.9. *See also* closet(s)
Carter, Charles, 38, 40, 58–59, 98, 99
Cartwright, Charlotte, 59
carving, 51, 78, 138–41, 145, 157, 161–62
Catchmay, Frances, 191, 192
Cater, Anne, 143–44, 230, 236, 238
Cavendish, Margaret, 176
celebrity status, 5, 36, 40, 55–56
chefs, 35–47
Child, Lydia Maria, 167
chocolate, 193, 196
Christ-cross (crisscross), 151
citational structure of recipes, 11–12, 229–33
civilizing process, 4, 57, 60–61, 117, 122, 160–61
class. *See* social classification
Clifford, Lady Anne, 30, 116–17
closet, 22–35, 260 n.7; as endowing value/status, 23–24, 32–33; eroticized, 23, 65, 82–83; as library, 26–28; recoded in mid-seventeenth century, 33–35; as sites of "repair," 29; "use" generated by, 28–31; Woolley's redefinition/critique of, 40–41, 43–44
A Closet for Ladies and Gentlewomen, 24, 71, 90, 151–52
Cockaigne, myth of, 102–4
cockwater recipe, 176, 215
Comley, William, 143, 144, 146
communities: domestic in relation to scientific, 219–50; memorialized, 189–90, 192–94; national, 44–48; recipe representations of, 2–3, 20–64. *See also* taste communities
The Compleat Servant-Maid, 41, 52, 120–23, 138, 139, 176
conceits, 7, 17, 65–69, 74–97; essence in relation to form in, 68, 79–80, 86, 90–91; ideological issues in, 67, 93–97; pliable food substances for, 74; problem of simulation/parody in, 92–96; problem of the raw and the cooked in, 79–80, 83–85; problem of the "real" in, 85–92; recipes as, 66–69; religious, 80, 92–93, 265 n.41; as "thoughtful practice," 84–85
Conrad, Joseph, 69, 264 n.9
consumption. *See* taste communities
Cook, Ann, 54, 55
cookery: as connected to aesthetics, 58–64, 66, 78–79; as pleasure, 65–74; as imaginative play, 74–101, 109; as memorialization, 167–208; as part of female-managed domesticity, 40–58; separation of housewifery from, 35–39; as shaping national identification, 44–51, 56–58; as shaping status, 20–33, 49–58; as site for experimentation, 209–50; as site for literacy-acquisition, 112–66; violence around, 8, 105, 175–76, 273 n.17
Coote, Edmunde, 118
Corlyon, Mrs., 178
Cormack, Bradin, 30–31
Coryat, Thomas, 154–55
creams, 74, 98, 113
Cromwell, Elizabeth, 34, 160
Crooke, Helkiah, 118
Crowne, John, 174–75
Cruso, Mary, 16
cuisine: international/national, ix–x, 9, 22, 33, 34, 40, 45–51, 56–57, 68, 106, 260 n.6; transmutationalist/purist, x, 68
cultural capital, 7, 21, 27–28, 32–33, 95–96. *See also* social classification
cutting/cutwork, 119–20, 137–41, 156–57, 161–62
Cymbeline (Shakespeare), 146

Daston, Lorraine, 211, 228
Davies, John, 139
Dawson, Thomas, 14, 25, 26, 32, 67, 219
Daybell, James, 268 n.21, 268 n.29
de Acosta, José, 93
Dear, Peter, 211, 228, 233–34, 241, 280 n.61, 280 n.62
death, 8, 18; autopsy report, 203; masks, 157; elegiac ode, 159, 204; personified, 176; recorded in genealogies, 199–207. *See also* mortality

deer, 97, 102; artificial venison, 98, 125; pastry/pie, 79–80, 84; potted, 131, 135
Delany, Mary (Granville), 192–94
Delightes for Ladies (Plat), 31, 68, 71, 88–89, 91–92, 145–46, 170–71, 183–85, 186–87, 229
Denbigh, Hester, 12, 131
desserts, 8, 81, 90, 98–99, 152–53, 264 n.23
diet: housewife's responsibility for, 25, 40–58; and humoral physiology, 7–8; national/international, ix–xi, 33, 40, 45–48, 56–57. *See also* cookery, cuisine, food
Digby, Elizabeth, 238–39
Digby, Sir Kenelm, 34, 248, 280 n.54
DiMeo, Michelle, 2, 3, 190
Disraeli, Isaac, ix
distillation/distilling, 85–86, 171, 173–74, 183–89, 222, 274 n.44, 274 n.45
dog bite cure, 214, 241
Dogget, Mary, 15, 171, 173
Dolan, Frances, 5, 114–15, 267 n.6
domestication, 160–62, 266 n.51
Donne, John, 89, 140, 154–55, 159
doodle/doodling, 113, 132, 133, 163
Dorset, Lady Marquess, 171, 224
Dr. Stephen's water, 25, 230
dropsy (swelling) cure, 126, 173, 230, 281 n.73

Eamon, William, 211, 228, 258 n.8, 280 n.49
Egerton, Ann, 243
Elias, Norbert, 122, 160–61
empiricism, 209–10, 220, 221, 228, 229, 231, 239–44
Englishness, ix–xii, 9, 22, 34, 45–51, 56–57, 68, 106, 260 n.6
epilepsy (or falling sickness) recipes, 174, 176, 222, 229–30
Erasmus, 122, 151, 161
eroticism. *See* pleasure
Evelyn, John, 210, 228, 246
experience (as basis for knowledge), 9, 212–18, 220–21, 227–46
experimental cultures, 209–55
Eyton, Amy, 127, 165
Ezell, Margaret, 115–16

Fairfax, Rhoda, 126–27, 209
fall narratives, 101–9

Fanshawe, Lady Ann, 112, 131, 191, 241
Farley, John, 99
Fenwick, Diana Matilda, 216
Ferguson, Margaret, 115, 267 n.9
Ferguson, Priscilla, 20, 190
Fettiplace, Elinor Poole, 191
Field, Catherine, 272 n.106
Finch, Anne, 204
fistula cures, 178
Flandrin, Jean-Louis, 98, 257 n.5
Fleming, Juliet, 116–17, 127
food: as cultural capital, 7, 21, 27–28, 32–33, 95–96; as fantasy/artifice, 70–97; foreign, ix–xi, 33, 44–47, 56–57; in healthcare, 7–8, 25, 172–77; "live," 75, 79–80, 83, 85, 86, 89; mythologies of, 49, 61–63, 101–9; and religious iconography, 80, 91–93, 263 n.75, 265 n.41; and time, 3, 81, 167–89. *See also* cookery; conceits; diet
Foucault, Michel, 230
Fowler, Elizabeth, 131–33, 169, 243–44
Freke, Elizabeth, 212, 230, 235–36
Friedman, Alice, 23
front matter (of recipe books), 20–21, 49–51; commendatory poems, 28, 37–39; dedicatory epistles, 26–27; as encouraging female use, 22–31; frontispieces, 26, 41, 52, 53, 55, 102, 103; as promoting male authors/chefs, 36–40; prefaces, 106–8; tables of contents, 71, 73, 99; title pages, 37, 41–43, 61–63, 99
Frye, Susan, 117, 119, 159
Fuller, Elizabeth, 157–58
Fumerton, Patricia, 82, 94, 97, 177

gardens/gardening, 62–63, 72–74, 86–88, 107, 119, 142–43, 171, 221, 249, 270n67, 270n68, 282n80
Gascoigne, George, 66
genealogies, 192, 195–207
The Genteel House-Keepers Pastime, 140
The Gentlewomans Companion, 65, 118–20, 140, 161–62, 268 n.22
Gigante, Denise, 60–62
Girouard, Mark, 23
Glasse, Hannah, 48–49, 51, 54, 98, 99, 165–66
Glyd (Glydd), Ann, 198, 204–7, 212, 240–41
Godfrey, Elizabeth, 6, 14, 216

Goldberg, Jonathan, 112, 122, 161, 271–72 n.103
Goldstein, David, 46, 62, 231, 272 n.10
Goodenough, Ann, 85, 170
A Good Huswifes Handmaide for the Kitchin, 25, 32, 67
Gopnik, Adam, 252–53
graffiti, 113, 116, 127, 163, 267 n.2
Granville, Anne, 192–94
Granville, Mary, 16, 135, 173–74, 192, 194, 244
Greville, Fulke, 66
Grey, Elizabeth, Countess of Kent, 34, 221
Guarini, Battista, *Il pastor fido*, 174
Guillory, John, 115
gum arabic, 74, 147, 223, 224
gum tragacanth, 74
"gusto," 36

Hall, Augusta, Baroness Llanover, 194–95, 275 n.69
Hall, Constance, 139, 147
Hall, Kim, 45, 260 n.9, 264 n.19
Halpern, Richard, 274 n.44
Hamlet (Shakespeare), 162, 172
handiwork, as literacy, 137–58
handwriting, 118–37
Harkness, Deborah, 211, 221, 222
Harrison, Sarah, 47, 48, 101
Harrison, William, 96–97
Hartlib, Samuel, 1, 210, 221, 228
Haynes, Cisilia, 130
Haywood, Eliza, 21, 51–53, 57
health care. *See* medical care; food
Heldke, Lisa, 84
Henderson, William, 51, 52
Henrietta Maria, Queen, 34, 141
Herbert, George: 93 ("The Banquet"); 110–11 ("Faith")
Hill, Thomas, 142
Hirst, Elizabeth, 133, 135, 212–14, 224, 230, 241
Hoby, Lady Margaret, 29, 221
Hogarth, William (*The Gates of Calais*), xi
Holland, Mary, 51, 53
home schooling, 118
honey (distilled) recipe, 173–74
Hooke, Mary, 190
Hooke, Robert, 210, 228
hornbooks, 151

Horsington, Sarah, 222
housekeepers, 10, 22, 40–47, 53–58, 110
housewife/housewifery (ideal) 25, 44–45, 49–51, 56–58, 81, 161
Hudson, Sarah, 207–8
Hughes, Sarah, 159
Hull, Suzanne, 260 n.11
humoral physiology, xi, 7–9, 172–76, 183
Hunter, Lynette, 211, 221, 222, 248
Hussey, Rhoda, 209
Hyrde, Richard, 161

illiterate/illiteracy, 112–15, 213
inheritance, recipe books as, 189–98, 275 n.71
ink recipes, 141, 223–25
isinglass, 74, 90

Jackson, Jane, 135, 137
jelly/jellies, 32, 39, 74, 95–98, 176, 201, 204, 212, 218, 241
Jephson, Penelope Patrick, 163, 165
jokes, 16, 63, 93, 123, 159–60, 174, 177, 250, 273 n.22
Jones, Ann Rosalind, 191
Jones, Katherine, Lady Ranelagh, 221, 224, 247, 248
Jones, Richard, 24, 25
Jonson, Ben, 37; *Bartholomew Fayre*, 93; "Inviting a Friend to Supper," 153–54, 155; *Neptune's Triumph for the Returne of Albion*, 65, 78–79, 264 n.20; "To Penshurst," 102, 104; *The Staple of News*, 77–78, 109, 264 n.20
Juana Inés de la Cruz, Sor, 226
jumbals (jumbles), 74, 95, 141

Kant, Immanuel, 61
Kavey, Allison, 279 n.41
keeping, 167–76, 184
Kendall, Rose, 143–45, 230, 236, 238
kidney stone recipes, 125, 229, 281 n.69
King, William, 20, 59–60
kitchen, 35–58; as culinary art studio, 74–101; as home laboratory, 219–26; and nation, 22, 44–58; in relation to scientific laboratory, 246–49; as site of memory, 168–83, 189–208; as site of violence, 8, 105, 139–41, 175–76; and writing utensils, 141

Knight, Mrs., 15
Knoppers, Laura, 34, 261 n.33
knots, 74, 95, 141–48, 270 n.63
knowledge, 2–5, 209–55; and circulation of texts, 226–46; in domestic locales, 22–58, 246–49; "maker's," 8–9, 220, 221; and lexicons of proof, 212–18, 226–46; vernacular, 219–25

laboratories, 219–26, 247–50
The Ladies Cabinet Enlarged and Opened, 24, 71–75, 86
ladies (as class category), 49–58
Lamb, Patrick, 39
Land of Cockaigne (Breughel), 102
Laroche, Rebecca, 116, 211
La Varenne, Pierre, x
Lawson, William, 142–43
Lehmann, Gilly, 25
Leigh, Dorothy, 118
Leong, Elaine, 258 n.9
letters, 2. *See* literacy/literacies
Lévi-Strauss, Claude, 79
literacy/literacies, 9, 17–18, 112–66; and cutting, 137–41, 156–57, 161–62; edible literacy, 145–58; sites of acquisition, 118; problem in defining/calibrating, 112–16; tactile, 115, 117, 149–50
Loewenstein, Joseph, 153
Long, Pamela, 211
Lowdham, Caleb, 222, 224
Lowdham, Jane, 222, 224
Lupton, Julia, 81, 257 n.4, 264 n.23

Maddison Family Recipe Book, 123, 124, 126
"maker's knowledge," 8–9, 220, 221
making, 3, 13, 16–17, 66, 85, 90, 109, 121–22, 157, 163, 165, 241; knowledge making, 212–46; *poeisis*, 3, 165; world making, 3, 78–79
manicules, 134–35, 137
manners, 4, 42, 57–58, 122, 160–62
Marchitello, Howard, 226
marginalia. *See* annotations
Markham, Gervase: defining ideal housewife, 21, 44–46; and conceits/foodplay, 91, 94–96; on distillation, 187, 188; *The English Housewife*, 8, 21, 25, 29, 44–46, 91, 94–96, 105, 171, 173, 187, 188, 221, 258–59 n.15, 261 n.44; on nations and markets, 44–46
marking, 30–31, 35
Martino, Maestro, 2
marzipan (or marchpane), 28, 74, 81–82, 86, 90, 92, 93, 97, 146, 149, 151, 154
masques, 76–79
Masten, Jeffrey, 155–56, 271 n.89
matter/materiality, 29, 66, 111, 116–17, 141, 150–53, 159, 165, 168, 186–87, 189, 191, 218, 220
May, Robert, 36–38, 75–77, 79–84, 101, 275 n.69
Mayerne, Theodore, 167, 168, 261 n.43
Mayne, Jasper, 93
Mazzio, Carla, 30–31
medical/health care, 4, 7–8, 14, 16, 18, 25, 33, 42, 172–83, 203, 207, 211, 229–30
memento mori, 199
memorialization, 189–208
The Merchant of Venice (Shakespeare), 171
The Merry Wives of Windsor (Shakespeare), 151, 162
Michel, Elizabeth, 112–14
Middleton, Thomas, 29
Mildmay, Lady Grace, 229–30, 237
Miller, Mary, 127–28
Milton, John, 61–63
Moorat, S. A. J., 112–14
mortality, 175–83, 273 n.17
Moxon, Elizabeth, 54, 99
Murrell, John, 15, 25, 26, 32, 67, 71, 72, 74–75, 84–85, 96, 137, 140, 146–151, 265 n.34
mutton, 91 (outlandish), 96 (meatloaf), 98 (marinated), 108 (roasted with pickled herring), 125 (as faux venison), 140 (carved), 204 (with cauliflower)

Nagy, Doreen, 211
Nashe, Thomas, 81–82
national identity. *See* Englishness
Natura Exenterata, 209, 229, 240
"nature" (v. food/artifice), x–xi, 3, 68, 79–80, 85–92, 98, 101–9, 170–72, 183–89, 225–26; and aesthetics, 58, 60; and "affections," 94–95; feminized concept of, 225; in production of scientific knowledge, 8–9, 228
Newton, Jane, 15, 133–34, 223–24
Nott, John, 99, 102, 103, 105–7, 262–63 n.68

Oates, Joyce Carol, 176
Okeover, Elizabeth, 12–13, 30, 123, 127, 164, 165, 171, 214–16, 225, 230, 241, 277 n.13, 281 n.70
Oldenberg, Henry, 233
Orlin, Lena Cowen, 23
ownership marks, 11, 13, 25, 113, 123, 125–27, 131, 134, 150, 195, 200, 201, 214, 225, 243, 250, 269 n.34, 269 n.35

Packe, Susanna, 8, 169–70, 212–13, 216–18, 241, 258 n.14
Painter, William, 242
Palmer, Archdale, 178, 224
Palmer, Katherine, 56–57
Paradise Lost (Milton), 61–63
Parker, Bridget, 159
Parry, James, 77
Partridge, John, 6, 9–10, 22–33, 67, 71, 73, 92–94, 171, 223
Peckham, Ann, 47, 51, 53–54, 68, 110
pen/penknives, 119, 138, 139, 141
penmanship. *See* handwriting
Pennell, Sara, 2, 3, 5–6, 14, 190, 211, 213, 227, 232–34, 236
pepper, cayenne, 56
Percy, Lady Anne, 134–36
Pérez-Ramos, Antonio, 8, 220
Pharmacopeia, 33
Philosophical Transactions, 233–34, 240, 249
Pine, John, 102–5
Plat, Hugh, 25, 31, 67, 68, 71, 88–92, 145–46, 152, 170–71, 175, 183–87, 189, 221, 222, 229, 244, 248; on domestic preservation, 183–85; and edible letters, 145–46, 152; and women as intellectual sources, 222
Plato, 69
pleasure, 7, 17, 25–26, 65–111; in early modern v. modern recipes, 70–74; and eroticized domesticity, 162, 174–75, 181, 185–86, 274 n.44; in food-play, 74–96; recipes as technologies of, 67–68, 75, 97; "use" as, 71–74
poeisis, 3, 165. *See also* making
poems (in recipe collections), 16, 56–57, 159, 204
Pollock, Linda, 221
posies, 151–53
posset, 15, 56–57, 197, 225
Power, Henry, 233

practice/*praxis*, 28–31, 51, 75, 109, 160–61, 227–46, 249–50; recipes as documenting, 2, 4, 5, 21–22, 213–18; thoughtful, 84, 89, 105
Presbyterian (recipe for making one), 16, 159–60
preserves/preservation, 18, 89, 93, 167–208, 272, n.10, 274 n.44. *See also* keeping; and family traditions/genealogies, 18, 192, 195–205; and health maintenance, 16, 18, 44–45, 173–78, 181, 207; through writing, 183–86, 189–208
print: as a domestic activity, 75, 92, 122, 139–40, 152, 157; market for recipe books, 20–64, 82, 97; book as print artifacts, 71, 99–100
probatum est, 16, 212–18, 227, 229, 239–40, 250, 281 n.70
professional kitchen staff, 35–58
proof, 18–19, 212–18; and distributed verification, 238; in/of home experimentations, 226–46; and witnessing, 231–37, 242–43. *See also* approval
pudding, 91 (faux mutton), 96 ("fond"), 190 (almond), 197 (hogspudding)
Pudsey, Lettice, 14, 124–26, 150, 173, 225
Puleston, Mary Egerton, 190
Puttenham, George, 152

The Queen-Like Closet, 41, 43–44
The Queens Closet Opened, 34, 178, 188
The Queens Delight, 141–42
quills, 138–39, 141, 165–66
quince, 5 (King Edward's preserved), 32 (Lady Grey Clement's jelly), 74 (syrup), 95 (paste), 141 (jumbles), 170 (preserved without sugar), 197 (cake), 208 (preserved), 226 (for liquefying sugar)

rabbit, 14 (boiled), 32 (sauced, King Henry VIII's way), 92 (tail), 125 (fricasseed), 136 ("smeared" the French way), 139 (carved)
Rabisha, William, 38–39, 108
Raffald, Elizabeth, 48, 55–56
Rand, Abigail, 152
Randolph, Grace Blome, 135, 136, 159, 201–4
Randolph, Mary Castillion, 204
Ranelagh, Lady. *See* Jones, Katherine
readership (of recipes), 6–7, 9–10, 24–25, 33, 48, 57–58, 97

Index

reading, 2; detached from labor, 49–56; locales for, 20–58; as marking, 30–31, 35; as opposed to apprenticeship, 38, 46–47; physical/embodied dimension of, 31, 115–16, 151–54, 175, 184; as pleasure, 71–74, 77; as truth-testing, 228–29, 237–38, 250; as "use," 28–31. *See also* literacy(-ies)

"receipts," 3–4, 13–14, 67, 111, 227, 266 n.53.

recipe(s): for artistry/creativity, 65–111; as bids for status, 28, 32; for combating temporal cycles, 167–208; for defining social identities, 20–64; as documentary/ fictive, 5–6, 251; and experimental cultures, 208–50; as escape from suffering, 254–55; formal characteristics of, 13–14, 227, 237–38; illustrations in, 99, 100; as inheritances/bequests, 189–98, 275 n.71; large-scale scholarly narratives about, 4–5; as memorialization, 189–208; as mobilizing desire, 253; readerships of, 6–7, 9–10, 24–25, 33, 48, 57–58, 97; as sites for household "writing," 112–66; and taste communities, 17–18, 20–64

recipere, 3, 227

recycled books, 153–55

religious iconography, 80, 91–93, 263 n.75, 265 n.41

Roper, Margaret, 161

Rose, Giles, 140

roses (preserved), 85, 149, 169, 174–75, 185–87, 229

rosewater (as ingredient), 74, 86, 92, 96, 128, 147, 148, 187

Rotton, Elisabeth, 150

Rowley, William, 29

Royal Society, 210, 211, 231–34, 241, 246

salmon ball recipe, 219

Schoenfeldt, Michael, 62

Schwarz, Kathryn, 182

science, rise of modern, 210–12, 220–22, 225–26, 228, 231–32

scientific revolution, 210–12

Scott-Warren, Jason, 113, 150, 267 n.2

scribal communities, 11–13, 115–16, 229–31, 234–36

scribes, 130–33

scrofula, 215

seasoning, 168, 172; as flavoring, ix–xi, 58, 108, 177, 258 n.14; as a knowledge, 20, 171–72, 215; as quality of a material, 175, 177, 182; as a relational process, 173; as temporal, 168–83, 188–89

servants 9–10, 22, 40–41, 48–58, 81–82, 117, 120–23, 140, 153, 161, 165–66

Shackleford, Ann, 61–63

Shakespeare, William: *All's Well That Ends Well*, 18, 168–69, 177–83, 207, 242–46, 272 n.2, 273 n.36, 274 n.38; on art and nature, 86–87; on "carving," 162; *Cymbeline*, 146; on distillation, 185–87; on edible letters, 146; on gall in ink, 223; *Hamlet*, 162, 172; *The Merchant of Venice*, 171; *The Merry Wives of Windsor*, 151, 162; on proving, 237, 242–46; on seasoning, 168–69, 177–83; *Sonnets*, 185–87, 237; *The Tempest*, 91; *Titus Andronicus*, 176; *Troilus and Cressida*, 177; *Twelfth Night*, 150, 169, 223; *The Winter's Tale*, 86–87

Shapin, Steven, 231–32, 239, 246–48

Shenstone, William, 101

Sherman, Sandra, 36, 56, 249

Sherman, William, 30, 135

Shirley, John, 139

Sidney, Philip, 66, 165

Sillyard, Lady, 144

skulls, 97, 176, 199, 214, 225

Sleigh, Lady Elizabeth, 250

Smith, Ann, 131

Smith, Eliza, 58, 106–9

Smith, Pamela, 115, 220, 228, 248

Smith, Robert, 39–40

Smollett, Tobias, 57

social class, 10, 21–22, 25–29, 31–33, 39–40, 51–58, 130. *See also* cultural capital

Socrates, 69, 70

Sommers, Abraham, 130

Spenser, Edmund, 66, 87–88 (*The Faerie Queene*); 165 (*The Shepheardes Calendar*)

spices, ix–xi, 45–46, 56–57, 82, 108, 155, 177, 257 n.5

Spiller, Elizabeth, 5, 6, 33, 211, 221, 228–29, 241, 279 n.41

Sprat, Thomas, 220

Springatt, Frances (Ayshford), 198, 200–201

Stallybrass, Peter, 191

Stanhope, Philip, Earl of Chesterfield, 134, 212, 234–35
Staveley, Jane, 127
Still Life with Letter Pastries, 149–50
Stubbes, Philip, 90–91
suckets, 74, 89, 97
sugar paste, 74–75, 84–85

table layouts, 99, 100
tables of contents, 71, 73, 99
Talbot, Aletheia, Countess of Arundel, 221, 229
taste, 2, 16–17, 20–22, 26, 39–40, 58–64, 98, 101, 115, 263 n.69
taste acts/communities, 17–18, 20–64
The Tempest (Shakespeare), 91
temporalities, 18, 167–208
tenting, 178
testimony, 230–32, 240
Thacker, John, xi
Thatcher, Katherine, 130
Theophano, Janet, 56, 123, 126, 197
time. *See* temporalities
title pages. *See* front matter
Titus Andronicus (Shakespeare), 176
Town, John, 37, 101
The Treasurie of Commodious Conceits, 10, 22–33, 67, 71, 73, 92–94, 171
Trevelyon, Thomas, 156
Troilus and Cressida (Shakespeare), 177
trompe l'oeil food, 7, 82, 87–90
Tusser, Thomas, 150, 187–88
Twelfth Night (Shakespeare), 150, 169, 223

use, 28–31, 54–55, 71–74

Vaughan, Thomas, 225
verification. *See* proof
violets, 85, 86, 197, 218
Vives, Juan, 112, 116
Voltaire, 21, 58

Warwick, Countess of, 144, 230
waxwork, 42, 119, 157
Wentworth, Anne, 230
Westcombe, Martin, 192, 193
Wheaton, Barbara Ketcham, 10
White, John, 67
Whitfield, Felicia, 250
Whitney, Geoffrey, 31
Whitney, Isabella, 175
Williams, Raymond, 259 n.5
The Winter's Tale (Shakespeare), 86–87
wit, 5, 68, 80, 82, 85, 90–92. *See also* conceits
witnessing, 231, 232, 234–37, 242–43
Woolley (Wolley), Hannah, 40–44, 46–47, 118–24, 190; attribution of books, 40–41, 268 n.22; *The Compleat Servant-Maid*, 41, 52, 120–23, 138, 139, 176; *The Cook's Guide*, 40, 99; *The Ladies Directory*, 40–43, 47; *The Queen-Like Closet*, 24, 40, 41, 43, 189; reclaiming recipes/cookery for women, 40–47; *A Supplement to the Queen-Like Closet*, 24, 46–47, 65, 119, 157, 244; on writing as domestic work, 118–24, 157
world making, 3, 78–79
Wright, Thomas, 85

Yates, Julian, 176

ACKNOWLEDGMENTS

They say that too many cooks in the kitchen spoil the broth, but this was never the case with *Recipes for Thought*. In fact, I welcomed them all.

I am fortunate to work with a cadre of exceptionally dynamic and generous early modern colleagues at Northwestern. Special thanks to Will West, for sitting in Crowe courtyard and talking me out of a particularly hair-brained idea for this book; Kasey Evans, for insight especially about a Jonson poem that spurred me to rethink edible writing; Laurie Shannon, for continual reminders about the importance of intellectual mono-tasking; Susie Phillips, for her unbridled enthusiasm always, but in this case, about the ambiguities of culinary parodies; and Jeff Masten, whose thinking about materiality has become part of the intellectual air that I breathe.

As I've presented my research, I have benefited from numerous fruitful conversations. Peter Stallybrass and Chris Castiglia had a startlingly similar insight, posed from different perspectives, about how recipe writers coyly withheld information from readers. Fran Dolan and Margaret Ferguson, in person and in writing, insisted that I refine claims about literacy and gender. Mary Floyd Wilson was productively dubious about what scholars tended to count as science. David Goldstein and Amy Tigner altered my frame of reference by gloriously welcoming me into food studies collaborations. I was astounded to find out how much Rebecca Laroche knows about violet syrup, snail water, and experiential learning. As she always does, Gail Paster nimbly moved between detailed archival suggestions and a demand to see the big picture.

Other astute responses echoed in my mind as I stared at my computer screen during Chicago winters. David Baker, Crystal Bartolovich, Dympna Callaghan, Margaret Ezell, Lena Orlin, Jennifer Richards, Fred Schurink, Bill Sherman, Helen Smith, Elizabeth Spiller, Garrett Sullivan, and Valerie Traub all asked shrewd questions about the wacky world of recipes. I owe much as well to Meghan Daly-Costa, Becky Fall, Jeff Knight, Liz Rodriguez, and Will Pierce for allowing me to draw on their impressive research skills.

The Kaplan Institute for the Humanities at Northwestern helped me to finish work nurtured by librarians at the Wellcome Library, Folger Library, New York Public Library, University of Pennsylvania Library, and Huntington Library. I am especially grateful to David Schoonover for ushering me through the treasures of the Szathmary Collection at the University of Iowa Library. As many do, I rely on Georgianna Ziegler at the Folger to steer me in the right direction. Allyson Booth's generous D.C. hospitality doubled my pleasure in exploring the archives at the Folger.

It's fitting that I would become enthralled to the nexus of cooking and thinking, because my beloved partner in crime, Jules Law, does both with such flair and style.

I dedicate this work to my daughter, Leah Wall, whose passion for food artistry is only one of her many astonishing gifts.

www.ingramcontent.com/pod-product-compliance
Lightning Source LLC
Chambersburg PA
CBHW020331240426
43665CB00043B/214